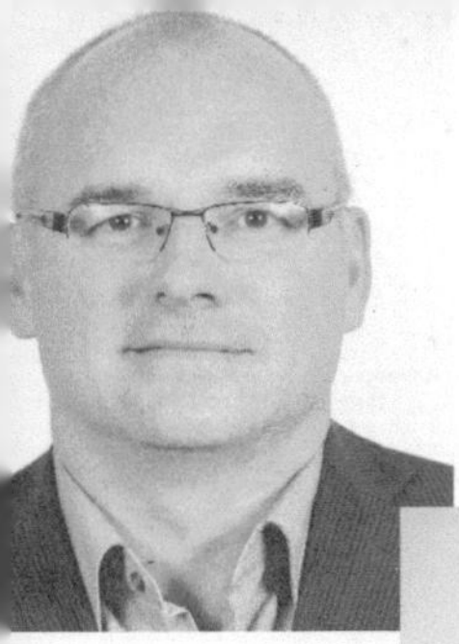

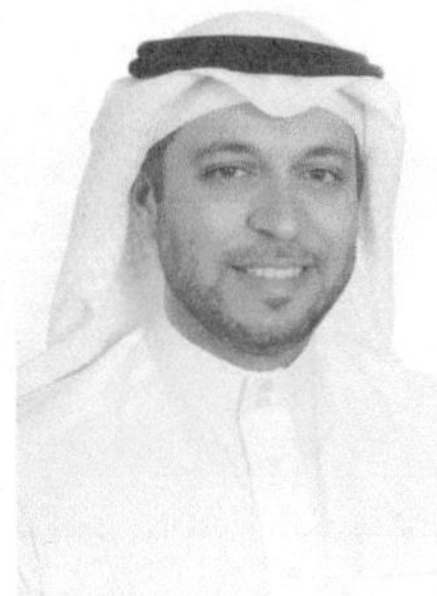

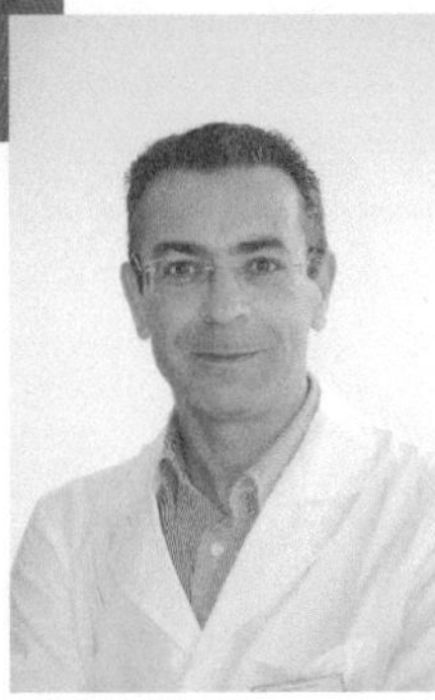

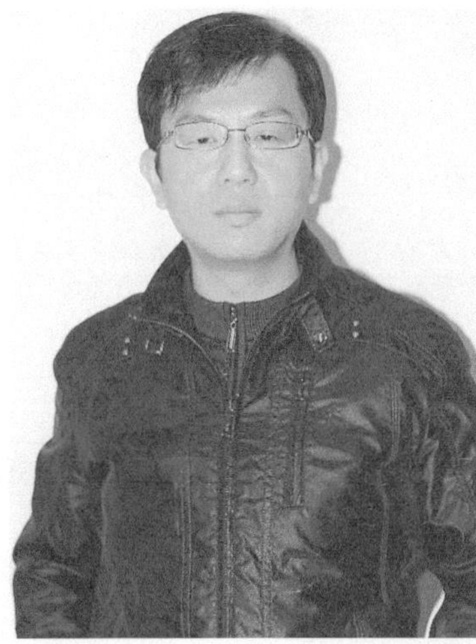

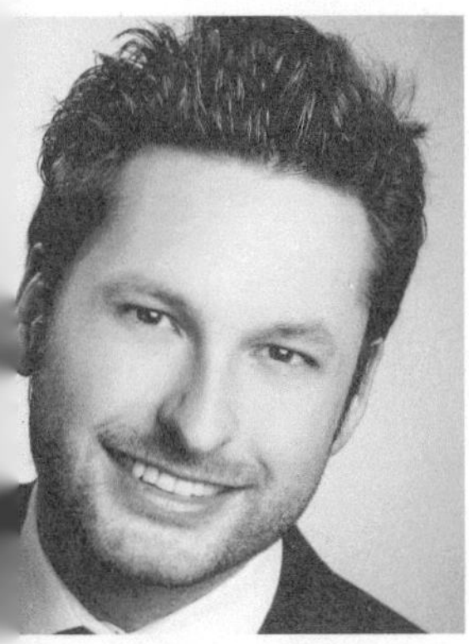

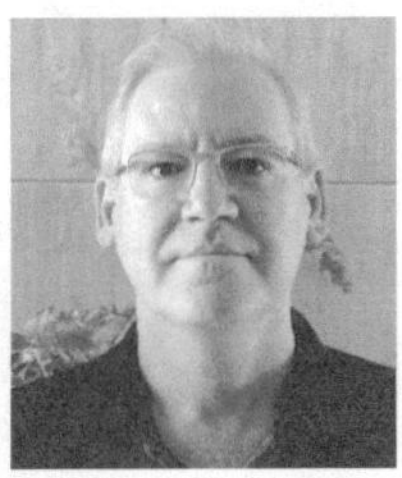

IntechOpen

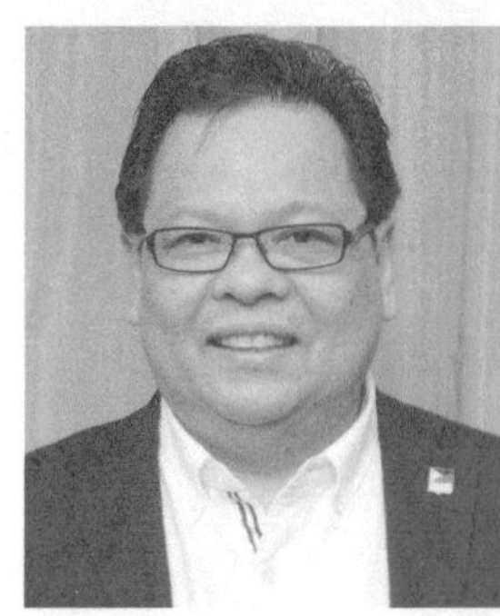

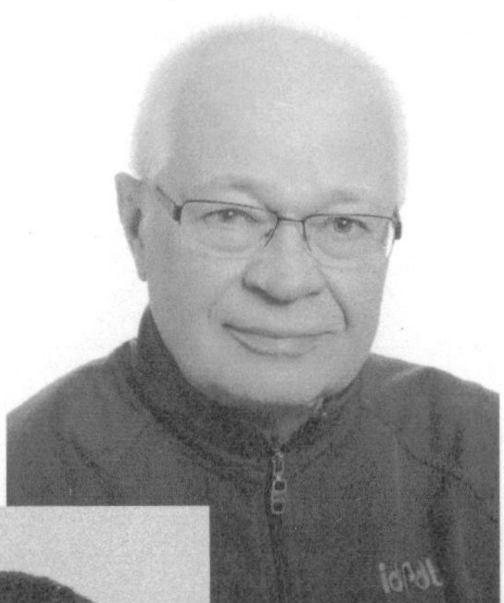

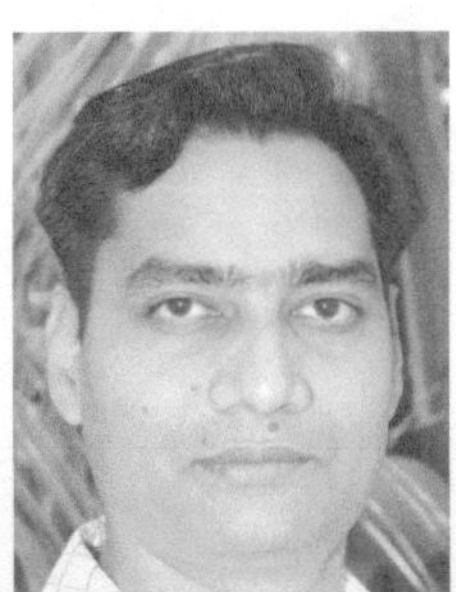

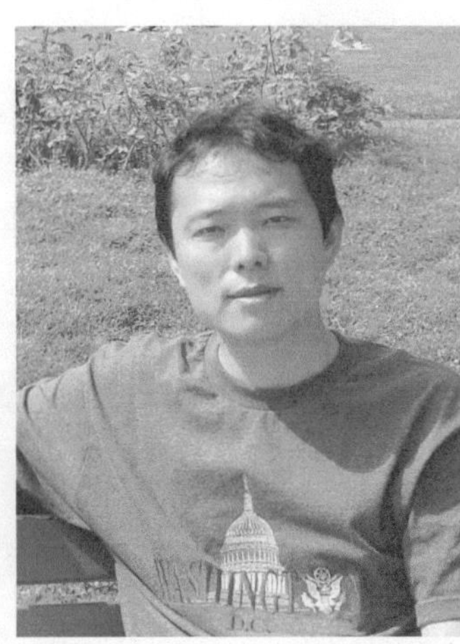

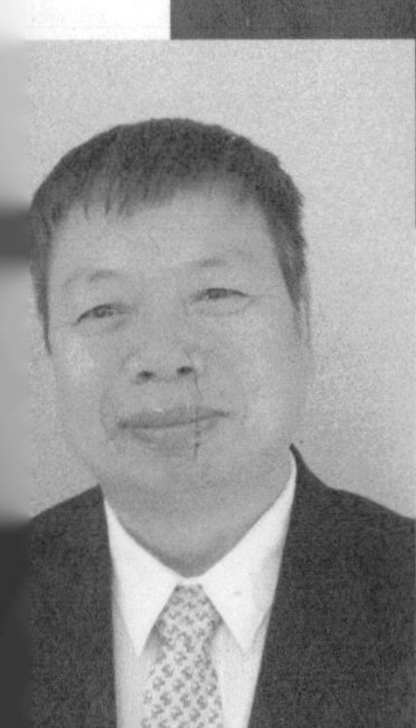

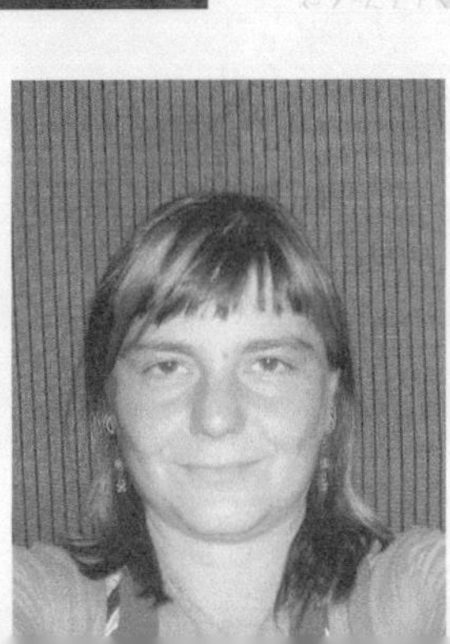

Infertility and Assisted Reproduction

Edited by Wei-Hua Wang

Published in London, United Kingdom

Preface

Infertility affects approximately 15% of couples of reproductive ages, and this percentage keeps increasing. Current infertility treatment through in vitro fertilization (IVF) can achieve approximately 80% of accumulated live birth rates, with even greater rates in young patients and patients who use donor egg IVF. High live birth rates rely on many advanced technologies in infertility treatment, including more accurate clinical diagnosis and patient management as well as state-of-the-art IVF technologies. Even though new treatment options are available, there are still many unknown factors affecting laboratory and clinical outcomes and thus improvements are still needed. This book focuses on such topics as recurrent failed embryo implantation, non-invasive preimplantation genetic diagnosis (PGT), oocyte cryopreservation, cryopreservation of small numbers of sperm, and embryo culture technologies.

This book contains thirteen chapters on five topics. The first section includes Chapters 1–5 and discusses recurrent failed implantation. The chapters review the general reasons and mechanisms of recurrent failed implantation, the effects of anatomy abnormalities in the uterus (e.g., fibroids) on infertility, endometrial receptivity in patients with polycystic ovary syndrome (PCOS), and current PGT technologies, emphasizing non-invasive PGT and its benefits to IVF patients.

The second topic includes two chapters related to oocyte cryopreservation. During the past decade, oocyte cryopreservation has been added to human-assisted reproduction technologies and has benefited many women. Chapter 6 reviews and discusses the ethical issues of oocyte cryopreservation, while Chapter 7 reports clinical outcomes of oocyte cryopreservation in different categories of patients.

The third topic includes four chapters. Chapter 8 discusses male infertility and Chapter 9 examines the molecular mechanisms of heavy metals on male infertility, with a focus on sperm capacitation and fertilization. Chapter 10 reviews literature on rare sperm cryopreservation and Chapter 11 presents a very efficient method of cryopreservation of small numbers of spermatozoa.

The fourth topic includes Chapter 12, which discusses the potential role of kisspeptins in human reproduction.

The final topic includes Chapter 13, which reports the authors' research results on different incubators for embryo development and their effectiveness to maintain temperature and pH during embryo culture.

Although this book does not cover all interesting topics in infertility and assisted reproduction, the collected chapters certainly deliver new information and data valuable to clinicians, embryologists, and others in infertility treatment.

I would like to thank the contributors who shared their intellectual and practical laboratory expertise and experiences with infertility treatment and with those who will enter the field in the future. I also want to thank Ms. Jasna Bozic at IntechOpen for her assistance, without which publication of this book would not have been possible.

Wei-Hua Wang
Prelude Fertility,
Houston, USA

Chapter 1

Reasons and Mechanisms of Recurrent Failed Implantation in IVF

Violeta Fodina, Alesja Dudorova and Juris Erenpreiss

Abstract

Recurrent pregnancy loss (RPL) and recurrent implantation failure (RIF) are serious problems in IVF and ICSI cycles. Different factors are showed to be responsible for these clinical challenges – such as paternal, maternal, embryonic, immunological, infectious, hormonal, and others. In this chapter we have tried to review the available data on reasons for the RIF, and systematize them into: 1) uterine factors; 2) embryo factors; 3) immunological factors; 4) other factors. Interplay between all these factors play a role in RIF, and further investigations are needed to elucidate their significance and interactions – in order to elaborate more definite suggestions or guidelines for the clinicians dealing with artificial reproductive techniques and facing RPL and RIF.

Keywords: IVF, failed implantation, embryo loss, pregnancy loss

1. Introduction

1978 was the year when the first IVF baby Louise Brown was born. From that time reproductive technology progress grew exponentially as well as the experience in current field. In the next years after Louise Brown birth initial implantation rates were < 5% per embryo [1]. As ART technology progressed, many clinics replaced cleavage-stage embryos to blastocyst-stage embryos, and switched from multiple embryo transfers to double- or single-embryo transfers. Each of those achievements led to the point where modern reproductology stands.

Despite the accumulated experience and knowledge, there are many medical questions that need to be answered, because recurrent pregnancy loss (RPL) and recurrent implantation failure (RIF) still exist.

RPL is a disorder defined by the American Society for Reproductive Medicine (ASRM) as the loss of two or more consecutive clinical pregnancies until 20 weeks of gestation [2]. It is known that around 5% of all women are experiencing two consecutive pregnancy losses, 75% of which are implantation failures [3]. In the case of RIF, because of rapidly changing field of ART there has been always a lack of consensus on the definition of RIF, and up till today the definition of RIF is still not unanimous.

One of the first attempts to define RIF was done by Coulam twenty years ago. He defined RIF as a failure to achieve pregnancy with more than 12 embryos transferred in several procedures [4]. During the consecutive 20 years, more and criteria have been added. A parameter of the blastocyst in the definition of RIF was introduced in 2007: it has been stated that for RIF to be diagnosed, in the patients history there should be the transfer of ≥8 of the 8-cell embryos, the transfer or ≥ 5 blastocysts without achieving the pregnancy [5]. After that the researchers started to specify that good-quality embryos is also a significant factor that should be taken into account [6]. Good-quality embryo was defined as having the correct number of cells corresponding to the day of its development and day-5 embryos (blastocysts) were graded according to expansion and quality of the inner cell mass and trophectoderm [7]. Coughlan with colleagues in 2014 proposed definition in which they also added the age of women [8]. About the same time, Lukasz with co-workers stated that RIF should be defined as the absence of implantation defined by a negative serum hCG 14 days after oocyte collection, after two consecutive cycles of IVF, ICSI or frozen embryo transfer, where the cumulative number of transferred embryos was no less than four for cleavage-stage embryos and no less than two for blastocysts, with all embryos being of good quality and of appropriate developmental stage [9]. The PGD Consortium, a specialized group of European Society of Human Reproduction and Embryology, suggested one of the last definitions of RIF: it is a failure to achieve pregnancy after ≥3 embryo transfers (ET) of high-quality embryos in women <40 years, or transfers of ≥10 embryos in total in multiple transfers. Presence or absence of pregnancy is diagnosed by an ultrasound examination after the 5th week [8, 10, 11]. Implantation failure can depend on different factors. Successful embryo implantation is an interactive process between the blastocyst and the uterus. Synchronized development of embryos with uterine differentiation to a receptive state is necessary to complete pregnancy. Implantation failure may occur even on early stages during the embryo attachment or migration. As a result, there will be no objective evidence of a pregnancy, i.e. negative urine or blood pregnancy tests (negative hCG) [12]. Another scenario - embryo can migrate through the luminal surface of the endometrium and start to produce hCG, which may be detected in the blood or urine. But even on this stage the process could be disrupted before the formation of an intrauterine gestational sac. In general, implantation failure is usually distinguished into two groups. The first group included women who never shown quantifiable signs of implantation, such as increased levels of hCG. The second group include women who have an evidence of implantation (detectable hCG production) but it did not proceed beyond the formation of a gestational sac visible on ultrasonography 2 weeks later [8]. From the clinical point of view, as defined by the ASRM, implantation is considered successful when there is ultrasonographic evidence of an intrauterine gestational sac or by histopathological examination [2]. With vast numbers of potential causes to consider, to diagnose an etiology of implantation failure is still a complex task for every reproductologist. Some researchers attempted to present summarized reasons of RIF. For example, Timeva et al. have divided RIF causes in three main groups: 1) multifactorial RIF with the subgroups of maternal or paternal factors, hormonal or metabolic disorders, infections and thrombophilias; 2) endometrial RIF that is caused due to thin (≤6 mm) endometrium, with or without variations in vascularity; 3) idiopathic RIF, which is unexplained failure to achieve pregnancy after transfer of good quality embryos, without any anatomical and histological changes in uterine cavity and endometrium, without any other disturbances in patient, patient-partner and embryos [13]. Some other authors, in turn, have distinguished etiologic groups such as decreased endometrial receptivity, defective embryonic development and also multifactorial effectors, including into the multifactorial group endometriosis, hydrosalpinges and suboptimal ovarian stimulation [6]. However, there are two main causes of implantation failure that are always present in the majority of all the classifications: uterine and embryo factors. Therefore, we will shortly review these two, and will also add some data on the immunological and other factors of interest in the context of RIF.

2. Uterine factors

2.1 Endometrial receptivity

Endometrial environment plays a crucial role in embryo implantation and early placental development. There is a certain period of endometrial maturation during which the trophectoderm of the blastocyst can attach to the endometrial epithelial cells and subsequently proceed to invade the endometrial stroma, which is called endometrial receptivity [14]. This complex process provides the embryo with the opportunity to normally attach, implant and develop.

There is a short period of time during the menstrual cycle, when the endometrial receptivity is optimal and embryo implantation is possible. This period is called "window of implantation" (WOI). Studies with donor embryos in humans have shown that this receptive period starts at day 6 post ovulation and continues 4–5 days (or 3–6 days) within the secretory phase (day 20–24 of the menstrual cycle) in most healthy women [15, 16]. Endometrium is unique in its ability to block embryos from implanting, except during this narrow window of receptivity, where endometrium undergoes morphological, cytoskeletal, biochemical, and genetic changes [17]. As shown in the mouse models (and is also true in the other species), WOI is regulated by ovarian steroid hormones. In the receptive endometrium, crucial hormones are progesterone and 17β-estradiol [18, 19]. In certain pathologic conditions, this window is narrowed or shifted, which disrupts normal implantation, leading to infertility or pregnancy loss [15, 16].

2.2 Human endometrium transcriptomics

The transcriptome reflects the genes that are actively expressed at any given time within a specific cell population or tissue [20]. Human endometrial receptivity transcriptome is a rather complex issue because the quantity of crucial genes that plays a main role in receptivity is still a debatable question. Despite so many publications that revealed hundreds of simultaneously up- and down-regulated genes, the number of selected genes usually differs from one publication to another.

The early search using mouse models started with a few identified genes of receptivity, such as leukemia inhibitory factor-LIF, Homeobox protein X3, genes of embryo response- Cyclooxygenase 2-COX 2; and decidualization -Interleukin 11 Receptor-IL-11R [20]. In 2003 from comparing the gene expression pattern of 375 human cytokines, chemokines, and related factors in receptive and prereceptive human endometrium identified IGF-1 (insulin-like growth factor-binding protein) as a new endometrial receptivity gene [21]. Furthermore, Zhang et al. proposed 148 receptivity biomarkers [22]. Tapia et al. suggested a list of 61 receptivity biomarkers [23]. Bhagwat et al. found 179 genes that have the potential to be called Receptivity Associated Genes [24]. In an enrichment analysis used to identify a meta-signature of highly presumed biomarkers of endometrial receptivity, a statistically significant meta-signature of 52 up-regulated and five down-regulated genes was identified [25]. The highest scores in receptive-phase endometrium reserved 5 up-regulated transcripts - GADD45A, SPP1, PAEP, GPX3 and MAOA. The five down-regulated transcripts receptivity-associated genes were SFRP4, EDN3, OLFM1, CRABP2 and MMP7 [22–24, 26, 27]. Interestingly, commercial Endometrial receptivity array (ERA test) by Igenomix [28, 29] shares 47 genes in common with the identified 57 putative receptivity biomarkers.

As the potential biomarkers for endometrial receptivity, many other molecules have been also studied - like mucin (MUC-1), trophinin, L-selectin, Wingless (Wnt) family members, etc. [30].

2.3 Endometrial receptivity Array

Endometrial receptivity array was developed and patented in 2009. The group of Garrido Gomez from Igenomix have developed a clinical algorithm with a computational predictor which test results are based on the expression analysis of 248 genes [29]. Expression profiling is accomplished by assaying mRNA levels with microarrays or next-generation sequencing technologies (RNA-seq), that allowed identification of the transcriptomic signature of the window of implantation [31]. The idea is to detect a specific point in time of endometrial cycle in which the WOI starts, allowing physicians to perform personalized embryo transfer (pET). The accuracy and consistency of the ERA test had been demonstrated in several trials, that showed that the ERA test is a reliable and reproducible method for determination of the exact time of the WOI that can be used with better results in comparison to histological dating of endometrial receptivity [32]. A pilot study was conducted by Igenomix of 17 RIF patients, who underwent oocyte donation and routine embryo transfer (ET) but were then treated with pET after the personalized diagnosis of their WOI. This study demonstrated that embryo-endometrial synchronization within an optimal time-frame increases the chances of success in an assisted reproductive treatment [33]. The same group showed that patients with at least three previous failed oocyte donation cycles, and IVF patients aged <40 years, with at least three failed IVF cycles with a receptive ERA diagnosis resulted in a 62.8% pregnancy rate [20]. Other groups also showed increased probability of having successful implantation and pregnancy after performed pET in accordance to the ERA result. Results in the Indian population revealed an endometrial factor in 27.5% of the RIF patients, which was significantly greater than 15% in the non-RIF group [17]. Increased percentages of non-receptive ERA test in women with RIF have been also demonstrated [17, 28, 34]. However, the data on the ability of the ERA test to improve the implantation chances in RIF patients are conflicting, with some studies showing no beneficial effect of the test [35, 36]. Also, some studies failed to demonstrated concordance between the ERA test and histological dating of the endometrial biopsies [37].

2.4 Uterine microbiome

Normal microbiome in healthy women primarily consists of hydrogen peroxide-producing Lactobacilli species [38]. During infancy the vaginal flora consists of aerobic and anaerobic bacterial populations, including Streptococcus and Staphylococcus, Prevotella and Enterobacteria species [39]. When puberty comes, the estrogen production causes glycogen to rise and pH to decrease with subsequent domination by Lactobacilli species. Microbiomes of all reproductive organs (vagina, cervix, Fallopian tubes, and ovaries) are significantly correlated [40]. It has been suggested that instead of a single most frequent microbiome, there are multiple core microbiomes: either dominated by variety of Lactobacillus species, or with a lower percentage of Lactobacilli and dominance of anaerobic bacteria [38].

Studies indicate that lower diversity in the microbiome show better outcomes [41–43]. It seems that gravid vaginal microbiome tends to be more stable and less diverse through all the period of pregnancy [44] with major change such as an increase in the dominance of four Lactobacillus spp. (*L. crispatus*, L. jensenii, L. gasseri, and *L. vaginalis*) and a decrease in the amount of anaerobic species [45].

Regarding the endometrial microbiome of women with RIF, Bacteroides and Proteobacteria seem to be the most represented [46]. Meta-analysis that was done in 2013 also proved that dysbiotic shifts are more frequent in subfertile population [47]. Also, a contamination from the transfer catheter tip by Enterobacteriaceae, Streptococcus, Staphylococcus, *Escherichia coli* and Gram-negative bacteria has a negative effect on implantation and pregnancy rates [48–52].

3. Embryo factors

3.1 Embryo quality

Blastocysts (day-5 embryos) are graded according to expansion and quality of the inner cell mass and trophectoderm. Other criteria include blastomeres of equal size and regular in distribution, distribution of cytoplasm without granularity and less than 10% fragmentation [7]. Good-quality embryo needs to have the correct number of cells corresponding to the day of its development. To make this statement and describe all the pathological elements in development, at least 4 decades of research was needed to achieve the modern stage of embryo evaluation such as time-lapse imaging.

At early stages a morphological evaluation of the embryo was the only criteria for estimating developmental potential of embryo and predicting the probability of achieving pregnancy [53]. The history behind the science of current time-lapse embryo imaging goes back to 1997 when Payne et al. documented the use of time-lapse video cinematography in order to observe the initial events in 38 normally fertilized human oocytes and compare these events with the day 3 embryo development [54]. After ten years based on Payne et al. work, Mio and Maeda extended the analysis period to blastocyst stage and obtained 286 images of human oocytes and embryos [55]. At the same year, Lemmen and colleagues analyzed the events that occur during the first day of the development after fertilization of 102 oocytes by using a microscope with an enclosed camera system [56]. They were the first group that paid attention to embryo kinetic properties, by establishing a link between the early disappearance of pronuclei after fertilization, early first cleavage, and many blastomeres on day 2 of the development. After some period of time many authors started suggesting that kinetic properties need to be added to the morphological evaluation, like timing of embryonic cell divisions [57, 58].

At first the main focus was on time of first embryonic division or early cell division after which embryo becomes 2-cell organism. Correlation between pregnancy rate and time of early cell division was first studied by Edwards group [59]. They concluded that the transfer of embryos that cleaved 24–26 h after fertilization results in higher implantation and pregnancy rates compared to embryos with delayed division. Later many other publications showed that to fast or to slow cleavage has a negative impact on embryo development [60–62].

Modern time-lapse observation systems are developed for more optimized and accurate selection of viable embryos that includes morphological grading with the possibility to register kinetic parameters [60]. Time-lapse imaging has its own benefits, like low light exposure in relation to traditional morphology observation methods [63] and possibility of observing embryo inside incubator without moving it, which provides stable and uninterrupted conditions that could be beneficial for the final result [64].

Several statistical models were created to predict parameters like blastocyst stage development and quality. Morphokinetic algorithms that could predict successful implantation, biochemical or clinical pregnancy were described [60, 65, 66].

3.2 Embryo aneuploidy

Throughout the life a human body and their cells are affected by many negative life-style and external environment factors. Adding the aging and cellular senescence, it results in errors in chromosome segregation during meiosis I and II [67]. Due to the aging of the oocytes, these errors lead to increase of embryos with abnormal chromosome number. The reasons behind these chromosome segregation errors are due to many factors, like incorrect formation of bivalents, derogation of cohesins, sister kinetochores separation by large distances and incorrect attachment of spindle microtubules to kinetochores during meiosis. Despite the well-known fact of decreasing quality of oocytes with aging, many women in the modern age delay having their first child until later in their life [68].

One of the largest studies on the impact of age on the aneuploidy rates was performed in 2011. More than 20 000 oocytes were obtained from 2830 patients with an average age of 38.8 years, and their polar bodies were examined using FISH method. A study detected 20% of aneuploidies in women at the age of 35 that increased to the nearly 60% aneuploidy oocytes in women over 43 years of age. Of all the tested oocytes, almost half of them (46.8%) were aneuploid [69].

Detection and management of embryo anomalies that occur due to the age, poor quality oocytes or sperm abnormalities may be accomplished by performing preimplantation genetic testing (PGT) that allows to pick up and transfer blastocysts with normal genetic constitution.

The history of PGT goes back to 1989 when Handyside performed first preimplantation genetic diagnostic (PGD) cases detecting a Y chromosome-specific region with PCR in case of X-linked adrenoleukodystrophy and X-linked mental retardation [70]. Defining embryo gender can complement to genetic testing of monogenic disorders linked to the sex chromosomes.

With time PGT underwent significant methodological changes, starting from the polar body testing and blastomere analysis to adapting trophectoderm biopsy with subsequent blastocyst freezing [71]. In early days the blastomeres were analyzed using FISH method for chromosomes X, Y, 18, 13, and 21 [72]. The analysis of more than a single cell has led to a more robust downstream molecular investigation [73]. Molecular genetic testing started as analysis of single loci by PCR method and grew to sophisticated single cell whole genome amplification [74]. Also, instead of PGT many groups have tried to develop algorithms to detect ploidy based on morphokinetic properties. There were several attempts to create such algorithms using time-lapse monitoring. The idea was based on assumption, that embryos display different cleavage dynamics depending on their genetic material, but this have not been fully proved [75, 76].

PGT consists of two main tests: PGT-M and PGT-A. PGT-M is a pre-implantation genetic testing of embryos for monogenic (or single gene) diseases. PGT-M is used on as a part of IVF process in couples with hereditary genetic disorders.

PGT-A (preimplantation genetic testing for aneuploidy) is a procedure that allows determining the chromosomal status of IVF embryos by screening all 23 pairs of human chromosomes including sex chromosomes. Many different methods are used, which includes array comparative genomic hybridization (aCGH), quantitative PCR (qPCR), single nucleotide polymorphism array (SNP array) and next-generation sequencing (high and low resolution) (NGS). The difference between those methods is in quantity of genomic amplification, ability to detect balanced or unbalanced translocations, partial aneuploidies, polyploidy, and mosaicism. For example, Array CGH, SNP array, and high resolution NGS utilize whole genome amplification of genomic DNA but at the same time can introduce an artifact. Quantitative PCR and low resolution NGS are not able to amplify the whole genome and because of their low genomic coverage small deletions or duplications could not be detected [72].

In the PGT-A results embryos can be diagnosed three ways: as euploid with the normal number of chromosomes; as aneuploid with abnormal number of chromosomes, or mosaic - where 2 different cell lines are present within the same embryo (often one euploid cell line and one aneuploid cell line). Regarding mosaic embryos, it has been shown that mosaicism rates decrease with extended embryo culture. This could happen due to embryos ability to self-correct or because euploid cell lines predominate at later developmental stages [77].

However, the data on the ability of the PGT-A to improve the implantation and live birth rates in RIF patients is also still a controversial issue [36, 78–80].

4. Immunologic factors

4.1 Lymphocytes Th1/Th2 profile and Th17

T lymphocytes are types of immune cells that originate from bone marrow and mature in thymus cortex. One of those mature populations of lymphocytes are T-helpers, which express antigens CD4. CD4+ T cells are divided into two major types: T helper 1 (Th1) and T helper 2 (Th2) cells. Th1and Th2 are characterized by cytokines that they secrete and are important in cellular and humoral immunity function. Th1 in general tends to be proinflammatory and secrete such cytokines as interferon-γ, TNF-α and interleukins (ILs) 1, 2, 6, 12, 15 providing help to other T cells and macrophages. Th2 on the other hand, cancel out the Th1 subpopulation and serve as anti-inflammatory agents that secrete ILs 4, 5, 10 and provide help to B cells, in the production of antibodies [81, 82].

During pregnancy, the milieu of Th cells in normal circumstances shifts towards the prevalence of Th2 subpopulation. It happens due to rise of Progesterone, which inhibits the secretion of Th1 cytokines. In immunologic profiles the levels of IL-4 and IL-10 goes up and levels of IL-2, TNF-α and interferon-γ goes down. When the child is born, he/she also has a Th2-dominant cytokine milieu, which quickly changes because of the microbial colonization [83]. If the milieu reverses towards the Th1 cell dominance, it could impact pregnancy by causing cytokine-triggered abortion due to thrombotic/inflammatory processes in maternal uteroplacental blood vessels.

It has been demonstrated on mice that injection of Th1 cytokines, i.e., TNF-a or IFN-gamma mediates abortion, while the administration of TNF-a antagonists reduces the fetal loss [84]. However, Th1 prevalence in the peripheral blood during peri-implantation period is normal in healthy women, also, there is no correlation between cytokine expression and serum hormone levels, which makes screening tests difficult to use in predicting imbalance in future pregnancies [85, 86].

Liang et al. compared the ratios of pro- and anti-inflammatory cytokines IFN-c/IL-4, IFN-c/IL-10, IFN-c/TGF-b1, TNF-a/TGF- b1 in the RIF patients and women with successful pregnancies. They discovered the shift towards pro-inflammation in RIF group [87]. Another group also indicated that without any difference in gestational age, the pro-inflammatory cytokine levels such as TNFα, IFNγ, are significantly higher in euploid miscarriages, than in healthy pregnant women at 10–14 weeks of pregnancy [88].

As the role of Th1/Th2 population gain more and more evidence of their relevance in fertility, the role of third population of cells like Th17 also gained attention. Th17 cells are types of T-helper lymphocytes that are characterized by pro-inflammatory cytokine IL-17 production. Signals such as transforming growth factor beta (TGF-β), interleukin 6 (IL-6), interleukin 21 (IL-21) and interleukin 23 (IL-23) cause the Th17 formation in mice and humans while at the same time these signals inhibit regulatory T cell differentiation [89, 90]. IL-17 is a cytokine which promotes the expression of various mediators of inflammation while playing an important role in maintaining mucosal surfaces pathogen free. The loss of Th17 cell populations at mucosal surfaces is related to chronic inflammation and microbial translocation. It has been demonstrated that the levels of Th17 cells in peripheral blood lymphocytes do not change in women with normal pregnancy [91] but proportion of Th17 cells in the peripheral blood and decidua significantly increases in unexplained recurrent spontaneous abortion patients [92, 93].

4.2 TNF-a

Overproduction of TNF-a could have toxic effect of pregnancy despite its necessity to assure endometrial receptivity. By analyzing cytokine profile of 210 women undergoing IVF with the endometrial secretion analysis technique, higher TNF-a and IL-1b levels have been detected in patients with the previous history of implantation failure that achieved clinical pregnancy [94]. This could emphasize, that proinflammatory cytokines are also needed for successful transfer, pregnancy to occur.

4.3 Regulatory T cells

Regulatory T cells, formally known as suppressor T cells or Tregs express the CD4, FOXP3, and CD25 biomarkers and develop from the same lineage as T-helpers [95]. These cells are best known for their function to generally suppress Th1- and Th17-mediated immunity, or in other words - to suppress autoreactive and alloreactive immune responses, thereby preventing autoimmune diseases and allograft rejection [96]. These cells also modulate the immune system and downregulate induction and proliferation of effector T cells (CD8+). Tregs are involved in the regulation of local maternal tolerance towards the fetus, their concentration increases within 2 days of conception in normal human pregnancy [97]. Expression of IL-10 and TGF-b by Tregs and its suppression potential is significantly reduced in patients with unexplained recurrent spontaneous miscarriage in comparison to fertile patients [98]. Tregs also regulate the CD8(+) T cell differentiation by significantly reducing the expression of perforin and granzyme B in the decidua compared to peripheral blood EM CD8(+) T cells, which may also play a crucial role in establishing the maternal immune tolerance cells [99]. It has been demonstrated that patients with recurrent miscarriages and cellular immune imbalance could be treated with intravenous immunoglobulin G given it increases the of Th17 and Foxp3(+) Treg cell numbers [100].

4.4 Natural killers (NK) and uterine NK (uNK)

Parents wishing for a pregnancy are not tissue-matched, therefore, a mother's immune system has to be suppressed. NK cells seem to play an important role in this process [101].

Natural killer cells, or NK cells, are a type of cytotoxic lymphocytes. In the uterus there are a special type of Natural Killers that consists of two main subsets: CD56 + CD16+ cells (10% of uNK) with dim phenotype, and CD56 + CD16-cells

(90% of uNK) with bright phenotype [102]. The bright type that should be dominant cell subset, has low cytotoxic ability and are potent in secreting the cytokines [101].

IL-15 and IL-18 are involved in the maturation of uNK. As the potential markers of uNK activity, levels of IL-15 and IL-18 are positively correlated with uNK levels in patients with implantation failure [103]. uNK cells increase in numbers from about 70% up to 83.2% of the uterine leukocytes during the mid- to late luteal phase, and first trimester of pregnancy [104, 105]. In some studies, it has been established that uterine NK play a role in decidual vascularization. This elevation of uNK CD56 cells density could contribute to increased angiogenesis in pre-implantation period leading to reduced uterine artery resistance to blood flow, endometrial oedema and as a result to implantation failure [106, 107]. Abnormal decidual vascularization and the increase in angiogenic factors contribute to the development of miscarriages and implantation failures.

4.5 Altered expression of associated molecules

4.5.1 Prostaglandins

Prostaglandins are group of physiologically active lipid compounds called eicosanoids. Prostaglandins are synthetized from Arachidonic acid by the action of cyclooxygenase (COX) isoenzymes [108]. Their function is to sustain homeostasis, mediate pathogenic mechanisms by stimulating a reaction in one tissue (inflammatory response) and inhibiting the same reaction in another tissue. The type of the receptor to which the prostaglandins bind determines these reactions.

Decidual cells also secrete prostaglandins that latter interacts in complex reactions with other cytokines, growth factors and hormones like progesterone, prolactin, relaxin.

Achache et al. suggested that decreased prostaglandin synthesis might be a key factor in altered endometrial receptivity, therefore plays a role in implantation failure. Levels of cytosolic phospholipase A2 (cPLA2a) and COX-2 that was measured by PCR and Western blot tests were found to be decreased in patients with RIF in comparison to the fertile group. It was suggested that it might be detrimental to implantation only when both enzymes are missing. Interestingly, in response to the decreased function and presence of these enzymes, secretory phospholipase A2 (sPLA2-IIA) was overexpressed. This overexpression most likely is a form of compensation to maintain release of arachidonic acid [109].

Another data on RIF patients show that they express defective endometrial PG on the days 21–24 of the cycle. It has been estimated at both mRNA and protein level that already mentioned enzymes such as cyclooxygenase-2 (COX-2), secretory phospholipase A2 group (sPLA2-IIA, sPLA2-V, sPLA2-IB), and other molecules like glypican-1, PG-E synthase, PG-E receptors, and lysophosphatidic acid receptor 3 (LPA3), play an important role in PG synthesis and are found in very low concentrations in 85% of RIF patients [109].

4.5.2 HOX-a and E-cadherin

Certain type of transcription factors, such as HOXA-10 and E-Cadherin, could also play the potential role in the implantation process. HOXA-10 and E-Cadherin are localized in the glandular epithelium cells of endometrium. Specifically, HOXA-10 in the nuclei of stroma cells and E-Cadherin the cytoplasm of glandular epithelium cells. Regarding HOXA-10 and E-cadherin expression, positive correlation was established between significantly reduced levels of HOXA-10 and E-cadherin expression in women with the history RIF, as compared with a control group [110].

4.5.3 Leukemia inhibitory factor (LIF)

LIF primarily was identified as macrophage differentiation inductor of the myeloid leukemia M1 cell line [111]. Later LIF started to be considered as the first cytokine that is shown to play critical role in mice blastocyst development and implantation [112]. The other functions of LIF included proliferation, differentiation and cell survival [113]. Given the fact that LIFs mRNA is expressed during days 18–28 of the menstrual cycle in the endometrium of the fertile women, it also suggests it has a role in human implantation [114]. LIF expression is regulated by Progesterone. Treating women with the progesterone receptor antagonist immediately after ovulation, it reduces immunoreactivity of LIF at the expected time of implantation [115].

Evidence for LIF role in human fertility was described several authors showing that low concentrations of LIF in the uterine flushing fluid at day 26 may be a good predictor of successful implantation, while at the same time endometrial explants from infertile women and women with recurrent miscarriages secrete less LIF than those from fertile women [116–119].

4.5.4 Apolipoprotein A-I

From the proteomic analysis of the endometrial biopsies, a new molecule was found that could be a potential predictor of the endometriosis and even of the RIF patients.

Apolipoprotein A-I (Apo A-I) was identified as an anti-implantation protein, that is secreted by differentiating endometrium. It seems that higher expression of Apo A-I can be found in ectopic secretory endometrium in patients with endometriosis. This statement implies that dysregulation of certain molecule secretion might be a significant factor in pathogenesis of endometriosis and a crucial point for RIF [120]. But more date on this “fingerprint” is needed to apply it to the diagnostics.

4.6 Antiphospholipid antibodies (APL)

Antiphospholipid syndrome (APS) is an autoimmune condition that is associated with thrombosis and morbidity in pregnancy [121]. The pathogenic pathway by which whose conditions occur are not yet fully understood but it is known that mechanisms may be heterogeneous. The main Antiphospholipid Antibodies (aPLs) that is found in APS are lupus anticoagulant (LA), anticardiolipin antibodies (aCLs) and anti-β2glycoprotein I antibodies (aβ2GPI) [122].

APS is diagnosed if at least one of three antiphospholipid antibodies are detected on two or more occasions within a 12-weeks interval, and is associated with a clinical condition such as thrombosis or morbidity in pregnancy. Morbidity in pregnancy includes preterm delivery due to eclampsia, preeclampsia, unexplained stillbirths at≥10 weeks of gestation, or placental insufficiency, and three or more consecutive miscarriages [123]. Recurrent early miscarriage is one of antiphospholipid syndrome (APS) obstetrical features with the incidence of aPLs in 15–20% of the patients with recurrent miscarriages [122]. However, the link between APS and RIF should be further investigated.

5. Other factors

5.1 Body mass index (BMI)

Obesity is defined as BMI equal to or more than 30. According to the WHO, more than 1.9 billion adults of the world population are suffering from the extra body mass (BMI >25), and more than 650 million are obese [124].

A significantly lower ongoing pregnancy rate and implantation rate in obese women have been reported [125, 126]. The implantation rate, pregnancy and live birth rate are shown to be lower in obese women with the tendency to progressively go down with each unit of BMI (kilograms per square meter) [127]. It has been also found that higher BMI is associated with lower clinical pregnancy rates especially in women under age 35 using their own oocytes [128].

5.2 Ovarian response to stimulation

The goal of ovarian stimulation is the collection of multiple dominant follicles in an effort to compensate for the inefficiencies of embryology culture, embryo selection, thus improving chances for successful conception in IVF [129]. The definition of poor ovarian response (POR) should be understood as an essential inability of woman's ovaries to properly react to the selected stimulation [130]. At least two of the following three features must be present for the POR to be diagnosed: 1) advanced maternal age (≥40 years), or any other risk factor for POR; 2) a previous POR (≤3 oocytes with a conventional stimulation protocol); 3) an abnormal ovarian reserve test (antral follicle count: 5–7 follicles, or Anti-Mullerian hormone 0.5–1.1 ng/ml) [131–133].

There are many risk factors that may cause poor ovarian response: short menstrual cycle, single ovary, ovarian cystectomy, smoking, unexplained infertility, previous chemotherapy and/or radiotherapy treatment, family history of premature menopause, pelvic infection, etc. Further studies are needed to elucidate the role of these factors in RIF.

5.3 Male factor

Many studies have emphasized the role of sperm DNA integrity on the fertility of a couple, also reporting the relationship of the increased sperm DNA damage and pregnancy loss after IVF and ICSI [134]. However, some studies have failed to support a hypothesis that sperm DNA integrity is an important factor in RIF [135], therefore, also this important question needs to be further investigated.

6. Conclusion

We have described that recurrent implantation failure in IVF cycles depends on the interplay of many factors - female factors (different aspects of the uterine health), embryo factors (embryo quality and aneuploidy), possibly male factors (sperm DNA integrity), immunological factors, and probably many more. More investigations are needed before the clinicians can be clearly advised what diagnostic and treatment approaches must be implemented in the cases of RIF.

Acknowledgements

Authors are grateful to Anna Dorondo for her technical help.

Author details

Violeta Fodina[1], Alesja Dudorova[1] and Juris Erenpreiss[1,2]*

1 Clinic "IVF-Riga", Riga, Latvia

2 Riga Stradins University, Riga, Latvia

*Address all correspondence to: jerenpreiss@gmail.com

References

[1] Niederberger C, Pellicer A, Cohen J, Gardner DK, Palermo GD, O'Neill CL, et al. Forty years of IVF. Fertil Steril. 2018;110(2):185-324.e5.

[2] Bashiri A, Halper KI, Orvieto R. Recurrent Implantation Failure-update overview on etiology, diagnosis, treatment and future directions 11 Medical and Health Sciences 1114 Paediatrics and Reproductive Medicine. Reprod Biol Endocrinol. 2018;16(1):4-7.

[3] Comins Boo A, Segovia AG, del Prado NN, Fuente L de la, Alonso J, Ramon SS. Evidence-based Update: Immunological Evaluation of Recurrent Implantation Failure. Reprod Immunol Open Access. 2016;01(04).

[4] Coulam CB. Implantation failure and immunotherapy. Hum Reprod [Internet]. 1995 Jun 1;10(6):1338-40. Available from: https://doi.org/10.1093/HUMREP/10.6.1338

[5] Rinehart J. Recurrent implantation failure: Definition. J Assist Reprod Genet. 2007;24(7):284-287.

[6] Margalioth EJ, Ben-Chetrit A, Gal M, Eldar-Geva T. Investigation and treatment of repeated implantation failure following IVF-ET. Hum Reprod. 2006;21(12):3036-3043.

[7] Cutting R, Morroll D, Roberts SA, Pickering S, Rutherford A, ACE on behalf of the BFS and. Elective Single Embryo Transfer: Guidelines for Practice British Fertility Society and Association of Clinical Embryologists. Hum Fertil [Internet]. 2008 Jan 1;11(3):131-46. Available from: https://doi.org/10.1080/14647270802302629

[8] Coughlan C, Ledger W, Wang Q, Liu F, Demirol A, Gurgan T, et al. Recurrent implantation failure: Definition and management. Reprod Biomed Online. 2014;28(1):14-38.

[9] Polanski LT, Baumgarten MN, Quenby S, Brosens J, Campbell BK, Raine-Fenning NJ. What exactly do we mean by "recurrent implantation failure"? A systematic review and opinion. Reprod Biomed Online [Internet]. 2014;28(4):409-423. Available from: http://dx.doi.org/10.1016/j.rbmo.2013.12.006

[10] Thornhill AR, deDie-Smulders CE, Geraedts JP, Harper JC, Harton GL, Lavery SA, et al. ESHRE PGD Consortium "Best practice guidelines for clinical preimplantation genetic diagnosis (PGD) and preimplantation genetic screening (PGS)." Hum Reprod. 2005;20(1):35-48.

[11] Geyser PJ, Siebert IT. Early Recurrent Pregnancy Loss. Obstet Gynaecol Forum. 2015;25(1):28-31.

[12] Maesawa Y, Yamada H, Deguchi M, Ebina Y. History of biochemical pregnancy was associated with the subsequent reproductive failure among women with recurrent spontaneous abortion. Gynecol Endocrinol [Internet]. 2015 Apr 3;31(4):306-8. Available from: https://doi.org/10.3109/09513590.2014.994601

[13] Timeva T, Shterev A, Kyurkchiev S. Recurrent implantation failure: The role of the endometrium. Vol. 15, Journal of Reproduction and Infertility. 2014.

[14] Lessey BA, Young SL. Structure, Function, and Evaluation of the Female Reproductive Tract [Internet]. Eighth Edi. Yen & Jaffe's Reproductive Endocrinology: Physiology, Pathophysiology, and Clinical Management: Eighth Edition. Elsevier Inc.; 2019. 206-247.e13 p. Available from: https://doi.org/10.1016/B978-0-323-47912-7.00009-3

[15] Lessey BA, Young SL. What exactly is endometrial receptivity? Fertil Steril

[Internet]. 2019;111(4):611-7. Available from: https://doi.org/10.1016/j.fertnstert.2019.02.009

[16] Bergh PA, Navot D. The impact of embryonic development and endometrial maturity on the timing of implantation. Fertil Steril. 1992 Sep 1;58(3):537-542.

[17] Mahajan N. Endometrial receptivity array: Clinical application. J Hum Reprod Sci. 2015;8(3):121-129.

[18] Tan J, Paria BC, Dey SK, Das SK. Differential uterine expression of estrogen and progesterone receptors correlates with uterine preparation for implantation and decidualization in the mouse. Endocrinology. 1999;140(11):5310-5321.

[19] Paria BC, Huet-Hudsont YM, Dey SK. Blastocyst's state of activity determines the "window" of implantation in the receptive mouse uterus. Vol. 90, Proc. Natl. Acad. Sci. USA. 1993.

[20] Garrido-Gómez T, Ruiz-Alonso M, Blesa D, Diaz-Gimeno P, Vilella F, Simón C. Profiling the gene signature of endometrial receptivity: Clinical results. Fertil Steril. 2013;99(4):1078-1085.

[21] Dominguez F, Avila S, Cervero A, Martin J, Pellicer A, Castrillo JL, et al. A Combined Approach for Gene Discovery Identifies Insulin-Like Growth Factor-Binding Protein-Related Protein 1 as a New Gene Implicated in Human Endometrial Receptivity. J Clin Endocrinol Metab [Internet]. 2003; 88:1849-57. Available from: https://academic.oup.com/jcem/article/88/4/1849/2845539

[22] Zhang D, Sun C, Ma C, Dai H, Zhang W. Data mining of spatial-temporal expression of genes in the human endometrium during the window of implantation. Reprod Sci. 2012;19(10).

[23] Tapia A, Vilos C, Marín JC, Croxatto HB, Devoto L. Bioinformatic detection of E47, E2F1 and SREBP1 transcription factors as potential regulators of genes associated to acquisition of endometrial receptivity. Reprod Biol Endocrinol [Internet]. 2011;9(1):14. Available from: http://www.rbej.com/content/9/1/14

[24] Bhagwat SR, Chandrashekar DS, Kakar R, Davuluri S, Bajpai AK, Nayak S, et al. Endometrial Receptivity: A Revisit to Functional Genomics Studies on Human Endometrium and Creation of HGEx-ERdb. PLoS One. 2013;8(3).

[25] Altmäe S, Koel M, Võsa U, Adler P, Suhorutšenko M, Laisk-Podar T, et al. Meta-signature of human endometrial receptivity: A meta-analysis and validation study of transcriptomic biomarkers. Sci Rep. 2017;7(1):1-16.

[26] Horcajadas JA, Pellicer A, Simón C. Wide genomic analysis of human endometrial receptivity: new times, new opportunities. Hum Reprod Update [Internet]. 2007;13(1):77-86. Available from: https://academic.oup.com/humupd/article/13/1/77/751486

[27] Tseng LH, Chen I, Chen MY, Yan H, Wang CN, Lee CL. Genome-based expression profiling as a single standardized microarray platform for the diagnosis of endometrial disorder: an array of 126-gene model. Fertil Steril [Internet]. 2010;94(1):114-119. Available from: http://dx.doi.org/10.1016/j.fertnstert.2009.01.130

[28] Ruiz-Alonso M, Blesa D, Díaz-Gimeno P, Gómez E, Fernández-Sánchez M, Carranza F, et al. The endometrial receptivity array for diagnosis and personalized embryo transfer as a treatment for patients with repeated implantation failure. Fertil Steril. 2013;100(3):818-824.

[29] Díaz-Gimeno P, Horcajadas JA, Martínez-Conejero JA, Esteban FJ,

Alamá P, Pellicer A, et al. A genomic diagnostic tool for human endometrial receptivity based on the transcriptomic signature. Fertil Steril. 2011;95(1).

[30] Lessey BA. Assessment of endometrial receptivity. Fertil Steril [Internet]. 2011;96(3):522-529. Available from: http://dx.doi.org/10.1016/j.fertnstert.2011.07.1095

[31] Hung J-H, Deng Z. Analysis of Microarray and RNA-seq Expression Profiling Data. Cold Spring Harb Protoc. 2016 Aug 29;2017.

[32] Díaz-Gimeno P, Ruiz-Alonso M, Blesa D, Bosch N, Martínez-Conejero JA, Alamá P, et al. The accuracy and reproducibility of the endometrial receptivity array is superior to histology as a diagnostic method for endometrial receptivity. Fertil Steril. 2013;99(2):508-517.

[33] Ruiz-Alonso M, Galindo N, Pellicer A, Simó C. What a difference two days make: "personalized" embryo transfer (pET) paradigm: A case report and pilot study. Available from: https://academic.oup.com/humrep/article/29/6/1244/627046

[34] Tan J, Kan & A, Hitkari & J, Taylor & B, Tallon & N, Warraich & G, et al. The role of the endometrial receptivity array (ERA) in patients who have failed euploid embryo transfers. Assist Reprod Technol [Internet]. 2018;35:683-92. Available from: https://doi.org/10.1007/s10815-017-1112-2

[35] Hashimoto T, Koizumi M, Doshida M, Toya M, Sagara E, Oka N, et al. Efficacy of the endometrial receptivity array for repeated implantation failure in Japan: A retrospective, two-centers study. Reprod Med Biol. 2017;16(3):290-296.

[36] Cozzolino M, Diaz-Gimeno P, Pellicer A, Garrido N. Evaluation of the endometrial receptivity assay and the preimplantation genetic test for aneuploidy in overcoming recurrent implantation failure. J Assist Reprod Genet [Internet]. 2020;37(12):2989-97. Available from: https://doi.org/10.1007/s10815-020-01948-7

[37] Cohen A, Ye X, Colgan T, Greenblatt E, Chan C. Comparing endometrial receptivity array to histologic dating of the endometrium in women with a history of implantation failure. Syst Biol Reprod Med. 2020 Sep 30;66.

[38] Ravel J, Gajer P, Abdo Z, Schneider GM, Koenig SSK, Mcculle SL, et al. Vaginal microbiome of reproductive-age women. Available from: www.pnas.org/cgi/doi/10.1073/pnas.1002611107

[39] Huang B, Fettweis JM, Brooks JP, Jefferson KK, Buck GA. The Changing Landscape of the Vaginal Microbiome. 2014;

[40] Walther-António MRS, Chen J, Multinu F, Hokenstad A, Distad TJ, Cheek EH, et al. Potential contribution of the uterine microbiome in the development of endometrial cancer. Genome Med [Internet]. 2016;8(1):1-15. Available from: http://dx.doi.org/10.1186/s13073-016-0368-y

[41] Prince AL, Chu DM, Seferovic MD, Antony KM, Ma J, Aagaard KM. The Perinatal Microbiome and Pregnancy: Moving Beyond the Vaginal Microbiome. Available from: http://perspectivesinmedicine.cshlp.org/

[42] Prince AL, Antony KM, Chu DM, Aagaard KM. The Microbiome, Parturition, and Timing of Birth: More questions than answers. 2014;

[43] Aagaard K, Riehle K, Ma J, Segata N, Mistretta T-A. A Metagenomic Approach to Characterization of the Vaginal Microbiome Signature in Pregnancy. PLoS One [Internet].

2012;7(6):36466. Available from: www.plosone.org

[44] Romero R, Hassan SS, Gajer P. The composition and stability of the vaginal microbiota of normal pregnant women is different from that of non-pregnant women. Microbiome. 2014 Jan 1;2.

[45] Romero R, Hassan SS, Gajer P, Tarca AL, Fadrosh DW, Bieda J, et al. The vaginal microbiota of pregnant women who subsequently have spontaneous preterm labor and delivery and those with a normal delivery at term. Microbiome. 2014;2(1):1-15.

[46] Verstraelen H, Vilchez-Vargas R, Desimpel F, Jauregui R, Vankeirsbilck N, Weyers S, et al. Characterisation of the human uterine microbiome in non-pregnant women through deep sequencing of the V1-2 region of the 16S rRNA gene.

[47] Van Oostrum N, De Sutter P, Meys J, Verstraelen H. META-ANALYSIS Infertility Risks associated with bacterial vaginosis in infertility patients: a systematic review and meta-analysis. Hum Reprod [Internet]. 2013;28(7):1809-1815. Available from: https://academic.oup.com/humrep/article/28/7/1809/611205

[48] Egbase PE, Al-Sharhan M, Al-Othman S, Al-Mutawa M, Udo EE, Grudzinskas JG. Incidence of microbial growth from the tip of the embryo transfer catheter after embryo transfer in relation to clinical pregnancy rate following in-vitro fertilization and embryo transfer [Internet]. Vol. 11, Human Reproduction. 1996. Available from: https://academic.oup.com/humrep/article/11/8/1687/598119

[49] Fanchin R, Harmas A, Benaoudia F, Lundkvist U, Olivennes F, Frydman R. Microbial flora of the cervix assessed at the time of embryo transfer adversely affects in vitro fertilization outcome. Fertil Steril. 1998 Nov 1;70(5):866-870.

[50] Egbase PE, Udo EE, Al-Sharhan M, Grudzinskas JG. Prophylactic antibiotics and endocervical microbial inoculation of the endometrium at embryo transfer. Lancet. 1999 Aug 21;354(9179):651-652.

[51] Moore DE, Soules MR, Klein NA, Fujimoto VY, Agnew KJ, Eschenbach DA. Bacteria in the transfer catheter tip influence the live-birth rate after in vitro fertilization. Fertil Steril. 2000 Dec 1;74(6):1118-1124.

[52] Selman H, Mariani M, Barnocchi N, Mencacci A, Bistoni F, Arena S, et al. Examination of bacterial contamination at the time of embryo transfer, and its impact on the IVF/ pregnancy outcome. 2007;

[53] Baczkowski T, Kurzawa R, Głabowski W. Methods of embryo scoring in in vitro fertilization. Reprod Biol. 2004;4(1):5-22.

[54] Payne D, Flaherty SP, Barry MF, Matthews CD. Preliminary observations on polar body extrusion and pronuclear formation in human oocytes using time-lapse video cinematography. Hum Reprod. 1997;12(3):532-541.

[55] Mio Y, Maeda K. Time-lapse cinematography of dynamic changes occurring during in vitro development of human embryos. Am J Obstet Gynecol. 2008;199(6):660.e1-660.e5.

[56] Lemmen JG, Agerholm I, Ziebe S. Kinetic markers of human embryo quality using time-lapse recordings of IVF/ICSI-fertilized oocytes. Reprod Biomed Online. 2008;17(3).

[57] Sakkas D, Shoukir Y, Chardonnens D, Bianchi PG, Campana A. Early cleavage of human embryos to the two-cell stage after intracytoplasmic sperm injection as an indicator of embryo viability. Hum Reprod. 1998;13(1).

[58] Lundin K, Bergh C, Hardarson T. Early embryo cleavage is a strong

indicator of embryo quality in human IVF. Hum Reprod. 2001;16(12).

[59] Edwards RG, Fishel SB, Cohen J, Fehilly CB, Purdy JM, Slater JM, et al. Factors influencing the success of in vitro fertilization for alleviating human infertility. J Vitr Fertil Embryo Transf. 1984;1(1).

[60] Meseguer M, Herrero J, Tejera A, Hilligsøe KM, Ramsing NB, Remoh J. The use of morphokinetics as a predictor of embryo implantation. Hum Reprod. 2011;26(10).

[61] Cruz M, Garrido N, Herrero J, Pérez-Cano I, Muñoz M, Meseguer M. Timing of cell division in human cleavage-stage embryos is linked with blastocyst formation and quality. Reprod Biomed Online. 2012;25(4).

[62] Basile N, Meseguer M. Time-lapse technology: Evaluation of embryo quality and new markers for embryo selection. Vol. 7, Expert Review of Obstetrics and Gynecology. 2012.

[63] Ottosen LDM, Hindkjær J, Ingerslev J. Light exposure of the ovum and preimplantation embryo during ART procedures. J Assist Reprod Genet. 2007;24(2-3).

[64] Meseguer M, Rubio I, Cruz M, Basile N, Marcos J, Requena A. Embryo incubation and selection in a time-lapse monitoring system improves pregnancy outcome compared with a standard incubator: A retrospective cohort study. Fertil Steril. 2012;98(6).

[65] Motato Y, de los Santos MJ, Escriba MJ, Ruiz BA, Remohí J, Meseguer M. Morphokinetic analysis and embryonic prediction for blastocyst formation through an integrated time-lapse system. Fertil Steril. 2016;105(2).

[66] Yang ST, Shi JX, Gong F, Zhang SP, Lu CF, Tan K, et al. Cleavage pattern predicts developmental potential of day 3 human embryos produced by IVF. Reprod Biomed Online. 2015;30(6).

[67] Handyside AH, Montag M, Magli MC, Repping S, Harper J, Schmutzler A, et al. Multiple meiotic errors caused by predivision of chromatids in women of advanced maternal age undergoing in vitro fertilisation. Eur J Hum Genet. 2012;20(7).

[68] Webster A, Schuh M. Mechanisms of Aneuploidy in Human Eggs. Vol. 27, Trends in Cell Biology. 2017.

[69] Kuliev A, Zlatopolsky Z, Kirillova I, Spivakova J, Cieslak Janzen J. Meiosis errors in over 20,000 oocytes studied in the practice of preimplantation aneuploidy testing. Vol. 22, Reproductive BioMedicine Online. 2011.

[70] Handyside AH, Kontogianni EH, Hardy K, Winston RML. Pregnancies from biopsied human preimplantation embryos sexed by Y-specific DNA amplification. Nature. 1990;344(6268).

[71] Renwick PJ, Trussler J, Ostad-Saffari E, Fassihi H, Black C, Braude P, et al. Proof of principle and first cases using preimplantation genetic haplotyping - A paradigm shift for embryo diagnosis. Reprod Biomed Online. 2006;13(1).

[72] Maxwell SM, Grifo JA. Should every embryo undergo preimplantation genetic testing for aneuploidy? A review of the modern approach to in vitro fertilization. Vol. 53, Best Practice and Research: Clinical Obstetrics and Gynaecology. 2018.

[73] Cimadomo D, Capalbo A, Ubaldi FM, Scarica C, Palagiano A, Canipari R, et al. The Impact of Biopsy on Human Embryo Developmental Potential during Preimplantation Genetic Diagnosis. Vol. 2016, BioMed Research International. 2016.

[74] Fiorentino F. Molecular genetic analysis of single cells. Semin Reprod Med. 2012;30(4).

[75] Chavez SL, Loewke KE, Han J, Moussavi F, Colls P, Munne S, et al. Dynamic blastomere behaviour reflects human embryo ploidy by the four-cell stage. Nat Commun. 2012;3.

[76] Vera-Rodriguez M, Chavez SL, Rubio C, Reijo Pera RA, Simon C. Prediction model for aneuploidy in early human embryo development revealed by single-cell analysis. Nat Commun. 2015;6.

[77] Santos MA, Teklenburg G, MacKlon NS, Van Opstal D, Schuring-Blom GH, Krijtenburg PJ, et al. The fate of the mosaic embryo: Chromosomal constitution and development of Day 4, 5 and 8 human embryos. Hum Reprod. 2010;25(8).

[78] Sato T, Sugiura-Ogasawara M, Ozawa F, Yamamoto T, Kato T, Kurahashi H, et al. Preimplantation genetic testing for aneuploidy: A comparison of live birth rates in patients with recurrent pregnancy loss due to embryonic aneuploidy or recurrent implantation failure. Hum Reprod. 2019;34(12).

[79] Rubio C, Bellver J, Rodrigo L, Bosch E, Mercader A, Vidal C, et al. Preimplantation genetic screening using fluorescence in situ hybridization in patients with repetitive implantation failure and advanced maternal age: Two randomized trials. Fertil Steril. 2013;99(5).

[80] Hatirnaz S, Ozer A, Hatirnaz E, Atasever M, Başaranoglu S, Kanat-Pektas M, et al. Pre-implantation genetic screening among women experiencing recurrent failure of in vitro fertilization. Int J Gynecol Obstet. 2017;137(3).

[81] Wegmann TG, Lin H, Guilbert L, Mosmann TR. Bidirectional cytokine interactions in the maternal-fetal relationship: is successful pregnancy a TH2 phenomenon? Vol. 14, Immunology Today. 1993.

[82] Kalu E, Bhaskaran S, Thum MY, Vishwanatha R, Croucher C, Sherriff E, et al. Serial estimation of Th1:Th2 cytokines profile in women undergoing in-vitro fertilization-embryo transfer. Am J Reprod Immunol. 2008;59(3).

[83] Raghupathy R. Th1-type immunity is incompatible with successful pregnancy. Vol. 18, Immunology Today. 1997.

[84] Clark DA, Chaouat G, Arck PC, Mittruecker HW, Levy GA. Cytokine-dependent abortion in CBA x DBA/2 mice is mediated by the procoagulant fgl2 prothrombinase [correction of prothombinase]. J Immunol [Internet]. 1998;160(2):545-9. Available from: http://www.ncbi.nlm.nih.gov/pubmed/9551885

[85] Macklon N. Recurrent implantation failure is a pathology with a specific transcriptomic signature. Vol. 108, Fertility and Sterility. 2017.

[86] Lim KJH, Odukoya OA, Ajjan RA, Li TC, Weetman AP, Cooke ID. The role of T-helper cytokines in human reproduction. Fertil Steril. 2000;73(1).

[87] Liang PY, Diao LH, Huang CY, Lian RC, Chen X, Li GG, et al. The pro-inflammatory and anti-inflammatory cytokine profile in peripheral blood of women with recurrent implantation failure. Reprod Biomed Online. 2015;31(6).

[88] Calleja-Agius J, Jauniaux E, Pizzey AR, Muttukrishna S. Investigation of systemic inflammatory response in first trimester pregnancy failure. Hum Reprod. 2012;27(2):349-357.

[89] Ivanov II, McKenzie BS, Zhou L, Tadokoro CE, Lepelley A, Lafaille JJ, et

al. The Orphan Nuclear Receptor RORγt Directs the Differentiation Program of Proinflammatory IL-17+ T Helper Cells. Cell. 2006;126(6).

[90] Hartigan-O'Connor DJ, Hirao LA, McCune JM, Dandekar S. Th17 cells and regulatory T cells in elite control over HIV and SIV. Curr Opin HIV AIDS. 2011;6(3).

[91] Nakashima A, Ito M, Yoneda S, Shiozaki A, Hidaka T, Saito S. Circulating and decidual Th17 cell levels in healthy pregnancy. Am J Reprod Immunol. 2010;63(2).

[92] Wang WJ, Hao CF, Yi-Lin, Yin GJ, Bao SH, Qiu LH, et al. Increased prevalence of T helper 17 (Th17) cells in peripheral blood and decidua in unexplained recurrent spontaneous abortion patients. J Reprod Immunol. 2010;84(2).

[93] Lee SK, Kim JY, Hur SE, Kim CJ, Na BJ, Lee M, et al. An imbalance in interleukin-17-producing T and Foxp3 regulatory T cells in women with idiopathic recurrent pregnancy loss. Hum Reprod. 2011;26(11).

[94] Boomsma CM, Kavelaars A, Eijkemans MJC, Lentjes EG, Fauser BCJM, Heijnen CJ, et al. Endometrial secretion analysis identifies a cytokine profile predictive of pregnancy in IVF. Hum Reprod. 2009;24(6).

[95] Curiel TJ. Tregs and rethinking cancer immunotherapy. Vol. 117, Journal of Clinical Investigation. 2007.

[96] Sakaguchi S, Sakaguchi N, Asano M, Itoh M, Toda M. Immunologic self-tolerance maintained by activated T cells expressing IL-2 receptor alpha-chains (CD25). Breakdown of a single mechanism of self-tolerance causes various autoimmune diseases. J Immunol. 1995;155(3).

[97] Schumacher A, Zenclussen AC. Regulatory T cells: Regulators of life. Vol. 72, American Journal of Reproductive Immunology. 2014.

[98] Bao SH, Wang XP, De Lin Q, Wang WJ, Yin GJ, Qiu LH. Decidual CD4 + CD25 + CD127 dim/- regulatory T cells in patients with unexplained recurrent spontaneous miscarriage. Eur J Obstet Gynecol Reprod Biol. 2011 Mar 1;155(1):94-98.

[99] Tilburgs T, Schonkeren D, Eikmans M, Nagtzaam NM, Datema G, Swings GM, et al. Human Decidual Tissue Contains Differentiated CD8 + Effector-Memory T Cells with Unique Properties . J Immunol. 2010;185(7).

[100] Kim DJ, Lee SK, Kim JY, Na BJ, Hur SE, Lee M, et al. Intravenous immunoglobulin G modulates peripheral blood Th17 and Foxp3+ regulatory T cells in pregnant women with recurrent pregnancy loss. Am J Reprod Immunol. 2014;71(5).

[101] Lash GE, Robson SC, Bulmer JN. Review: Functional role of uterine natural killer (uNK) cells in human early pregnancy decidua. Placenta. 2010;31(SUPPL.).

[102] Lachapelle MH, Miron P, Hemmings R, Roy DC. Endometrial T, B, and NK cells in patients with recurrent spontaneous abortion. Altered profile and pregnancy outcome. J Immunol. 1996;156(10).

[103] Lédée N, Petitbarat M, Rahmati M, Dubanchet S, Chaouat G, Sandra O, et al. New pre-conception immune biomarkers for clinical practice: Interleukin-18, interleukin-15 and TWEAK on the endometrial side, G-CSF on the follicular side. J Reprod Immunol. 2011;88(2).

[104] Nishikawa K, Salto S, Morii T, Hamada K, Ako H, Narita N, et al. Accumulation of cd16-cd56+ natural

killer cells with high affinity interleukin 2 receptors in human early pregnancy decidua. Int Immunol. 1991;3(8).

[105] Flynn L, Byrne B, Carton J, Kelehan P, O'Herlihy C, O'Farrelly C. Menstrual cycle dependent fluctuations in NK and T-lymphocyte subsets from non-pregnant human endometrium. Am J Reprod Immunol. 2000;43(4).

[106] Tuckerman E, Mariee N, Prakash A, Li TC, Laird S. Uterine natural killer cells in peri-implantation endometrium from women with repeated implantation failure after IVF. J Reprod Immunol. 2010;87(1-2).

[107] Quenby S, Nik H, Innes B, Lash G, Turner M, Drury J, et al. Uterine natural killer cells and angiogenesis in recurrent reproductive failure. Hum Reprod. 2009;24(1).

[108] Ricciotti E, Fitzgerald GA. Prostaglandins and inflammation. Arterioscler Thromb Vasc Biol. 2011;31(5).

[109] Achache H, Tsafrir A, Prus D, Reich R, Revel A. Defective endometrial prostaglandin synthesis identified in patients with repeated implantation failure undergoing in vitro fertilization. Fertil Steril. 2010;94(4).

[110] Yang Y, Chen X, Saravelos SH, Liu Y, Huang J, Zhang J, et al. HOXA-10 and E-cadherin expression in the endometrium of women with recurrent implantation failure and recurrent miscarriage. Fertil Steril. 2017;107(1).

[111] Hilton DJ, Nicola NA, Metcalf D. Purification of a murine leukemia inhibitory factor from Krebs ascites cells. Anal Biochem. 1988;173(2).

[112] Stewart CL, Kaspar P, Brunet LJ, Bhatt H, Gadi I, Köntgen F, et al. Blastocyst implantation depends on maternal expression of leukaemia inhibitory factor. Nature. 1992;359(6390).

[113] Metcalf D. Leukemia inhibitory factor-a puzzling polyfunctional regulator. Vol. 7, Growth Factors. 1992.

[114] Dimitriadis E, Salamonsen LA, Robb L. Expression of interleukin-11 during the human menstrual cycle: Coincidence with stromal cell decidualization and relationship to leukaemia inhibitory factor and prolactin. Mol Hum Reprod. 2000;6(10).

[115] Gemzell Danielsson K, Swahn ML, Bygdeman M. The effect of various doses of mifepristone on endometrial leukaemia inhibitory factor expression in the midluteal phase - An immunohistochemical study. Hum Reprod. 1997;12(6).

[116] Dimitriadis E, White CA, Jones RL, Salamonsen LA. Cytokines, chemokines and growth factors in endometrium related to implantation. Vol. 11, Human Reproduction Update. 2005.

[117] Laird SM, Tuckerman EM, Dalton CF, Dunphy BC, Li TC, Zhang X. The production of leukaemia inhibitory factor by human endometrium: Presence in uterine flushings and production by cells in culture. Hum Reprod. 1997;12(3).

[118] Lédée-Bataille N, Laprée-Delage G, Taupin JL, Dubanchet S, Frydman R, Chaouat G. Concentration of leukaemia inhibitory factor (LIF) in uterine flushing fluid is highly predictive of embryo implantation. Hum Reprod. 2002;17(1).

[119] Guzeloglu-Kayisli O, Kayisli UA, Taylor HS. The Role of Growth Factors and Cytokines during Implantation. Semin Reprod Med. 2009;27(1):62-79.

[120] Brosens JJ, Hodgetts A, Feroze-Zaidi F, Sherwin JRA, Fusi L, Salker MS,

et al. Proteomic analysis of endometrium from fertile and infertile patients suggests a role for apolipoprotein A-I in embryo implantation failure and endometriosis. Mol Hum Reprod. 2009;16(4).

[121] Santos T da S, Ieque AL, de Carvalho HC, Sell AM, Lonardoni MVC, Demarchi IG, et al. Antiphospholipid syndrome and recurrent miscarriage: A systematic review and meta-analysis. Vol. 123, Journal of Reproductive Immunology. 2017.

[122] Kutteh WH, Hinote CD. Antiphospholipid Antibody Syndrome. Vol. 41, Obstetrics and Gynecology Clinics of North America. Elsevier; 2014. p. 113-132.

[123] Miyakis S, Lockshin MD, Atsumi T, Branch DW, Brey RL, Cervera R, et al. International consensus statement on an update of the classification criteria for definite antiphospholipid syndrome (APS). J Thromb Haemost. 2006;4(2).

[124] World OH. World Health Organisation Obesity and Overweight Fact Sheet. World Health Organisation. 2016. p. https://www.who.int/news-room/fact-sheets/detail/o.

[125] DOODY K. Morbid obesity adversely impacts outcomes with IVF. Fertil Steril. 2003;80.

[126] Ryley DA, Bayer SR, Eaton J, Zimon A, Klipstein S, Reindollar R. Influence of body mass index (BMI) on the outcome of 6,827 IVF cycles. Fertil Steril. 2004;82.

[127] Bellver J, Ayllón Y, Ferrando M, Melo M, Goyri E, Pellicer A, et al. Female obesity impairs in vitro fertilization outcome without affecting embryo quality. Fertil Steril. 2010;93(2).

[128] Luke B, Brown MB, Stern JE, Missmer SA, Fujimoto VY, Leach R. Female obesity adversely affects assisted reproductive technology (ART) pregnancy and live birth rates. Hum Reprod. 2011;26(1).

[129] Macklon NS, Stouffer RL, Giudice LC, Fauser BCJM. The science behind 25 years of ovarian stimulation for in vitro fertilization. Vol. 27, Endocrine Reviews. 2006.

[130] De Geyter C, Calhaz-Jorge C, Kupka MS, Wyns C, Mocanu E, Motrenko T, et al. ART in Europe, 2014: Results generated from European registries by ESHRE. Hum Reprod. 2018;33(9).

[131] Ferraretti AP, La Marca A, Fauser BCJM, Tarlatzis B, Nargund G, Gianaroli L. ESHRE consensus on the definition of 'poor response to ovarian stimulation for in vitro fertilization: The Bologna criteria. Hum Reprod. 2011;26(7).

[132] Broer SL, Mol BWJ, Hendriks D, Broekmans FJM. The role of antimullerian hormone in prediction of outcome after IVF: comparison with the antral follicle count. Fertil Steril. 2009;91(3).

[133] La Marca A, Sighinolfi G, Radi D, Argento C, Baraldi E, Artenisio AC, et al. Anti-Müllerian hormone (AMH) as a predictive marker in assisted reproductive technology (ART). Vol. 16, Human Reproduction Update. 2009.

[134] Zini A, Boman JM, Belzile E, Ciampi A. Sperm DNA damage is associated with and increased risk of pregnancy loss after IVF and ICSI: systematic review and meta-analysis. Human Reproduction. 2008;23:2663-2668.

[135] Coughlan C, Clarke H, Cutting R, Saxton J, Waite S, Ledger W, Li T, Pacey AA. Sperm DNA fragmentation, recurent implantation failure and recurent miscarriage. Asian J Androl. 2015;17(4):681-685.

Chapter 2

Recurrent Implantation Failure: The Role of Anatomical Causes

Mariana Fonseca Roller Barcelos, Aluisio M. da Rocha Filho, Amanda Evelyn C. Goulart, Anna Luiza M. Souza, Daniely T. Costa, Gabriela Galdino de F. Barros, Isadora Manzi N. Theodoro, Jean Pierre B. Brasileiro, Murilo Cezar S. Oliveira, Natalia I. Zavattiero Tierno, Tatianna Quintas F. Ribeiro, Valeria L. Mathias Castro and Vinicius M. Lopes

Abstract

Recurrent implantation failure (RIF) is one of the great challenges of current reproductive medicine. The term refers to the failure of repeated transfers of embryos of good morphological quality. Embryo implantation is a crucial moment in *in vitro* fertilization (IVF) treatments. A successful pregnancy depends on a synchronized interaction between a good quality embryo and a receptive endometrium. Its failure may be a consequence of embryo quality, anatomical or immunological factors. The anatomic causes constitute an important factor for RIF, although they are usually manageable. Fibroids, polyps and adhesions that develop after a surgical procedure or infection can hamper the embryo - endometrium attachment process. In addition, Mullerian abnormalities and hydrosalpinx can cause a negative impact on implantation rates and should also be taken into account in patients with RIF. In this chapter, we will address the main anatomical causes that may impact the implantation rates of patients undergoing IVF, as well as recommendations on management and its treatment.

Keywords: implantation failure, fibroids, endometrial polyps, adhesions, uterine septum, mullerian abnormalities, hydrosalpinx

1. Introduction

Recurrent implantation failure (RIF) is one of the biggest challenges of the current reproductive medicine. Firstly, it is difficult to find its clinical standardized definition, despite the various articles on the topic. There is no agreement on issues, such as the number of embryo transfer failures, the embryo development stage, its morphology and aneuploidy, in order to define RIF [1]. There are also inconsistencies on the definition of implantation. Some authors consider it a failure when the gestational sac is not seen after the embryo transfer. Others claim that it happens when the β-hCG test is negative [1]. In 2014, some researchers proposed the following definition: it is the transfer of at least four good morphologic quality embryos, with at least three fresh or frozen transfers to women below 40 years old. This is the most accepted definition up to date [2]. However, an international common understanding is necessary to standardize the definition in order to create more consistent scientific studies.

The embryo implantation is a key stage during *in vitro* fertilization (IVF) treatment. A successful pregnancy relies on a synchronized interaction between a good quality embryo and a receptive endometrium for implantation. Its failure can be a consequence of embryonic, anatomic or immunologic factors.

The anatomic causes constitute an important factor for RIF, although they are usually manageable. Fibroids and polyps can cause endometrial cavity distortion. Adhesions that form after surgery or infection can hinder the process of embryo implantation. Besides that, mullerian abnormalities such as septate or bicornuate uterus should be considered in patients with RIF.

According to the American Society of Reproductive Medicine (ASRM), the presence of hydrosalpinx can negatively affect implantation rates, either by alteration on the fluid nutrients or even by mechanically affecting embryo implantation.

In this chapter, we will address the main anatomic causes that can affect the implantation rates in patients undergoing to IVF as well as recommendations on the management and treatment.

2. Uterine fibroids

Submucosal fibroids can affect embryo implantation due to different mechanisms, resulting in subsequent increased uterine contractility, abnormal endometrial vascularity, chronic endometrial inflammatory response and changes in local cytokines profile.

Fibroids which distort the endometrial cavity are associated with lower implantation and pregnancy rates among women who tried a natural pregnancy as well as among those who are undergoing IVF treatment [2].

2.1 Diagnosis

Uterine fibroids investigation among women with RIF can be done through the following methods:

- Transvaginal ultrasound scan: non-invasive method performed routinely in women undergoing IVF treatment [2, 3].

- Hysteroscopy procedure: it is considered a gold standard method in the diagnosis and treatment of intrauterine pathologies which cannot be seen during a transvaginal ultrasound scan, such as for example submucosal fibroids. A guideline published recently shows that the incidence of abnormal hysteroscopic findings in women with RIF ranges from 14–51%, including the submucosal fibroids. The author mentions a large and well conducted multicenter randomized clinical trial (RCT) - the TROPHY study - which discusses the role of hysteroscopy in RIF investigation among women with normal basal transvaginal ultrasound scan results. He found uterine alterations in 24% of women in the hysteroscopy group. However, only 4% showed an incidence of surgically treated alterations. Besides that, there was no statistical difference in live births rate among the two groups after surgical correction. Therefore, the above-mentioned guideline states that the routine hysteroscopy among RIF patients with normal basal transvaginal ultrasound scan is not recommended (recommendation strength: strong; evidence level: high) [1, 4]. Hysteroscopy must be considered before a new treatment cycle if the basal transvaginal ultrasound scan shows uterine pathology.

- Hysterosonography: although studies about cavity evaluation in RIF patients refer mainly to hysteroscopy, hysterosonography is a recommended and acceptable choice [1].

- Hysterosalpingography: it has a limited value for detection of intrauterine pathology and should not be used routinely for this purpose [2].

2.2 Treatment

Regarding the management of submucosal fibroids in women with RIF, one advocates their surgical removal, regardless the size, since evidence shows that their removal can improve clinical pregnancy rates [2, 3].

Prior to the surgery, the size and number of fibroids and the depth of intramural extension should be carefully assessed. Resection of a solitary submucous fibroid less than 5 cm in diameter and with little intramural extension should not pose significant difficulties. However, a submucous fibroid more than 5 cm in diameter or more than 50% embedded in the intramural part of the uterus may require removal in two stages. In the case of multiple submucosal fibroids, there is an increased risk of intrauterine adhesion formation after the procedure. Some surgeons advocate the removal of the anterior wall and posterior wall fibroids on separate occasions to reduce the risk of intrauterine adhesions [2, 3].

Unlike what happens to fibroids that distort the uterine cavity, there is no consensus regarding the removal of intramural fibroids in women with RIF. Some authors suggest adverse effects of intramural fibroids on implantation and pregnancy rates in women undergoing to IVF, particularly those larger than 4 cm, while other authors could not demonstrate such association [2].

The meta-analysis papers on the topic agree that women with intramural fibroids seem to have decreased implantation rates compared to those without intramural fibroids. However, the myomectomy did not seem to significantly increase clinical pregnancy and live births rates [3]. Therefore, the pros and cons of the myomectomy must be individually assessed. The patients must be aware of the possible complications caused by the procedure such as bladder and bowel injury, hemorrhage, risk of blood transfusion and hysterectomy that occurs in 1% of cases. Other consequences would be the formation of pelvic adhesions leading to infertility due to peritoneal tube factor, and the risk of uterine rupture in subsequent pregnancies. However, one must acknowledge that intramural fibroids can cause not only implantation failure but also some obstetric complications, such as increased risk of premature delivery, premature placental abruption, intrauterine growth restriction, abnormal fetal presentation and intrapartum hemorrhage. The decision-making must be individualized, and it is strongly recommended that an experienced surgeon takes part in the definition of the treatment [2].

In RIF cases with no determinant factors, the surgical removal of large or multiples fibroids is a choice [5]. After all explanations, the decision about the procedure to be taken - expectant conduct or myomectomy – is shared with the patient.

3. Endometrial polyps

Endometrial polyps are common, affecting more than 25% of women. They can be found within all ages [6, 7], and are common among infertile women with a prevalence up to 32% [8].

The potential mechanisms in which endometrial polyps can adversely affect fertility comprise mechanical interference and the release of molecules which adversely affect the spermatozoid transportation or the embryo implantation. Evidence shows increased levels of aromatase and glycodelin, a glycoprotein which inhibits the Natural Killer (NK) cells activity, resulting in a less receptive endometrium to implantation, inflammatory markers and decreased levels of HOXA-10 and 11 messenger RNA, which are known markers for endometrial receptivity [8, 9].

3.1 Diagnosis

The investigation of polyps in women with RIF can be done through some of the following methods:

- Transvaginal ultrasound scan: An endometrial polyp normally shows as a hyperechoic endometrial mass with regular borders partially or completely occupying the uterine cavity [1]. The ultrasound scan performed in the proliferative phase of the menstrual cycle generally shows more accurate results [10].

- Hysterosonography: The addition of intrauterine contrast agent (saline solution or ultrasound gel) increases transvaginal ultrasound diagnostic accuracy [11].

- Hysteroscopy: The hysteroscopy is gold standard for the diagnosis of endometrial polyps. They can be identified by hysteroscopy in 16–26% women with unexplained infertility. Hysteroscopy can also facilitate the assessment of several endometrial polyps features, such as size, number and vascular characteristics [11].

3.2 Treatment

Endometrial polyps surgical approach is controversial. The polyp size seems not to significantly affect pregnancy rates [12, 13]. Therefore, some studies have demonstrated that the resection of recently diagnosed polyps during ovarian stimulation cycle can decrease miscarriage rates and increase clinical pregnancy and live births rates, while others do not show such benefits. Lass et al. [14] showed that polyps smaller than 20 mm emerging during IVF can be expectantly managed without compromising clinical gestation and live births rates. However, in patients with RIF there is a recommendation for polypectomy prior to embryo transfer [3].

4. Congenital uterine anomalies

Congenital uterine anomalies come from failures along any step of the mullerian duct development process during embryo development, either in the formation, fusion or reabsorption. While an arcuate uterus shows a mild form of anomaly, a bicornuate uterus represents total failure. The actual uterine malformation prevalence is difficult to be determined since many of them are asymptomatic although they reach approximately 5.5% of the general population; 8% among infertile women and 13.5% among women with history of recurrent fetal loss [15]. A prospective observational study evaluated the prevalence of congenital uterine anomalies, including arcuate uterus, and their effect on the reproductive outcome among sub fertile women undergoing assisted reproduction. Clinical pregnancy and live births rates were similar among those with congenital uterine anomalies and the control group. There were no differences in the type of delivery, newborn gender or birthweight between the two groups. However, women with congenital uterine anomalies had more chance of premature delivery. After analysis of the anomalies subtypes, pregnancy and live birth rates were similar between arcuate and normal uterus groups. But the group with larger uterine anomalies showed worse reproductive outcomes [16].

Among the congenital uterine anomalies, the septate uterus is the most common and comprises 35% of the malformations. Its prevalence among infertile women (3%) seems to be comparable with the general population (2.3%) [15].

Women with septate uterus show increased risk of spontaneous abortion (2.9 relative risk [RR]; 95% confidence interval [95% CI] 2.0–4.1), premature delivery (2.1 RR; 95% CI 1.5–3.1) and abnormal fetal presentation (6.24 RR; 4.05–9.96 CI). They also have the lowest clinical pregnancy rates (0.86 RR; 95% CI 0.77–0.96) [17].

Little is known about the physiopathology responsible for the negative reproductive outcomes in women with septate uterus. According to a recent systematic literature review, all the eight studies which histologically investigated the septum showed that it consists of endometrial and myometrial tissue, and that most intrauterine septa are vascularized. One explanation for jeopardized reproductive outcomes of embryos implanted in the intrauterine septum could be the different histologic composition of the endometrial septum tissue. The glandular cells and the stroma have different morphologic characteristics: a smaller number of glandular cells and cilium, and incomplete cilium genesis.

Besides that, the endometrial septum contains the lowest levels of vascular endothelial growth fator (VEGF) receptors. It is believed that they have an important role in the early embryo implantation and placentation. In two studies, the HOXA10 gene expression, which is important for the early embryo implantation, seems to be altered in women with septate uterus. These findings can explain the disruptive development of the embryo implanted in the septum. However, since the studies' results on the issue are conflictive, a more detailed investigation is suggested [18].

4.1 Diagnosis

The definition of septate uterus has been discussed for a long time. Nowadays, there are three classification systems which are used worldwide. It's important to have a standardized classification system in order to prevent inappropriate or unnecessary surgical procedures and to compare reproductive results. The original classification system of the ASRM was modified and adapted. It currently uses morphometric criteria, such as the uterus internal indentation angle and internal midline cutout measurements to make a distinction between arcuated and septate uterus. It also uses the depth of uterus external surface to make a distinction between those and the bicornuate uterus. The uterus with indentation angle < 90°, length of midline internal cutout > 1.5 cm and uterine external cutout with less than 1 cm is defined as a septate uterus by the ASRM [19]. In 2012, the European Society of Human Reproduction and Embryology and the European Society for Gynecological Endoscopy (ESHRE/ESGE) published a classification system to replace the subjective criteria of the ASRM classification system by absolute morphometric criteria. Contrary to the American classification, the arcuate uterus is not mentioned and is considered a variant from normality. Septum is defined when the internal indentation is > 50% of the uterine wall thickness and the depth of the external fissure is < 50% of the wall thickness [20]. Women with previous diagnosis of arcuate uterus made by the ASRM (around 58%) would be classified as having a septate uterus when using the ESHRE/ESGE new classification. Thus, there would be an increase on the number of surgical procedures to fix uterine anomalies, with no evidence showing that this practice is beneficial to these women [21]. Recently, a simplified classification was proposed by the Congenital Uterine Malformations Experts (CUME), where the septum is defined as the depth of the internal indentation ≥ 10 mm [22]. It demonstrates the heterogeneity in the classification of mullerian malformations, making it difficult to produce scientific papers on these alterations in a homogeneous way.

4.2 Treatment

The uterine septum is the only malformation that can be corrected. There are many discussions about the impact of the septum resection on the reproductive results and if it improves natural conception rates and implantation rates after embryo transfer. Nowadays, the ASRM guidelines for septate uterus management recommend the hysteroscopic resection [18]. In contrast, the ESHRE, the National Institute for Health and Care Excellence (NICE) and the Royal College of Obstetricians and Gynecologists (RCOG) guidelines for recurrent fetal loss associated to septate uterus do not support this procedure until further studies can demonstrate its effectiveness [23–25]. Lavergne et al. found a retrospective multicentric study which shows that implantation rates after IVF cycle were significantly lower in patients with malformed uterus (septate, bicornuate or unicornuate) in comparison with patients with a normal uterus (6% vs. 12%, $p < 0.01$). There was significant improvement when the uterine anomaly was corrected (septate uterus) [26]. One study compared gestation and abortion rates after embryo transfer on an IVF cycle in patients with septate uterus before and after septum resection. They were compared to a control group, showing that pregnancy rates before hysteroscopic resection (both in women with septate or subseptate and arcuate uterus) were significantly lower in comparison to the patients in the normal control group [OR 2.9 ($P < 0.002$) and 2.2 ($P < 0.001$)], respectively. After surgery, pregnancy rate was comparable to the women with a normal uterus (OR 1.2 and 1.1). The uterine septum size did not influence pregnancy rate. The study conclusion recommends the hysteroscopic resection in order to improve the reproductive outcome, not limited to women with recurrent early fetal loss or premature labor, but it is also recommended to infertile women in order to improve pregnancy and live birth rates, especially if IVF is a choice [27]. Ozgur et al. showed that a history of abortion and IVF failure was frequent among women with untreated incomplete septate uterus in comparison to the infertile general population. After surgical correction of the septum, pregnancy rates in IVF cycle were similar to the group with normal uterine cavity [28]. In a recent article by the SWOT infertility group in Spain, the researchers stated that a septate uterus has been associated to a high prevalence of repeated implantation failure in assisted reproduction and abortion after IVF. In these cases, septum resection seems to be useful to improve IVF pregnancy rates [29]. These studies suggest that the correction of anatomical alterations which distort the uterine cavity, especially the septate uterus, can improve reproductive results.

In other studies, we saw that the septate uterus correction may not bring benefits. In an international multicentric cohort study with women with septate uterus and showing desire for pregnancy (which opted for septum resection or expectant approach), Rikken et al. showed that the septum resection did not increase the chance of live births nor reduced the risk of abortion or premature birth [30]. The only controlled randomized trial assessing the reproductive outcome after uterine septum resection was recently published. Women in reproductive age with a septate uterus and the wish to get pregnant and a history of subfertility, fetal loss or premature birth were selected. The results of this randomized clinical trial showed that the hysteroscopic resection of the septum did not improve live birth rates or other reproductive outcomes in women with septate uterus. In this study, one patient undergoing septum resection had a perioperative uterine perforation. The authors concluded that if there is no proven efficacy, they do not recommend septum resection as a routine procedure in clinical practice. Women with septate uterus need to be informed about this study data. After counseling and according to the principles of shared decision-making, an informed consent must be provided [31].

In relation to other malformations, except septate uterus, surgical correction seems not to bring benefits. Surrey et al. demonstrated that the arcuate uterus does not have an impact on the results of IVF cycle after euploid embryos transfer. Women undergoing IVF with indentation between 4 and 10 mm experience excellent results which are similar to those of women with internal indentation < 4 mm (live birth rate; 68.7% vs. 68.7%). Besides that, there were no differences in the reproductive outcome among those with arcuate or normal uterus, according to Salim et al. Criteria [32]. Chen et al. compared the reproductive outcome between unicornuate and morphologically normal uterus. There were no significant differences in the pregnancy, clinical pregnancy or live births rates. The abortion rates were similar. In single pregnancies, there were no differences in the preterm birth, birthweight or birth size rates. However, prematurity rates, lower birthweight and lower birth size rates as well as higher very low birth rates were found in twin pregnancies with unicornuate uterus. A single embryo transfer is recommended for unicornuate uterus [33].

The difficulty of having an agreement on the scientific studies is due to the impediments to unite mullerian malformations classification, differences on the definition of recurrent embryo implantation failure and a low prevalence of these events. Thus, we suggest the individualization of the cases in which mullerian malformations and recurrent implantation failure appear. Among all the malformations, the septate uterus is the one whose correction is possible in order to improve the reproductive outcome. Nevertheless, further studies are necessary to confirm this statement.

5. Intrauterine synechiae

Intrauterine synechiae, intrauterine adhesions or Asherman syndrome are names that define lesions on the endometrial tissue caused after aggressive curettage or any other intrauterine procedure that destroys the endometrium.

It is known that gestational complications such as missed or incomplete abortion and afterbirth bleeding are responsible for approximately 90% of the cases [34]. Nonetheless, infections in a non-pregnant uterus and surgeries such as myomectomies or septoplasty, for example, can lead to synechiae formation [35], causing or not secondary amenorrhea.

In terms of physiopathology, the assessment by electronic microscopy shows that the glandular cells have severe alterations in women with Asherman syndrome.

It is mainly due to ribosome metabolism which culminates in ATP depletion and subsequent tissue hypoxia. There is an abnormal expression of different growth factors which leads to the activation of cytokines related to the adhesion and a pro-inflammatory cascade [36]. There are also theories that associate the occurrence, severity and recurrence of intrauterine adhesions to an alteration of the endometrial microbiome, but they lack strong scientific evidence.

The presence of adhesions in the uterine walls can interfere in the embryo implantation impeding the embryo cellular fixation on the endometrial luminal layer. Demirol and Gurgaon found a prevalence of 8.5% of intrauterine synechiae in women with embryo implantation failure, which confirms the importance of a clinical investigation [37].

5.1 Diagnosis

For 20 years, the hysterosalpingography was the first line exam for the diagnosis of intrauterine synechiae. Today it is still used by many gynecologists for the evaluation of the uterine cavity, since it is a low-cost analysis showing 75% sensitivity [38]. It is similar to the hysterosonography whose sensitivity is of 82% [39]. The transvaginal ultrasound scan is also used to confirm a thin endometrium, but it has low accuracy for the diagnosis of synechiae [40], so that it is not considered the best method of investigation. The 3D hysterosonography has 91.1% sensitivity and 98.8% specificity, which makes it a good examination for the diagnosis of intra-uterine adhesions [41]. However, despite the data forementioned, the hysteroscopy is certainly a golden standard for the diagnosis of synechiae, once it allows direct visualization of the uterine cavity [42] and enables treatment. There is concrete evidence that the synechiae lysis during hysteroscopy improves the reproductive outcomes [43].

5.2 Treatment

Before hysteroscopy, cervix dilation and curettage associated with estrogenic therapy and use of IUD ensured 84% success rate in the treatment of Asherman syndrome. However, today we have the hysteroscopy as a golden standard in the diagnosis and treatment of this endometrial complication. It became necessary to define the site and severity of intrauterine adhesions. Classifying the disease process can be important once the severity imposes the prognosis after treatment [44]. The hysteroscopy enables the amplification and general observation of adhesions allowing the viewing of all structures, which decreases the risk of uterine perforation. However, there should be maximum care when using mechanic and electronic section since errors can bring undesirable repercussions [45].

The surgical treatment shows success rate after adhesiolysis ranging between 75 to 100% [46]. This rate can be evaluated by the return of menstrual periods, rates and pregnancy outcome. After a hysteroscopic surgery, around 92 to 96% of women returned to their bleeding pattern prior to the syndrome showing 63% pregnancy rate and 75% live births rate [44]. The most frequent complication in pregnancies after hysteroscopic treatment for uterine adhesions is the abnormal placentation [44].

The intraoperative fluoroscopy and transabdominal ultrasound scan or the laparoscopy are also efficient alternatives [45]. The fluoroscopic guidance enables the surgeon to see endometrium islands behind the scar tissue in an obliterated uterine cavity. The radio opaque dye is injected into a dense scar area in the place where the cavity is obliterated. Some endometrial adhesions can be identified using fluoroscopy. The area can be opened through acute dissection under hysteroscopy.

However, this technique is considered limited by the high cost, by technical difficulties or by the requirement for ionizing radiation [46].

The laparoscopic guidance for severe cases of intrauterine adhesiolysis has been advocated for the immediate recognition and treatment of uterine perforation, thus minimizing the extrauterine trauma. The intraoperative ultrasound scan, fluoroscopy or laparoscopy together with the hysteroscopy have been used as guidance to reduce the risk of perforation. Nevertheless, nowadays it is known that these interventions do not prevent uterine perforation or improve the outcome [46].

The stem cell therapy approach is much more efficient due to the potential for multiplication of a single cell and its transformation into undifferentiated forms (self-renovation) and into mature cells. Besides that, it can produce other types of cells, such as totipotent, pluripotent and multipotent cells [35].

In 2016, Tan et al. [47] investigated mesenchymal stem cells derived from bone marrow and stromal cells coming from the menstrual bleeding through transmiometral administration in the subendothelial area, direct installation of stromal cells in the uterine cavity and infusion of cells in spiral arteries through a catheter. Five out of six women with Asherman syndrome recovered their menstrual periods. Others reached adequate endometrial thickness and regular menstruation cycles and were able to get pregnant right after that. In this study, the authors compared some types of stem cells and could observe endometrial regeneration in most of the cases.

Thus, stem cells therapy has become a new method of treatment for the regenerative medicine, and more specifically, for the regeneration of endometrial diseases with Asherman syndrome and thin endometrium. However, stem cells transplant for Asherman syndrome is far from being common [46].

The biggest challenge for the treatment of Asherman syndrome is to prevent the recurrence of adhesions after the early treatment, which reaches 66% [46]. The treatment is defined by time. There are studies that evaluated the post-operative period comparing the use of intrauterine device (IUD) with intrauterine balloon catheter, Foley catheter, hormonal treatment and barriers such as amniotic membranes. The results are conflicting.

For instance, the copper IUD can provoke inflammation and is contraindicated [44]. Similarly, the hormone IUD have a small surface that limits its capacity to keep the endometrial cavity walls separated during healing [39]. The risk of infection after the insertion of an IUD after surgical resection of intrauterine adhesions is about 8% [44].

The placement of a Foley catheter with an IUD was assessed as a possible adjuvant treatment to prevent the formation of synechiae after hysteroscopy. The authors concluded that the Foley catheter placed one week and a half after adhesiolysis showed 81% success rate while the group which placed an IUD twelve weeks after the adhesiolysis showed 62% success rate [48]. The use of intrauterine hyaluronic gel after hysteroscopic treatment reduces adhesions recurrence [48], but further studies are needed for its incorporation into the treatment [44, 45].

Platelet-rich plasma (PRP) is a form of treatment for intrauterine adhesions after operative hysteroscopy and may be a substitute for the intrauterine balloon. However, randomized controlled trials with large sample sizes are warranted to further confirm the conclusions to compare the efficacy of intrauterine infusions of PRP with intrauterine balloons applied immediately after transcervical resection of the adhesions by hysteroscopy [49].

Clinical treatment with drugs such as aspirin, sildenafil and nitroglycerin have been done to increase endometrial blood flow in an attempt of stimulate cell regeneration. Successful pregnancies were reported after using them. However, more robust and well designed studies are required to confirm it [44].

Hormonal therapy with post-operative estrogen was not standardized in terms of dose, duration, route of administration or a combination with progesterone, Data about its efficacy are limited [44]. The American Association of Gynecologic Laparoscopists (AAGL) guidelines recommend hormonal therapy with estrogen after adhesiolysis, but there is no definition for dose or standard regimen [46]. The combination of this and adjuvant treatments is necessary for a maximum effect on patients with mild to severe adhesions.

As for the therapy with antibiotics, there is a lack of studies addressing the risks and benefits of those before, during and after surgical lysis of intrauterine adhesions. The American College of Obstetrics and Gynecology (ACOG) does not recommend the routine use of antibiotics with this objective [44, 46].

Hysteroscopic adhesiolysis cure infertility in mild, moderate and severe IUA in around 90, 70 and 30%, respectively [50]. Gestational surrogacy remains an alternative for those patients with intrauterine adhesions that stay infertile [51].

6. Adenomyosis

Adenomyosis is a benign uterine pathology known by the invasion of glandular endometrial tissue and myometrial stromal tissue which leads to disorders in the myometrial natural architecture [52].

There are some theories explaining the emergence of adenomyosis. The theory of tissue injury and repair (TIAR) as the main mechanism of myometrial invasion has been the most accepted hypothesis. Chronic peristaltic myometrial contractions can lead to micro lesions close to the endometrial-myometrial junction causing inflammation which in turn leads to an increase in local production of estrogen inducing a vicious cycle. Thus, the TIAR theory highlights the importance of tissue damages to the endometrial-myometrial interface supporting the common knowledge that the adenomyosis is associated with multiple births, previous cesarean section and previous uterine surgery [53]. However, it is known that there is a considerable number of macrophages in the ectopic endometrium of patients with endometriosis, fibroids and adenomyosis. Therefore, the potential for embryo implantation can be affected by adenomyosis [54]. This increase in the number of macrophages induced by adenomyosis can cause a hostile immunologic environment for embryos transferred during the implantation process. The interleukin-1 alpha tumor necrosis factor as well as reactive oxygen and nitrogen species are potentially toxic for embryos. It was demonstrated that an increased level of nitric oxygen is related to an adverse development of embryos and low pregnancy rates in the endometrial environment in patients with adenomyosis. Besides that, endometrial biopsies taken from adenomyosis showed that this tissue is composed of a high quantity of antioxidant enzymes as superoxide dismutase, catalase and glutathione peroxidase which are clear signs of oxidative stress caused by excessive ROS production [55].

Other risk factors are age over 40 years, multiple births, previous cesarean sections or other uterine surgeries. The disease is often diagnosed in young and infertile women or those with pain or abnormal uterine bleeding, or both [56].

Adenomyosis is associated with a great variety of symptoms. The common symptoms include pelvic pain (as dysmenorrhea, dyspareunia or chronic pelvic pain), abnormal uterine bleeding and impaired reproductive potential or even infertility itself. However, it is important to observe that 30% of women with adenomyosis have no symptoms [57]. In infertile women with adenomyosis, the topic endometrium shows a great variety of molecular alterations causing altered receptivity. That includes the alteration in the sexual steroid hormone via, increase of inflammatory markers and oxidative stress, decrease on the implantation markers expression, lack of adhesion molecular expression and altered gene function for the embryo development. Not only fertility outcomes are affected, but also pregnancy outcomes [58]. These include premature birth, premature rupture of membranes, postpartum hemorrhage, abnormal fetal presentation, increase on the risk of abortion in the second trimester and abnormal placental position [57].

6.1 Diagnosis

The diagnosis can be done after case history, clinical evaluation and image assessment with 2D/3D transvaginal ultrasound or magnetic resonance [52]. The transvaginal ultrasound for its facility of access and low cost in relation to other types of screenings has become a very useful tool to the diagnosis. Several ultrasographic criteria have been used to the adenomyosis diagnosis, including uterine size increase, anterior and posterior uterine walls thickness asymmetry, presence of heterogeneous myometrial areas, presence of myometrial anechoic areas, presence of sub endometrial echogenic striations, sub endometrial echogenic nodules, irregular endometrial-myometrial interface, poor definition and thickness of the junctional zone [57].

A meta-analysis about ultrasound accuracy in the diagnosis of adenomyosis demonstrated 82.5% sensitivity (95% CI), 77.5–87.9) and 84.6% specificity (95% CI, 79.8–89.8) with 4.7 positive likelihood ratio (3.1–7.0) and 0.26 negative likelihood ratio (0.18–0.39) which is comparable to the magnetic resonance [59].

The magnetic resonance is a precise and non-invasive technique used to the diagnostic of adenomyosis [60]. Its sensitivity and specificity in this diagnostic range from 88–93% and 67–91%, respectively [57]. The diagnosis of adenomyosis by magnetic resonance is essentially related to junctional zone characteristics, but can also include direct and indirect signs of endometrial glands inside the myometrium and smooth muscle cells hypertrophy [61, 62].

6.2 Treatment

Clinical pregnancy, implantation, and ongoing pregnancy rates were significantly higher in women undergoing frozen embryo transfer after long-term GnRH-analog therapy compared to those not pretreated with GnRH-analog [63].

Tremellen et al. reported that hypothalamic–pituitary- ovarian axis suppression therapy with GnRH agonist can produce a significant decrease in the number of endometrial macrophages, presumably interfering with the estradiol-mediated recruitment of macrophages to the endometrium and a subsequent normalization of embryo implantation rates [64]. Wang et al. showed that patients with normal ovarian reserve who underwent IVF/ICSI, adenomyosis seemed to negatively affect IVF/ICSI outcomes after a long GnRH agonist protocol (subcutaneous administration of short acting GnRH agonist on the dosage of 0.1 mg/day, for 10 days followed by 0.05 mg/day until the day of hCG injection which was started in the mid-luteal phase of the previous cycle), but patients with adenomyosis following an ultra-long GnRH-agonist protocol could experience stronger pituitary inhibition and lower ovarian responses but still could have a better IVF/ICSI outcomes. Ultra-long GnRH agonist protocol was considered the use of a depot injection of the long-acting GnRH agonist, triptorelin acetate (triptorelin) 3.75 mg, intramuscularly, every 28 days for at least 3 months before starting ovarian stimulation [65]. This therapy may produce a window of time with improved implantation rates [66].

The use of a levonorgestrel-releasing intrauterine device, danazol, or aromatase inhibitors may temporarily induce regression of adenomyosis and oral contraceptive pills, high-dose progestins, and selective progesterone receptor modulators can temporarily improve its symptoms, but these are not used in fertility treatments [66].

Patients with adenomyosis present a higher number of uterine contractions. Oxytocin (OT), a nonapeptide synthesized by neurons of the supraoptic nucleus and released from the posterior pituitary gland, has diverse effects on the female reproductive system. It is known to be a factor causing uterine contractions. It has also been shown in animal models that endometrial cells contain oxytocin receptors (OTRs) and that OT has the capacity to trigger the production of prostaglandin (PG) F2a from these cells. Atosiban, an OTR antagonist, treatment before ET in endometriosis is effective in the priming of the uterus, suitable for embryo implantation [67]. Since uterine contractions in IVF cycles are significantly increased following ovarian stimulation and women with frequent uterine contractions have a lower pregnancy rate, the use of atosiban around embryo transfer may resulted in higher pregnancy rates in women with RIF and adenomyosis. According to Hung Yu et al., the use of atosiban around embryo transfer did not improve the live birth rate in a general population of IVF patients [68].

7. Hydrosalpinx

Hydrosalpinx refers to a condition in which the fallopian tube is filled with fluids following infundibulum obstruction. It is a common condition among infertile women with 10–13% diagnosis rate after ultrasound scan. These numbers can be increased when other diagnostic methods such as hysterosalpingography or laparoscopy are used [69].

Perhaps the real cause for the implantation failure is not known, but studies suggest a decrease in live births rates in patients with hydrosalpinx [70].

The theories regarding hydrosalpinx and implantation failure are about a possible embryo toxicity, changes in the endometrium quality or even embryos washout mechanical effect [71].

The endometrial involvement secondary to hydrosalpinx is related to the presence of fluid inside the uterine cavity, altered endometrial flow, altered in inhibiting factors and increase in the inflammatory response. Besides the endometrial changes and a possible embryo toxicity, the implantation failure can be related to a negative effect on sperm motility and survival.

7.1 Diagnosis

A history of ectopic pregnancy, pelvic inflammatory disease, endometriosis or previous pelvic surgery increase the suspect of infertility by tubal factors [72]. For patients without risk factors, a negative antibody test for chlamydia indicates that there is less than 15% chance of tubal pathologies [73]. For an accurate diagnosis and an effective treatment of the tubal blockage it is necessary to do exams as the hysterosalpingography (HSG) which uses water or lipids soluble contrast medium. It is a golden standard method to evaluate tubal permeability and can bring some therapeutic benefits. The HSG can document tubal blockage in proximal and distal sites, show salpingitis isthmic nodosa, reveal fimbrial phimosis or peri tubal adhesions [74]. The HSG positive and negative predictive factors are 38% and 94%, respectively [75].

The laparoscopy with chromotubation with methylene blue test (dye test) injected thorough the cervix can demonstrate tubal permeability, proximal or distal tubal occlusion. This surgical route can also identify and correct peritoneal and tubal factors such as fimbriae or peri tubal adhesions which cannot be seen with less invasive methods as the HSG [74].

7.2 Treatment

The techniques used for the treatment of hydrosalpinx are many: laparoscopy or laparotomy for salpingectomy, salpingostomy or even uterine proximal occlusion.

A meta-analysis published in 2020 evaluated the effect of hydrosalpinx on the pregnancy rates, compared different types of treatment and the impact on the ovarian reserve after treatment for hydrosalpinx [70]. They reviewed 17 studies and observed that the hydrosalpinx was associated with a significant decrease in the implantation rate with embryo transfer with 0.41 OR [0.32–0.53]. Besides that, the clinical pregnancy rate per subject and per transference significantly decreased in women with hydrosalpinx (OR = 0.54; [0.32–0.89] and 0.44 [0.27–0.73], respectively) [70].

The hydrosalpinx removal with salpingectomy leads to an improvement of in vitro fertilization outcomes in comparison with no treatment, which turns it into a golden standard management before IVF. This evidence is replicated in other studies, such as Palagiano et al., where the pregnancy rates in patients with hydrosalpinx is lower than the control group [69]. There were negative effects either in fresh or frozen embryo transfers. An increase of two or threefold in abortions in women with hydrosalpinx was observed.

The hydrosalpinx mechanism action is still uncertain. Studies show a negative impact in IVF treatment outcomes, including a decrease in implantation rates, clinical pregnancy and in course pregnancies. Besides that, they show a risk of miscarriages (1.68 OR) and ectopic pregnancy (3.48 OR), according to Capmas et al. [70]. The salpingectomy is the treatment that increases success rate and prevents secondary aggressive factors. According to some authors, it is considered a golden standard. But it can be related to a decrease in the Anti-Mullerian Hormone average of 0.99 ng/ml, as shown the meta-analysis by Capmas et al. [70].

8. Conclusion

The recurrent implantation failure is a complex clinical condition with a wide variety of etiologies. Its criteria are not still well defined. Despite the lack of consensus, studies strongly show that anatomical factors affecting the uterine cavity contribute to implantation failure. Most of these factors are treatable, though.

Each patient approach must be individualized and offered to women with adequate RIF investigations to eliminate the possibility of all structural causes. The lack of success of an IVF can be devastating for some couples.

Uterine pathologies such as fibroids, adenomyosis, endometrial polyp, congenital abnormalities and synechiae must be considered in the diagnosis of RIF and must be excluded using image exams. Hydrosalpinx is known as a factor for implantation failure and a laparoscopy with salpingectomy or uterine proximal occlusion must be offered as a therapy option.

Even after more than 40 years of IVF procedures worldwide, the causes of RIF remain challenging and controversial. It is necessary to establish a consensus about diagnosis and therapeutic approaches to reduce expensive treatments which are not efficient and are time-consuming for infertile patients.

Conflict of interest

"The authors declare no conflict of interest."

Author details

Mariana Fonseca Roller Barcelos*, Aluisio M. da Rocha Filho,
Amanda Evelyn C. Goulart, Anna Luiza M. Souza, Daniely T. Costa,
Gabriela Galdino de F. Barros, Isadora Manzi N. Theodoro, Jean Pierre B. Brasileiro,
Murilo Cezar S. Oliveira, Natalia I. Zavattiero Tierno, Tatianna Quintas F. Ribeiro,
Valeria L. Mathias Castro and Vinicius M. Lopes
VERHUM Institute, Brasília, Brazil

*Address all correspondence to: marianaroller@gmail.com

References

[1] Shaulov T, Sierra S, Sylvestre C. Recurrent implantation failure in IVF: A Canadian Fertility and Andrology Society Clinical Practice Guideline. Reprod Biomed Online. 2020 Nov;41(5):819-833. DOI: 10.1016/j.rbmo.2020.08.007.

[2] Coughlan C, Ledger W, Wang Q, Liu F, Demirol A, Gurgan, Cutting R, Ong K, Sallam H, Li T.C. Recurrent implantation failure: Definition and management. *Reprod. Biomed. Online.* 2014; 28: 14-38. DOI: 10.1016/j.rbmo.2013.08.011.

[3] Coughlan C. What to do when good-quality embryos repeatedly fail to implant. Best Pract Res Clin Obstet Gynaecol. 2018 Nov;53:48-59. DOI: 10.1016/j.bpobgyn.2018.07.004.

[4] El-Toukhy T, Campo R, Khalaf Y, Tabanelli C, Gianaroli L, Gordts SS, Gordts S, Mestdagh G, Mardesic T, Voboril J, Marchino GL, Benedetto C, Al-Shawaf T, Sabatini L, Seed PT, Gergolet M, Grimbizis G, Harb H, Coomarasamy A. Hysteroscopy in recurrent in-vitro fertilisation failure (TROPHY): a multicentre, randomised controlled trial. Lancet. 2016 Jun 25;387(10038):2614-2621. DOI: 10.1016/S0140-6736(16)00258-0.

[5] Penzias AS. Recurrent IVF failure: other factors. Fertil Steril. 2012 May;97(5):1033-8. Erratum in: Fertil Steril. 2013 Jan;99(1):297. DOI: 10.1016/j.fertnstert.2012.03.017.

[6] Antunes A Jr, Costa-Paiva L, Arthuso M, Costa JV, Pinto-Neto AM. Endometrial polyps in pre- and postmenopausal women: factors associated with malignancy. Maturitas. 2007 Aug 20;57(4):415-21. DOI: 10.1016/j.maturitas.2007.04.010.

[7] Nijkang NP, Anderson L, Markham R, Manconi F. Endometrial polyps: Pathogenesis, sequelae and treatment. SAGE Open Med. 2019 May 2;7:2050312119848247. DOI: 10.1177/2050312119848247.

[8] Munro MG. Uterine polyps, adenomyosis, leiomyomas, and endometrial receptivity. Fertil Steril. 2019 Apr;111(4):629-640. DOI: 10.1016/j.fertnstert.2019.02.008.

[9] Richlin SS, Ramachandran S, Shanti A, Murphy AA, Parthasarathy S. Glycodelin levels in uterine flushings and in plasma of patients with leiomyomas and polyps: implications for implantation. Hum Reprod. 2002 Oct;17(10):2742-7. DOI: 10.1093/humrep/17.10.2742.

[10] Nalaboff KM, Pellerito JS, Ben-Levi E. Imaging the endometrium: disease and normal variants. Radiographics. 2001 Nov-Dec;21(6):1409-24. DOI: 10.1148/radiographics.21.6.g01nv211409.

[11] American Association of Gynecologic Laparoscopists. AAGL practice report: practice guidelines for the diagnosis and management of endometrial polyps. J Minim Invasive Gynecol. 2012 Jan-Feb;19(1):3-10. DOI: 10.1016/j.jmig.2011.09.003.

[12] Bozdag G, Aksan G, Esinler I, Yarali H. What is the role of office hysteroscopy in women with failed IVF cycles? Reprod Biomed Online. 2008 Sep;17(3):410-5. doi: 10.1016/s1472-6483(10)60226-x. PMID: 18765013. Bozdag G, Aksan G, Esinler I, Yarali H. What is the role of office hysteroscopy in women with failed IVF cycles? Reprod Biomed Online. 2008 Sep;17(3):410-5. DOI: 10.1016/s1472-6483(10)60226-x.

[13] Pérez-Medina T, Bajo-Arenas J, Salazar F, Redondo T, Sanfrutos L, Alvarez P, Engels V. Endometrial polyps

and their implication in the pregnancy rates of patients undergoing intrauterine insemination: a prospective, randomized study. Hum Reprod. 2005 Jun;20(6):1632-5. DOI: 10.1093/humrep/deh822.

[14] Lass A, Williams G, Abusheikha N, Brinsden P. The effect of endometrial polyps on outcomes of in vitro fertilization (IVF) cycles. J Assist Reprod Genet. 1999 Sep;16(8):410-5. DOI: 10.1023/a:1020513423948.

[15] Corroenne R, Legendre G, May-Panloup P, El Hachem H, Dreux C, Jeanneteau P, Boucret L, Ferré-L'Hotellier V, Descamps P, Bouet PE. Surgical treatment of septate uterus in cases of primary infertility and before assisted reproductive technologies. J Gynecol Obstet Hum Reprod. 2018 Nov;47(9):413-418. DOI: 10.1016/j.jogoh.2018.08.005.

[16] Prior M, Richardson A, Asif S, Polanski L, Parris-Larkin M, Chandler J, Fogg L, Jassal P, Thornton JG, Raine-Fenning NJ. Outcome of assisted reproduction in women with congenital uterine anomalies: a prospective observational study. Ultrasound Obstet Gynecol. 2018 Jan;51(1):110-117. DOI: 10.1002/uog.18935.

[17] Chan YY, Jayaprakasan K, Tan A, Thornton JG, Coomarasamy A, Raine-Fenning NJ. Reproductive outcomes in women with congenital uterine anomalies: a systematic review. Ultrasound Obstet Gynecol. 2011 Oct;38(4):371-82. DOI: 10.1002/uog.10056.

[18] Rikken J, Leeuwis-Fedorovich NE, Letteboer S, Emanuel MH, Limpens J, van der Veen F, Goddijn M, van Wely M. The pathophysiology of the septate uterus: a systematic review. BJOG. 2019 Sep;126(10):1192-1199. DOI: 10.1111/1471-0528.15798.

[19] Practice Committee of the American Society for Reproductive Medicine. Electronic address: ASRM@asrm.org; Practice Committee of the American Society for Reproductive Medicine. Uterine septum: a guideline. Fertil Steril. 2016 Sep 1;106(3):530-40. DOI: 10.1016/j.fertnstert.2016.05.014.

[20] Di Spiezio Sardo A, Campo R, Gordts S, Spinelli M, Cosimato C, Tanos V, Brucker S, Li TC, Gergolet M, De Angelis C, Gianaroli L, Grimbizis G. The comprehensiveness of the ESHRE/ESGE classification of female genital tract congenital anomalies: a systematic review of cases not classified by the AFS system. Hum Reprod. 2015 May;30(5):1046-58. DOI: 10.1093/humrep/dev061.

[21] Knez J, Saridogan E, Van Den Bosch T, Mavrelos D, Ambler G, Jurkovic D. ESHRE/ESGE female genital tract anomalies classification system-the potential impact of discarding arcuate uterus on clinical practice. Hum Reprod. 2018 Apr 1;33(4):600-606. DOI: 10.1093/humrep/dey043.

[22] Ludwin A, Ludwin I, Coelho Neto MA, Nastri CO, Bhagavath B, Lindheim SR, Martins WP. Septate uterus according to ESHRE/ESGE, ASRM and CUME definitions: association with infertility and miscarriage, cost and warnings for women and healthcare systems. Ultrasound Obstet Gynecol. 2019 Dec;54(6):800-814. DOI: 10.1002/uog.20291.

[23] RCOG. Guideline: The investigation and treatment of couples with recurrent first-trimester and second-trimester miscarriage. 2011: 1-18. Available from: https://www.rcog.org.uk/globalassets/documents/guidelines/gtg_17.pdf [Accessed: 2021-04-25]

[24] NICE. Guideline: Hysteroscopic metroplasty of a uterine septum for primary infertility.2015:1-8. Availablefrom: https://www.nice.org.uk/guidance/ipg509/resources/hysteroscopic-metroplasty-of-a-uterine-

septum-for-primary-infertility-pdf-1899871693326277 [Accessed: 2021-04-26]

[25] ESHRE Guideline Group on RPL, Bender Atik R, Christiansen OB, Elson J, Kolte AM, Lewis S, Middeldorp S, Nelen W, Peramo B, Quenby S, Vermeulen N, Goddijn M. ESHRE guideline: recurrent pregnancy loss. Hum Reprod Open 2018; DOI: 10.1093/hropen/ hoy004.

[26] Lavergne N, Aristizabal J, Zarka V, Erny R, Hedon B. Uterine anomalies and in vitro fertilization: what are the results? Eur J Obstet Gynecol Reprod Biol. 1996 Sep;68(1-2):29-34. DOI: 10.1016/0301-2115(96)02459-1.

[27] Tomaževič T, Ban-Frangež H, Virant-Klun I, Verdenik I, Požlep B, Vrtačnik-Bokal E. Septate, subseptate and arcuate uterus decrease pregnancy and live birth rates in IVF/ICSI. Reprod Biomed Online. 2010 Nov;21(5):700-5. DOI: 10.1016/j.rbmo.2010.06.028.

[28] Ozgur K, Isikoglu M, Donmez L, Oehninger S. Is hysteroscopic correction of an incomplete uterine septum justified prior to IVF? Reprod Biomed Online. 2007 Mar;14(3):335-40. DOI: 10.1016/s1472-6483(10)60876-0.

[29] Spanish Infertility SWOT Group (SISG), Checa MA, Bellver J, Bosch E, Espinós JJ, Fabregues F, Fontes J, García-Velasco J, Requena A. Hysteroscopic septum resection and reproductive medicine: A SWOT analysis. Reprod Biomed Online. 2018 Dec;37(6):709-715. DOI: 10.1016/j.rbmo.2018.09.013.

[30] Rikken JFW, Verhorstert KWJ, Emanuel MH, Bongers MY, Spinder T, Kuchenbecker WKH, Jansen FW, van der Steeg JW, Janssen CAH, Kapiteijn K, Schols WA, Torrenga B, Torrance HL, Verhoeve HR, Huirne JAF, Hoek A, Nieboer TE, van Rooij IAJ, Clark TJ, Robinson L, Stephenson MD, Mol BWJ, van der Veen F, van Wely M, Goddijn M. Septum resection in women with a septate uterus: a cohort study. Hum Reprod. 2020 Jul 1;35(7):1578-1588. DOI: 10.1093/humrep/dez284. Erratum in: Hum Reprod. 2020 Jul 1;35(7):1722.

[31] Rikken JFW, Kowalik CR, Emanuel MH, Bongers MY, Spinder T, Jansen FW, Mulders AGMGJ, Padmehr R, Clark TJ, van Vliet HA, Stephenson MD, van der Veen F, Mol BWJ, van Wely M, Goddijn M. Septum resection versus expectant management in women with a septate uterus: an international multicentre open-label randomized controlled trial. Hum Reprod. 2021 Apr 20;36(5):1260-1267. DOI: 10.1093/humrep/deab037.

[32] Surrey ES, Katz-Jaffe M, Surrey RL, Small AS, Gustofson RL, Schoolcraft WB. Arcuate uterus: is there an impact on in vitro fertilization outcomes after euploid embryo transfer? Fertil Steril. 2018 Apr;109(4): 638-643. DOI: 10.1016/j.fertnstert.2017.12.001.

[33] Chen X, Liu P, Sheng Y, Li W, Tang R, Ding L, Qin Y, Chen ZJ. The impact of unicornuate uterus on perinatal outcomes after IVF/ICSI cycles: a matched retrospective cohort study. J Matern Fetal Neonatal Med. 2019 Aug;32(15):2469-2474. DOI: 10.1080/14767058.2018.1438403.

[34] Hur C, Rehmer J, Flyckt R, Falcone T. Uterine Factor Infertility: A Clinical Review. Clin Obstet Gynecol. 2019 Jun;62(2):257-270. DOI: 10.1097/GRF.0000000000000448.

[35] Coughlan C, Ledger W, Wang Q, Liu F, Demirol A, Gurgan T, Cutting R, Ong K, Sallam H, Li TC. Recurrent implantation failure: definition and management. Reprod Biomed Online. 2014 Jan;28(1):14-38. DOI: 10.1016/j.rbmo.2013.08.011.

[36] Tao Z, Duan H. [Expression of adhesion-related cytokines in the

uterine fluid after transcervical resection of adhesion]. Zhonghua Fu Chan Ke Za Zhi. 2012 Oct;47(10):734-7. Chinese. PMID: 23302729.

[37] Demirol A, Gurgan T. Effect of treatment of intrauterine pathologies with office hysteroscopy in patients with recurrent IVF failure. Reprod Biomed Online. 2004 May;8(5):590-4. DOI: 10.1016/s1472-6483(10)61108-x.

[38] Doroftei B, Dabuleanu AM, Ilie OD, Maftei R, Anton E, Simionescu G, Matei T, Armeanu T. Mini-Review of the New Therapeutic Possibilities in Asherman Syndrome-Where Are We after One Hundred and Twenty-Six Years? Diagnostics (Basel). 2020 Sep 17;10(9):706. DOI: 10.3390/diagnostics10090706.

[39] Seshadri S, El-Toukhy T, Douiri A, Jayaprakasan K, Khalaf Y. Diagnostic accuracy of saline infusion sonography in the evaluation of uterine cavity abnormalities prior to assisted reproductive techniques: a systematic review and meta-analyses. Hum Reprod Update. 2015 Mar-Apr;21(2):262-74. DOI: 10.1093/humupd/dmu057.

[40] Sylvestre C, Child TJ, Tulandi T, Tan SL. A prospective study to evaluate the efficacy of two- and three-dimensional sonohysterography in women with intrauterine lesions. Fertil Steril. 2003 May;79(5):1222-5. DOI: 10.1016/s0015-0282(03)00154-7.

[41] Makris N, Kalmantis K, Skartados N, Papadimitriou A, Mantzaris G, Antsaklis A. Three-dimensional hysterosonography versus hysteroscopy for the detection of intracavitary uterine abnormalities. Int J Gynaecol Obstet. 2007 Apr;97(1):6-9. DOI: 10.1016/j.ijgo.2006.10.012.

[42] Yu D, Wong YM, Cheong Y, Xia E, Li TC. Asherman syndrome--one century later. Fertil Steril. 2008 Apr;89(4):759-79.DOI: 10.1016/j.fertnstert.2008.02.096.

[43] Zikopoulos KA, Kolibianakis EM, Platteau P, de Munck L, Tournaye H, Devroey P, Camus M. Live delivery rates in subfertile women with Asherman's syndrome after hysteroscopic adhesiolysis using the resectoscope or the Versapoint system. Reprod Biomed Online. 2004 Jun;8(6):720-5. DOI: 10.1016/s1472-6483(10)61654-9.

[44] Khan Z, Goldberg JM. Hysteroscopic Management of Asherman's Syndrome. J Minim Invasive Gynecol. 2018 Feb;25(2):218-228. DOI: 10.1016/j.jmig.2017.09.020.

[45] Doroftei B, Dabuleanu AM, Ilie OD, Maftei R, Anton E, Simionescu G, Matei T, Armeanu T. Mini-Review of the New Therapeutic Possibilities in Asherman Syndrome-Where Are We after One Hundred and Twenty-Six Years? Diagnostics (Basel). 2020 Sep 17;10(9):706. DOI: 10.3390/diagnostics10090706.

[46] Benor A, Gay S, DeCherney A. An update on stem cell therapy for Asherman syndrome. J Assist Reprod Genet. 2020 Jul;37(7):1511-1529. DOI: 10.1007/s10815-020-01801-x

[47] Tan J, Li P, Wang Q, Li Y, Li X, Zhao D, Xu X, Kong L. Autologous menstrual blood-derived stromal cells transplantation for severe Asherman's syndrome. Hum Reprod. 2016 Dec;31(12):2723-2729. DOI: 10.1093/humrep/dew235.

[48] Orhue AA, Aziken ME, Igbefoh JO. A comparison of two adjunctive treatments for intrauterine adhesions following lysis. Int J Gynaecol Obstet. 2003 Jul;82(1):49-56. DOI: 10.1016/s0020-7292(03)00030-4.

[49] Aghajanova L, Cedars MI, Huddleston HG. Platelet-rich plasma in the management of Asherman

syndrome: case report. J Assist Reprod Genet. 2018 May;35(5):771-775. DOI: 10.1007/s10815-018-1135-3.

[50] Fernandez H, Al-Najjar F, Chauveaud-Lambling A, Frydman R, Gervaise A. Fertility after treatment of Asherman's syndrome stage 3 and 4. J Minim Invasive Gynecol. 2006 Sep-Oct;13(5):398-402. DOI: 10.1016/j.jmig.2006.04.013.

[51] Brinsden PR. Gestational surrogacy. Hum Reprod Update. 2003 Sep-Oct;9(5):483-91. DOI: 10.1093/humupd/dmg033.

[52] Sharma S, Bathwal S, Agarwal N, Chattopadhyay R, Saha I, Chakravarty B. Does presence of adenomyosis affect reproductive outcome in IVF cycles? A retrospective analysis of 973 patients. Reprod Biomed Online. 2019 Jan;38(1):13-21. DOI: 10.1016/j.rbmo.2018.09.014.

[53] Upson K, Missmer SA. Epidemiology of Adenomyosis. Semin Reprod Med. 2020 May;38(2-03):89-107. DOI: 10.1055/s-0040-1718920. Epub 2020 Oct 26.

[54] Dueholm M. Uterine adenomyosis and infertility, review of reproductive outcome after in vitro fertilization and surgery. Acta Obstet Gynecol Scand. 2017 Jun;96(6):715-726. DOI: 10.1111/aogs.13158.

[55] Safari S, Faramarzi A, Agha-Rahimi A, Khalili MA. Live birth in a woman with recurrent implantation failure and adenomyosis following transfer of refrozen-warmed embryos. Clin Exp Reprod Med. 2016 Sep;43(3):181-4. DOI: 10.5653/cerm.2016.43.3.181

[56] Vannuccini S, Petraglia F. Recent advances in understanding and managing adenomyosis. F1000Res. 2019 Mar 13;8:F1000 Faculty Rev-283. DOI: 10.12688/f1000research.17242.1.

[57] Chapron C, Vannuccini S, Santulli P, Abrão MS, Carmona F, Fraser IS, Gordts S, Guo SW, Just PA, Noël JC, Pistofidis G, Van den Bosch T, Petraglia F. Diagnosing adenomyosis: an integrated clinical and imaging approach. Hum Reprod Update. 2020 Apr 15;26(3):392-411. DOI: 10.1093/humupd/dmz049.

[58] Tremellen KP, Russell P. The distribution of immune cells and macrophages in the endometrium of women with recurrent reproductive failure. II: adenomyosis and macrophages. J Reprod Immunol. 2012 Jan;93(1):58-63. DOI: 10.1016/j.jri.2011.12.001.

[59] Meredith SM, Sanchez-Ramos L, Kaunitz AM. Diagnostic accuracy of transvaginal sonography for the diagnosis of adenomyosis: systematic review and metaanalysis. Am J Obstet Gynecol. 2009 Jul;201(1):107.e1-6. DOI: 10.1016/j.ajog.2009.03.021.

[60] Bazot M, Daraï E. Role of transvaginal sonography and magnetic resonance imaging in the diagnosis of uterine adenomyosis. Fertil Steril. 2018 Mar;109(3):389-397. DOI: 10.1016/j.fertnstert.2018.01.024

[61] Tamai K, Koyama T, Umeoka S, Saga T, Fujii S, Togashi K. Spectrum of MR features in adenomyosis. Best Pract Res Clin Obstet Gynaecol. 2006 Aug;20(4):583-602. DOI: 10.1016/j.bpobgyn.2006.01.009.

[62] Exacoustos C, Manganaro L, Zupi E. Imaging for the evaluation of endometriosis and adenomyosis. Best Pract Res Clin Obstet Gynaecol. 2014 Jul;28(5):655-81. DOI: 10.1016/j.bpobgyn.2014.04.010.

[63] Yoldemir T. Adenomyosis and fertility outcomes. Gynecol Endocrinol. 2020 Jun;36(6):473-474. DOI: 10.1080/09513590.2020.1773426.

[64] Tremellen K, Russell P. Adenomyosis is a potential cause of recurrent implantation failure during IVF treatment. Aust N Z J Obstet Gynaecol. 2011 Jun;51(3):280-3. DOI: 10.1111/j.1479-828X.2010.01276.x.

[65] Hou X, Xing J, Shan H, Mei J, Sun Y, Yan G, Sun H, Wang J. The effect of adenomyosis on IVF after long or ultra-long GnRH agonist treatment. Reprod Biomed Online. 2020 Nov;41(5):845-853. DOI: 10.1016/j.rbmo.2020.07.027.

[66] Pontis A, D'Alterio MN, Pirarba S, de Angelis C, Tinelli R, Angioni S. Adenomyosis: a systematic review of medical treatment. Gynecol Endocrinol. 2016 Sep;32(9):696-700. DOI: 10.1080/09513590.2016.1197200.

[67] He Y, Wu H, He X, Xing Q, Zhou P, Cao Y, Wei Z. Administration of atosiban in patients with endometriosis undergoing frozen-thawed embryo transfer: a prospective, randomized study. Fertil Steril. 2016 Aug;106(2):416-22. DOI: 10.1016/j.fertnstert.2016.04.019.

[68] Ng EH, Li RH, Chen L, Lan VT, Tuong HM, Quan S. A randomized double blind comparison of atosiban in patients undergoing IVF treatment. Hum Reprod. 2014 Dec;29(12):2687-94. DOI: 10.1093/humrep/deu263.

[69] Palagiano A, Cozzolino M, Ubaldi FM, Palagiano C, Coccia ME. Effects of Hydrosalpinx on Endometrial Implantation Failures: Evaluating Salpingectomy in Women Undergoing in vitro fertilization. Rev Bras Ginecol Obstet. 2021 Apr;43(4):304-310. English. DOI: 10.1055/s-0040-1722155.

[70] Capmas P, Suarthana E, Tulandi T. Management of Hydrosalpinx in the Era of Assisted Reproductive Technology: A Systematic Review and Meta-analysis. J Minim Invasive Gynecol. 2021 Mar;28(3):418-441. DOI: 10.1016/j.jmig.2020.08.017.

[71] Strandell A, Lindhard A, Waldenström U, Thorburn J, Janson PO, Hamberger L. Hydrosalpinx and IVF outcome: a prospective, randomized multicentre trial in Scandinavia on salpingectomy prior to IVF. Hum Reprod. 1999 Nov;14(11):2762-9. DOI: 10.1093/humrep/14.11.2762.

[72] Practice Committee of the American Society for Reproductive Medicine. Committee opinion: role of tubal surgery in the era of assisted reproductive technology. Fertil Steril. 2012 Mar;97(3):539-45. DOI: 10.1016/j.fertnstert.2011.12.031.

[73] Den Hartog JE, Morré SA, Land JA. Chlamydia trachomatis-associated tubal factor subfertility: Immunogenetic aspects and serological screening. Hum Reprod Update. 2006 Nov-Dec;12(6):719-30. DOI: 10.1093/humupd/dml030.

[74] Practice Committee of the American Society for Reproductive Medicine. Diagnostic evaluation of the infertile female: a committee opinion. Fertil Steril. 2015 Jun;103(6):e44-50. DOI: 10.1016/j.fertnstert.2015.03.019. Epub 2015 Apr 30.

[75] Coppus SF, Opmeer BC, Logan S, van der Veen F, Bhattacharya S, Mol BW. The predictive value of medical history taking and Chlamydia IgG ELISA antibody testing (CAT) in the selection of subfertile women for diagnostic laparoscopy: a clinical prediction model approach. Hum Reprod. 2007 May;22(5):1353-8. DOI: 10.1093/humrep/del521.

Chapter 3

Fibroids and Infertility

Juan Luis Giraldo Moreno and Susana Salazar López

Abstract

Uterine fibroids (also known as leiomyomas or myomas) are the most common pelvic tumors, affecting more than 70% of women over 70 years of age and although most are asymptomatic, some women may experience symptoms, depending on their location and size, which can alter your quality of life, such as abnormal uterine bleeding, anemia, pelvic pain and pressure, dyspareunia, increased urinary frequency and constipation. Its relationship with infertility has been controversial and, although insignificant for subserous fibroids, it appears that submucosal and intramural fibroids that distort the endometrial cavity can affect embryo implantation and are associated with an increased risk of early pregnancy loss. Its treatment will depend on the patient's symptoms, size, location, whether it is one or multiple, and whether or not she suffers from infertility. It is clear that submucosal fibroids have a negative impact on fertility and with respect to intramural fibroids it is known that fibroids larger than 4 cm alter the probability of pregnancy, however there are studies that show that even smaller or multiple fibroids could affect pregnancy rates. There are multiple options for the treatment of fibroids; however, patients who are candidates for expectant, medical or surgical management should be individualized, and especially if they are going to be taken to surgery, an excellent mapping of fibroids prior to surgical intervention is recommended. Minimally invasive surgery continues to be the approach of choice, it should be left for the open approach in cases in which Laparoscopy is contraindicated or the patient with multiple myomatosis.

Keywords: Fibroids, leiomyoma, myomas, infertility, myomectomy, pregnancy

1. Introduction

Uterine fibroids are the most common benign tumors in women of reproductive age. They are monoclonal tumors of the myometrium or uterine smooth muscle and are composed of large amounts of extracellular matrix, containing fibronectin, collagen and proteoglycans [1]. Myomas are estrogen dependent tumors, which growth is clearly associated with exposure to circulating estrogen. They predictably decrease in size during menopause and under other hypoestrogenic conditions [2].

Fibroid's prevalence is variable and age dependent. They can be detected in up to 70% of white and 80% of black women by 50 years of age [2, 3]. Compared with Caucasian women with symptomatic myomas, women of African descent frequently present to their provider at a younger age and with a significantly worse myoma burden (larger size and number) and have a threefold higher risk of hysterectomy [4].

IntechOpen

Fibroids can have a negative impact on the reproductive system and can be single, but are more often multiple, causing significant morbidity and deterioration of quality of life [5].

2. Risk factors

2.1 Race

Race constitutes an important risk factor for fibroid development, studies conducted using ultrasound have confirmed that the myoma prevalence is lower in Europe than in the United States, probably due to racial differences (**Figure 1**). In addition to a having greater lifetime incidence of fibroids, black women have fibroids diagnosed at earlier ages, are more likely to be symptomatic and are likely to have different responses to medical treatment than white women [5, 6].

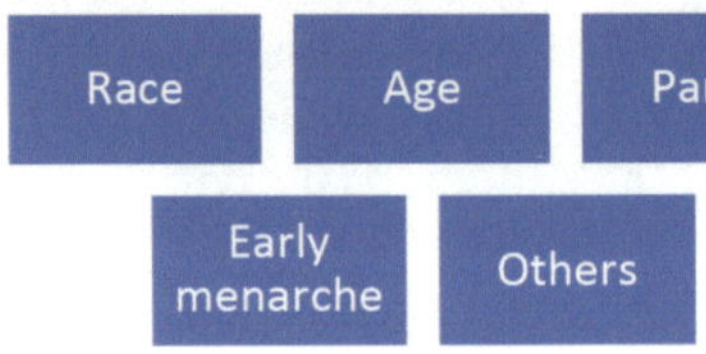

Figure 1.
Risk factors.

2.2 Age

Age is a significant risk factor for fibroid development. The incidence of pathologically diagnosed fibroids increases with age, reaching its maximum peak at age 50, is negligible before puberty, and also decreases with menopause [7].

2.3 Parity

Published evidence suggests that pregnancy is a protective factor against fibroid development, due to events that occur at the end of the pregnancy, at delivery or in the postpartum process [8]. Although a direct protective effect of pregnancy has been demonstrated, little is known of the mechanism. It has been suggested that fibroid tissue might be highly susceptible to ischemia during parturition and remodeling [9].

2.4 Genetic factors

Genetic factors can play an important role in myomas development, the growth of multiple myomas in the same uterus implies that heritage can cause some women to be more predisposed than others [5]. Leiomyomas are monoclonal in origin and 40% of the tumors have karyotypic abnormalities including deletions in chromosome 7, trisomy of chromosome 12 and rearrangements the HMGA1 (6p21) and HGMA2 (12q14) involving genes. Whole exome approaches have identified heterozygous somatic mutations in the mediator complex subunit 12 (MED12) [10]. Alterations of several genes, protooncogenes, signaling pathways and epigenetic mechanisms have been associated with its etiology, some of them are HOXA10, HOXA11, BMP2, among others [7].

Other factors: early menarche, late age for menopause, caffeine and alcohol, family history of uterine fibroids, obesity [1].

3. Clinical features

The majority of uterine myomas are asymptomatic. When symptomatic, uterine fibroids commonly present with abnormal uterine bleeding (heavy or irregular menstrual bleeding) which is the main reason for gynecologic consultations of women aged 40 to 50 years [11]. The mechanism of leiomyoma associated excessive menstrual bleeding is unknown. Increased endometrial surface area, vascular dysregulation, and interference with endometrial hemostasis have been offered as possible explanations [12]. Other less common symptoms include pelvic pressure, bowel dysfunction, urinary frequency and urgency, urinary retention, low back pain, constipation and dyspareunia [10]. This latest situations are generally determined by large fibroids; Urinary symptoms associated with anterior fibroids, constipation with posterior ones [13]. Pain as a symptom is relatively infrequent. It's usually associated with torsion of a pedunculated myoma, cervical dilatation by a submucous myoma protruding through the uterine segment or degeneration associated with pregnancy. This conditions cause acute pain and require immediate attention [2]. With respect to reproductive prognosis, the degree to which fibroids contribute to infertility is controversial, but they seem to be implicated as the sole factor during diagnostic workup in less than 10% of infertile couples [14].

3.1 Classification

There are many fibroid classifications in the literature. Many issues have been considered among these, including the leiomyoma's relationship with the endometrium and the serosa, their location within the uterus (upper segment, lower segment, cervix, anterior, posterior, lateral), the size and the number of lesions [15]. The primary classification system reflects only the presence of one or more leiomyomas; In the secondary system, focus on differentiation of fibroids that involve the endometrial cavity (submucosal or SM) from others is the main point because it's known that submucosal myomas are those that most likely contribute to the genesis of abnormal uterine bleeding [16].

The international Federation of Gynecology and Obstetrics (FIGO) classification system for abnormal uterine bleeding [17] is intended to help better categorize the causes of bleeding and treatment planning [18]. They describe eight types of fibroids as well as a hybrid presentation (a myoma that fulfills criteria for 2 different types among the classification). This classification offers a more representative "map" of fibroid distribution [19] and also includes the categorization of intramural and subserosal leiomyomas [20].

A myoma FIGO type 0 is pedunculated and 100% intracavitary, type 1 is submucosal with less than 50% intramural extension; type 2 is submucosal with 50% or more intramural extension, type 3 is intramural but in contact with the endometrium without disrupting it, type 4 is 100% intramural not in contact with the endometrium, type 5 is subserosal with 50% or more intramural extension, type 6 is subserosal with less than 50% intramural extension, type 7 is subserosal and pedunculated, type 8 are other types of myomas including cervical and parasitic fibroids. Hybrid fibroids are given two numbers, the first number refers to the relationship with the endometrium and the other with the serosa, e.g. 2–5 has submucosal and subserosal component (**Figure 2**) [19].

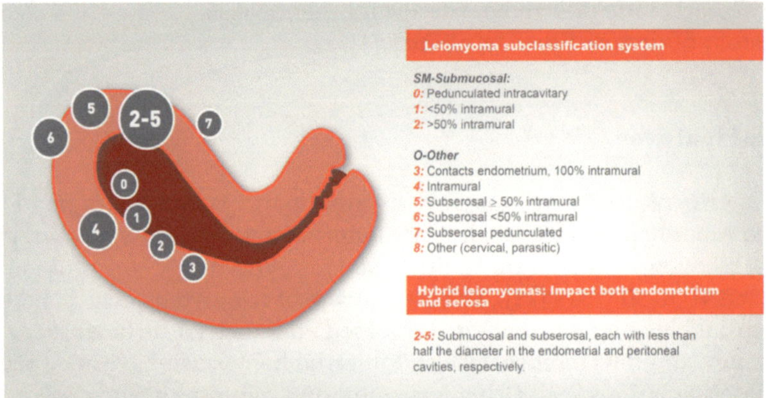

Figure 2.
Leimyoma subclassification system (FIGO). Image taken and edited from ref. [20].

4. Association of uterine fibroids and infertility

Uterine leiomyomas are associated as sole factor for infertility in <10% of infertility cases [14]. Many theories have been proposed to explain how myomas may cause infertility. They can cause clear anatomical disruption of the uterine architecture, also abnormal uterine contractility, hinder sperm transport [21], elongation of the uterine cavity and distortion of the vascularization [22]. In particular, submucosal leiomyomas may impact the endometrial cavity, altering embryo implantation and development [23]. Others have suggested that aberrant endometrial growth factors expression may also play a role [21] One of the sequences of signaling events in implantation has been defined with Hoxa-10, those genes are essential in the mouse for endometrial development and implantation, Matsuzai et al. reported Hoxa-10 mRNA and protein expression levels in endometrial stroma cells were significantly lower in infertile patients with endometriosis and in those with myomas and unexplained infertility compared with that in healthy fertile controls [24]. Hoxa-10 and Hoxa-11 are known factors to be necessary to the endometrial receptivity and are decreased in women with submucosal myomas [25].

Bone morphogenetic protein type II (BMP2) mediates HOXA10 expression and if there exists an increase endometrial resistance to BMP2, it may add up to a decreased expression of HOXA 10 in the endometrium of this patients [26].

In fertile women, glycodelin and glutathione peroxidasa3 genes expression rises during the luteal phase, more often during de implantation window and the expression of these genes decreased in women with myomas [27].

Many types of cytokines such as leukemia inhibitory factor (LIF), interleukin 1 and 11 are necessary for embryo implantation in mice. In humans LIF is expressed in the endometrial epithelium, and its maximum expression is observed in the middle late secretory phase of the menstrual cycle [28]. Pier et al. demonstrated decreased LIF in patients with non-cavity distorting leiomyomas greater than 3 cm compared to patients with a normal uterus [29].

The literature regarding uterine leiomyomas and their impact on reproductive outcome can be confusing. High heterogeneity of patient characteristics and clinical presentation of fibroids, as well as randomization difficulties related to remarkable emotional and economic considerations of fertility related treatments, have made evidence-based conclusions difficult to achieve. Current consensus is that submucosal leiomyomas and intramural/submucosal (intramural fibroids encroaching the endometrial cavity) affect implantation and diminish pregnancy rates. Besides, it's clear that subserosal fibroids have no effect on fertility prognosis. Controversy lies on the effect of exclusively intramural fibroids that do not distort the endometrial cavity, on reproductive outcome. Evidence suggests that in this issue, size is the determining factor, with intramural fibroids larger than 4 to 5 cm being associated with impaired embryo implantation and diminished pregnancy rates. There is fair evidence that myomectomy for cavity-distorting myomas (submucosal or intramural with submucosal component) improves pregnancy rates and reduces the risk of early pregnancy loss [22, 30–32].

In a systematic review published on 2009 in Fertility and Sterility by Pritts et al. with 23 studies included in the data analysis, when evaluating the outcomes of women with any location of fibroid, the relative risks of clinical pregnancy, implantation, and ongoing pregnancy/live birth were all significantly lower in women with myomas than in control subjects; When the effect of the fibroid was evaluated by location, the women with SM fibroids, compared with infertile women without fibroids, demonstrated a significantly lower clinical pregnancy rate (CPR), implantation rate, and ongoing pregnancy rate (OPR)/Live birth rate (LBR) and a significantly higher spontaneous abortion rate. No difference was seen in rate of preterm delivery. According to Pritts systematic review removal of submucosal fibroids appears likely to improve fertility. Although intramural fibroids appeared to be associated with decreased fertility and increased pregnancy loss risk, it's surgical treatment failed to show an increase in pregnancy and live birth rates [33].

Casini et al. reported a tendency to have a higher pregnancy rate among the women who underwent a surgical treatment for fibroid removal compared with those who were not treated, although the results were not statistically significant in the IM and submucosal-intramural fibroids [34].

Bulleti et al. reported laparoscopic myomectomy improved pregnancy rates over non-surgical management of fibroids [35].

The diversity of myomas and patient characteristics also hinders the ability to determine whether size and location impact reproductive outcomes. Some studies have demonstrated conflicting reproductive outcomes related to fibroid size, for example some data support the notion that myomas larger than 3 cm negatively impact reproduction, nevertheless other studies suggest that leiomyomas less than 5 cm do not [23].

4.1 Fibroids and likelihood of achieving spontaneous pregnancy

There are few data assessing the impact of myomas on the likelihood of spontaneous pregnancy. Johnson et al. published in 2012 one retrospective study where a cohort of 3000 women in early pregnancy were enrolled, patients retrospectively report time to conception, and leiomyomas characteristics were determined by the first trimester ultrasound. Of the 3000 patients, 89% did not have leiomyomas and 11% had one or more, the most common fibroids were intramural and subserous. They found no significant association between myomas and time to pregnancy, in this study of women who were able to conceive without medical intervention; The presence of leiomyomata did not alter the length of time to conception [36]. Although this is the only evidence available of likelihood of achieving a spontaneous pregnancy on untreated patients with fibroids, it has an important bias since patients with previous fertility treatments were excluded.

4.2 Fibroids and likelihood of achieving pregnancy in IVF treatments

4.2.1 Intramural fibroids

Sunkara et al. Published in 2010 a systematic review and meta-analysis with 19 articles included and 6087 cycles, they found that the presence of non-cavity distorting intramural fibroids on average reduces the LBR 21% and the CPR by 15% per IVF cycle compared with no fibroids. The relatively lower chance of achieving a live birth compared with clinical pregnancy probably reflects the adverse influence of intramural fibroids on the course of pregnancy. With respect to implantation rate (IR) it showed a statistically non-significant 13% reduction in IR in women with non-cavity distorting intramural fibroids. They also did not find statistically difference in miscarriage rate [37].

Xiaodan Wang et al. published in 2018 an updated meta-analysis about the impact of non-cavity distorting intramural fibroids on the efficacy of In Vitro fertilization, they included a total of 28 studies involving 9189 IVF cycles, and showed a significant reduction in LBR, CPR and implantation rate, and also have a significant increase in miscarriage rate compared with control group [38].

Eric et al. published a retrospective case controlled analysis in 2001 and they found that LBR was not affected by the presence of intramural leiomyomas in IVF patients with normal endometrial cavity visualized in the hysteroscopic [21].

Somigliana et al. concluded in their critical analysis of the evidence that evidence support the vision that myomas may alter fertility, from the detrimental effect on implantation in IVF, delivery rate is also reduced in patients with fibroids, and second even if a randomized studies are lacking, surgical treatment appears to increase the pregnancy rate [13].

Hart et al. did the large prospective controlled study of the effect of the fibroids on the outcome of assisted reproduction. Their results showed that small IM fibroids reduces the chance of an embryo implanting by half., the presence or absence of an intramural fibroid was a significant factor influencing a woman's chance of having an ongoing pregnancy after ART [39].

Raikhraj et al. found in the systematic review that patients with noncavity-distorting intramural fibroids undergoing IVF had 44% lower odds of live birth and 32% lower odds of clinical pregnancy than patients without fibroids. A trend was also found toward lower implantation rates and higher miscarriage rates.

4.2.2 Type 3 fibroid

FIGO type 3 fibroids are intramural extra cavitary lesions that abut the endometrium without distorting the uterine cavity [20]. Lei Yan et al. in a retrospective study with 228 women with type 3 fibroid undergoing IVF-ICSI cycles, reported that those myomas affect implantation, clinical pregnancy and live birth rates but do not significantly increase the clinical miscarriage rate, the deleterious impact of this type of fibroid was remarkable in women with single fibroid diameter or total reported fibroid diameter >2 mm [40].

Xi Bai et al. published in 2020 a retrospective case–control study about the impact of FIGO type 3 fibroids on the outcome of IVF cycles. They reported that type 3 fibroids ≥30 mm might exert deleterious impact on implantation, clinical pregnancy and live birth rates of IVF cycles [41].

Available evidence suggests that FIGO type 3 fibroids are a transition between submucosal and intramural fibroids, that are intramural location wise but behave as submucosal in terms of reproductive outcome, even when they are of limited size.

Localization	Number of studies included	Breslow-Day test (P-value)	Common OR(95% CI)
Clinical			
Pregnancy rate			
Submucosal	2	0.92	0.3 (0.1–0.7)
Intramural	7	0.38	0.8 (0.6–0.9)
Subserosal	3	0.92	1.2 (0.8–1.7)
Intramural and/or subserosal	11	0.30	1.0 (0.8–1.2)
All types	16	0.24	0.8 (0.7–1.0)
Delivery rate			
Submucosal	2	0.79	0.3 (0.1–0.8)
Intramural	7	0.09	0.7 (0.5–0.8)
Subserosal	3	0.94	1.0 (0.7–1.5)
Intramural and/or subserosal	11	0.68	0.9 (0.7–1.1)
All types	16	0.43	0.8 (0.6–0.9)

Table taken and edited from ref. [13].

Table 1.
Meta-analyses on the influence of fibroids on IVF outcome according to the localization of the lesion.

4.2.3 Intracavitary fibroids

Submucosal leiomyomas and intramural fibroids distorting the uterine cavity negatively impact assisted reproduction outcomes. Many retrospective and small prospective studies indicated that these tumors disrupt implantation by 33–70% and decrease clinical pregnancy by up to 67% [31].

Somigliana et al. reported in their meta-analysis that myomas negatively affect pregnancy rate, specially submucosal lesions appear to strongly interfere with the chance of pregnancy OR(95% IC) of conception and delivery is 0.3 (0.1–0.7) and 0.3 (0.1–0.8) respectively (**Table 1**) [13].

Klatsky et al. in their systematic review stated that patients with submucosal fibroids had the strongest association with lower ongoing pregnancy rates primarily through decreased implantation [42].

Pritts et al. investigated the effect of fibroids on fertility and published a systematic literature review and meta-analysis reporting that women with submucosal component led to decreased clinical pregnancy and implantation rates compared with infertile control subjects [33].

Many studies are focused on association between fibroids and IVF outcomes. The most extensively investigated factor is myoma location. There is a consensus that submucous uterine fibroids or intramural fibroids with submucosal component that distorts the uterine cavity are associated with lower clinical pregnancy and delivery rates and higher spontaneous miscarriage rate after IVF/ICSI treatment [26].

5. Treatment

The ideal treatment should satisfy three goals: relief of symptoms, sustained reduction of fibroid size, and maintenance or improvement of fertility [43]. Having into account the heterogeneity of the fibroid presenting patient population, the confounding evidence about fibroid effect on reproductive outcome and its relationship with assisted reproductive techniques for infertility treatment, the therapeutic decisions should be based on personalized and patient specific considerations.

5.1 Hormonal therapy

5.1.1 Ulipristal acetate

Ulipristal acetate (UPA) is the first selective progesterone receptor modulator (SPRM) to be approved for the treatment of uterine fibroids. It was initially allowed for preoperative treatment of moderate to severe uterine fibroid symptoms in women of reproductive age. Afterwards, the indication was extended in United States to include the intermittent treatment of moderate to severe symptoms [44]. UPA has shown to be effective in controlling uterine bleeding related to myomas, to reduce the size and to have a good safety profile [45]. The PEARL studies have shown that ulipristal acetate offers a good alternative treatment option for long term management of uterine fibroids associated with heavy uterine bleeding, it has been shown to be effective in reducing pain and fibroid volume [46].

Mathieu et al. reported a retrospective analysis of a series of 52 patients, 21 of them wished to conceived upon treatment with UPA completion with variable periods of time (from 3 to 12 months). Of these 21 patients, 19 (90.5%) underwent myomectomy at the end of therapy, according to the protocol; 2 patients did not require surgery because an almost complete disappearance of their fibroids. Fifteen women (71%) became pregnant, resulting in 18 pregnancies, 12 resulted in the delivery of 13 healthy babies, and 6 ended in early miscarriage. Of those 18 pregnancies, 12 were spontaneous and 6 by IVF [47].

Despite the good results that UPA has in the treatment of fibroids, it has been linked to some cases of liver damage, on 2018 European Medicine Agency (EMA) recommended that several measures should be put in place to minimize the risk of rare but serious liver injury with UPA and that UPA should only be used for treatment in patients who are not candidates for surgical fibroid resection.

Detailed review of the latest phase III trials showed isolated transient increases in several liver function tests before, during and/or after treatment in a very small number of patients, some individuals exposed to a therapeutic dose of UPA may go on develop idiosyncratic drug-induced liver injury (DILI), and there are no biomarkers to identify the individuals susceptible, nevertheless UPA is not recommended in patients with moderate or severe hepatic impairment [48].

In conclusion for patients with moderate to severe symptoms due to uterine fibroids who are to undergo surgery, treatment with UPA allows to have rapid relief from heavy bleeding with improvement in quality of life. The reduction of fibroid size and uterine volume may allow for an easier or less invasive surgery, and in some cases to avoid it [49].

5.1.2 GnRH agonists

Preoperative administration of aGnRH boosts hemoglobin levels and significantly reduces fibroid volume, but long term treatment is contraindicated because bone mineral density [50]. A rationale for the use of preoperative medical therapy before surgery for fibroids is to make surgery easier [51].

5.2 Surgical treatment

Women with infertility or pregnancy loss and myomas present a challenge because, in absence of symptoms, treatment recommendations are less clear given the quality of evidence regarding the impact of myomectomy on infertility outcomes [23].

Minimally invasive techniques allow careful dissection of tissues, causing minimal damage, while still removing the entirety of fibroid tumor [52].

5.2.1 Hysteroscopic myomectomy

This has been the standard minimally invasive surgical procedure for submucous myomas. Small fibroids less than 2 cm are routinely removed in outpatient setting, depending on personal experience and available equipment, the gynecologist has a choice of several alternative procedures [1]. Casini et al. reported in a prospective controlled study that women who underwent surgery of submucous fibroids had statistically significant higher pregnancy rates than women who were not treated surgically [34].

In a Cochrane review updated on 2018 they reported that in women with otherwise unexplained subfertility and submucous fibroids, it remains uncertain whether hysteroscopic myomectomy improves the clinical pregnancy rate compared to expectant management [53].

The ASRM reported in their guide published in 2017 there is fair evidence that hysteroscopic myomectomy for submucosal fibroids improves clinical pregnancy rate, and that there is insufficient evidence to conclude that hysteroscopic myomectomy reduces the likelihood of early pregnancy loss in women with infertility and submucous fibroid [23].

5.2.2 Surgical techniques

Hysteroscopic myomectomy is usually performed with a progressive slicing of the intracavitary portion of the submucosal fibroid, a subsequent cold loop pushing of the intramural part and finally a slicing resection of it [54]. The two steps resectoscopic surgery is the most widely performed surgical technique for submucosal fibroids with a difficult approach due to the deep or size of intramyometrial location, it consists of a partial myomectomy to resect the intracavitary portion of the myoma, followed by a second surgery to remove the remaining portion.

Hysteroscopic resection is the most popular technique to remove intrauterine abnormalities [55]. This technique can be performed only with a nonconducting electrolyte-free fluid to irrigate and distend the uterine cavity [56]. Another technique used for the intracavitary fibroids are the hysteroscopic tissue removal systems (HTRs), they opened a new scenario for hysteroscopic myomectomy, data suggest that morcellator is safe and does not increase the complication rate and postoperative adhesions with respect to resectoscopy [54].

Comparison between the resectoscope and the morcellator: The extent of successful myoma resection depends more on the type and size of the fibroid rather than the technique used, data remain unclear on which technique is truly superior [55].

Another technique is the blunt dissection with the tip of the hysteroscope under direct visualization. After complete enucleation cervical dilation must be performed and a new designed bilumen intracervical cannula is inserted at the dilated cervix. This device has two lumens through which the Bettochi's hysteroscope and a laparoscopic tenaculum forceps can be introduced into the uterine cavity simultaneously avoiding the retrograde fluid loss and allowing comfortable maneuvering with both instruments to perform previously enucleated fibroid removal under direct visualization. Absence of thermal damage to neighboring myometrium and the use of isotonic fluid distention media diminishes risks of surgical complications, offers a rapid recovery and efficiently restores the intrauterine microenvironment necessary to allow embryo implantation [57]. Besides, the need for second look hysteroscopy or additional surgical steps is less frequent.

Ideal hysteroscopic myomectomy should be done in one surgical session regardless of the intramural development of the myoma, Mazzon et al. reported 87% of completely resected fibroid in a single step procedure, and 12.3% needed multiple step procedures, the grading and the size of the myoma play a crucial role in completing the procedure in a single step, only the diameter greater than 3 cm in type 2 fibroids is correlated to a higher risk of multiple steps procedure [58].

Although complications from hysteroscopy are rare, they can be potentially life threatening. The most common complication are uterine perforation, fluid intravasation, metabolic complications and adhesion formation [53].

5.2.3 Open vs. laparoscopic myomectomy

Open myomectomy was frequently performed, however laparoscopic myomectomy has recently become more common because it's less invasive. Open surgery is used only in cases in which laparoscopy is contraindicated, including patients with multiple fibroids [59].

In infertile population, cumulative pregnancy rates by the laparoscopic and minilaparotomy approaches are similar, but laparoscopic approach is associated with a quicker recovery, less postoperative pain and less febrile morbidity [12].

Laparoscopic myomectomy is the gold standard treatment for the majority of myomas, with advantages over open myomectomy as reduced postoperative pain, faster return to activity, improved cosmetic results and less adhesion formation [12, 60]. The incidence of uterine rupture after laparoscopic myomectomy is not well defined. Although some report an incidence close to 1%, a clear publication bias probably makes this complication to be overestimated [61].

With respect to recurrence rate, Kotani et al. reported lower recurrence after open surgery, concluding that it was the result of manual fibroid removal with a more exhaustive extraction of smaller myomas as performed during laparoscopy. Fewer residual myomas left after open surgery contribute to a lower postsurgical recurrence rate [59].

Chelsea et al. determined the effects of fibroids and their removal on assisted reproductive treatment outcomes with a retrospective cohort study on infertility patients who underwent myomectomy prior IVF or IUI (intrauterine insemination). They found that among women undergoing IVF, the cumulative incidence of clinical pregnancy was significantly higher in the myomectomy group than in the in situ fibroid group [62].

Bulleti et al. reported in 1999 higher delivery rates (42%) in infertile women underwent myomectomy than women who did not (11%), $p < 0.001$ [35]. Then in 2004, this same group reported the beneficial role of laparoscopic surgery for myomas performed before attempting IVF programs, when intramural myomas were larger than 5 cm. They found statistically significant increase in cumulative pregnancy and delivery rates among patients who underwent surgery than in the group that underwent IVF without surgical removal of their myomas [63].

Oliveira et al. reported in their retrospective study that patients with subserosal or intramural fibroids <4 cm had IVF-ICSI outcomes similar to their controls, but patients with intramural fibroids >4 cm had lower pregnancy rates than patients with intramural fibroids <4 cm; Whether or not women with fibroids >4 cm could benefit from fibroid treatment remains to be determined [64].

In our center InSer Medellín we perform laparoscopic myomectomy on those patients undergoing IVF who have intramural fibroids larger than 4 cm. Smaller intramural myomas might also be considered for surgical treatment in patients with previous failed IVF attempts [65].

Robot assisted laparoscopic myomectomy (RALM).

The use of RALM has several advantages which allows the articulation of instruments by 540° as well as easier intracorporeal suturing. It also may considered in complex surgical cases for which traditional laparoscopy is not indicated [66]. It should be clearly stated that RALM constitutes the minimally invasive alternative to open myomectomy in those cases that cannot be adequately and consistently addressed with conventional minimally invasive surgery [52].

5.3 Other methods

Uterine artery embolization (UAE) technique has been studied as an alternative to myomectomy and hysterectomy mainly in women who no longer desire children, one of the contraindication is infertility or desire for future pregnancy because of lower pregnancy rates and higher miscarriage rates following UAE [12].

Magnetic resonance guided focused ultrasound (MRgFUS) was approved in 2004 by the FDA for leiomyoma treatment. Initial fertility studies were encouraging but randomized controlled trials need to be done [67]. This technique involves the destruction of uterine fibroid tissue through coagulative necrosis by heating tissue to over 70°C, focusing high frequency ultrasound beams on the target tissue [12].

Cryomyolisis is a variation on the laparoscopic technique in which the myoma tissue is coagulated rather than removed. It has the advantage of being minimally invasive and easier to perform than laparoscopic myomectomy and for this reason may present an alternative to myomectomy and hysterectomy for selected women with symptomatic intramural or subserous fibroids who wish to preserve their uterus but do not desire future fertility [68].

6. Conclusion

Myomatosis in infertility remains to be a challenge for clinician. It's management will depend on the symptoms and for infertile women, on fibroid location, number and size. A good ultrasound mapping of the fibroids determining the location, size and especially the degree of the endometrial involvement are essential to determine the treatment modality required. It's clear that intracavitary and intramural fibroids that deform the cavity have negative impact on ART.

The presence of intramural fibroids not distorting the endometrial cavity and their impact on fertility outcome is less clear, however there is also evidence of diminished clinical pregnancy and live birth rates in women who undergo IVF especially with intramural fibroids larger than 4 cm.

Treatment must be individualized according to the symptoms and whether or not there is infertility. Minimally invasive surgery continues to be the therapy of choice.

7. Take home points

When we talk about fibroids and infertility, we must take into account the age of the patient and the fibroid number, size and localization.

Type 0,1,2 fibroids can affect implantation and embryo development and hysteroscopic myomectomy may be considered.

Myomectomy should be considered for infertile patients with intramural fibroids that are larger than 4 cm, multiple or that distort the endometrial cavity. Previous failed IVF cycles should be taken into account when making a decision about surgical treatment.

Cumulative pregnancy rates are similar with laparoscopic and abdominal myomectomy approaches; however laparoscopy is associated with quicker recovery, less pain and less adhesion formation.

Subserosal fibroids do not appear to affect fertility outcome and do not require surgery to improve pregnancy rates.

Clinicians should wait 3 months after surgery prior to IVF, but in older women with low ovarian reserve, embryo cryopreservation and cryopreserved embryo transfer after appropriate uterine scarring should be considered.

Author details

Juan Luis Giraldo Moreno* and Susana Salazar López
InSer, CES University, University of Antioquia and University Pontificia Bolivariana, Medellín, Colombia

*Address all correspondence to: juangiraldo@inser.com.co

References

[1] Donnez J, Dolmans M-M. Uterine fibroid management: from the present to the future. Hum Reprod Update. noviembre de 2016;22(6):665-686.

[2] Wallach EE, Vlahos NF. Uterine Myomas: An Overview of Development, Clinical Features, and Management: Obstet Gynecol. agosto de 2004;104(2):393-406.

[3] Cook H. The Impact of Uterine Leiomyomas on Reproductive Outcomes. 2014;15.

[4] Peddada SD, Laughlin SK, Miner K, Guyon J-P, Haneke K, Vahdat HL, et al. Growth of uterine leiomyomata among premenopausal black and white women. Med Sci. :6.

[5] Sparic R, Mirkovic L, Malvasi A, Tinelli A. Epidemiology of Uterine Myomas: A Review. Int J Fertil Steril. 2016 Jan-Mar;9(4):424-35.

[6] Eltoukhi HM, Modi MN, Weston M, Armstrong AY, Stewart EA. The health disparities of uterine fibroid tumors for African American women: a public health issue. Am J Obstet Gynecol. marzo de 2014;210(3):194-199.

[7] Pavone D, Clemenza S, Sorbi F, Fambrini M, Petraglia F. Epidemiology and Risk Factors of Uterine Fibroids. Best Pract Res Clin Obstet Gynaecol. enero de 2018;46:3-11.

[8] Day Baird D, Dunson DB. Why is Parity Protective for Uterine Fibroids?: Epidemiology. marzo de 2003;14(2):247-250.

[9] Laughlin S, Schroeder J, Baird D. New Directions in the Epidemiology of Uterine Fibroids. Semin Reprod Med. mayo de 2010;28(03):204-217.

[10] Mittal P, Shin Y, Yatsenko SA, Castro CA, Surti U, Rajkovic A. Med12 gain-of-function mutation causes leiomyomas and genomic instability. J Clin Invest. 3 de agosto de 2015;125(8):3280-3284.

[11] Marret H, Fritel X, Ouldamer L, Bendifallah S, Brun J-L, De Jesus I, et al. Therapeutic management of uterine fibroid tumors: updated French guidelines. Eur J Obstet Gynecol Reprod Biol. diciembre de 2012;165(2):156-164.

[12] Vilos GA, Allaire C, Laberge P-Y, Leyland N, Vilos AG, Murji A, et al. The Management of Uterine Leiomyomas. J Obstet Gynaecol Can. febrero de 2015;37(2):157-178.

[13] Somigliana E, Vercellini P, Daguati R, Pasin R, De Giorgi O, Crosignani PG. Fibroids and female reproduction: a critical analysis of the evidence. Human Reproduction Update. 13(5):465-76.

[14] Bajekal N. Fibroids, infertility and pregnancy wastage. Hum Reprod Update. 1 de noviembre de 2000;6(6):614-620.

[15] Munro MG, Critchley HOD, Fraser IS, the FIGO Menstrual Disorders Committee. The two FIGO systems for normal and abnormal uterine bleeding symptoms and classification of causes of abnormal uterine bleeding in the reproductive years: 2018 revisions. Int J Gynecol Obstet. diciembre de 2018;143(3):393-408.

[16] Munro M, Critchley H, Fraser I. The Flexible FIGO Classification Concept for Underlying Causes of Abnormal Uterine Bleeding. Semin Reprod Med. septiembre de 2011;29(05):391-399.

[17] Fraser I, Critchley H, Broder M, Munro M. The FIGO Recommendations on Terminologies and Definitions for Normal and Abnormal Uterine Bleeding. Semin Reprod Med. septiembre de 2011;29(05):383-390.

[18] Laughlin-Tommaso SK, Hesley GK, Hopkins MR, Brandt KR, Zhu Y, Stewart EA. Clinical limitations of the International Federation of Gynecology and Obstetrics (FIGO) classification of uterine fibroids. Int J Gynecol Obstet. noviembre de 2017;139(2):143-148.

[19] Bosteels J, van Wessel S, Weyers S, Broekmans FJ, D'Hooghe TM, Bongers MY, et al. Hysteroscopy for treating subfertility associated with suspected major uterine cavity abnormalities. Cochrane Gynaecology and Fertility Group, editor. Cochrane Database of Systematic Reviews

[20] Munro MG, Critchley HOD, Broder MS, Fraser IS, for the FIGO Working Group on Menstrual Disorders. FIGO classification system (PALM-COEIN) for causes of abnormal uterine bleeding in nongravid women of reproductive age. Int J Gynecol Obstet. abril de 2011;113(1):3-13.

[21] Surrey ES, Lietz AK, Schoolcraft WB. Impact of intramural leiomyomata in patients with a normal endometrial cavity on in vitro fertilization–embryo transfer cycle outcome. Fertil Steril. febrero de 2001;75(2):405-410.

[22] Bul C, De Ziegler, Dominique, Polli, Valeria, Flamigni, Carlo. The Role of Leiomyomas in Infertility. J Am Assoc Gynecol Laparoscopists. noviembre de 1999;6(4):441-445.

[23] Penzias A, Bendikson K, Butts S, Coutifaris C, Falcone T, Fossum G, et al. Removal of myomas in asymptomatic patients to improve fertility and/or reduce miscarriage rate: a guideline. Fertil Steril. septiembre de 2017;108(3):416-425.

[24] Matsuzaki S, Canis M, Darcha C, Pouly J-L, Mage G. HOXA-10 expression in the mid-secretory endometrium of infertile patients with either endometriosis, uterine fibromas or unexplained infertility. Hum Reprod. 1 de diciembre de 2009;24(12):3180-3187.

[25] Doherty LF, Taylor HS. Leiomyoma-derived transforming growth factor-β impairs bone morphogenetic protein-2-mediated endometrial receptivity. Fertil Steril. marzo de 2015;103(3):845-852.

[26] Lisiecki M, Paszkowski M, Woźniak S. Fertility impairment associated with uterine fibroids – a review of literature. Menopausal Rev. 2017;16(4):137-140.

[27] Sanoee MF, Alizamir T, Shamila Faramarzi, Saidijam M, Yadegarazari R, Nooshin Shabab, et al. Effect of Myomectomy on Endometrial Glutathione Peroxidase 3 (GPx3) and Glycodelin mRNA Expression at the Time of the Implantation Window. Iran Biomed J IBJ ISSN 1028-852X [Internet]. 1996 [citado 11 de abril de 2021]; Disponible en: http://ibj.pasteur.ac.ir/browse.php?a_id=1110&sid=1&slc_lang=en

[28] Hasegawa E, Ito H, Hasegawa F, Hatano K, Kazuka M, Usuda S, et al. Expression of leukemia inhibitory factor in the endometrium in abnormal uterine cavities during the implantation window. Fertil Steril. abril de 2012;97(4):953-958.

[29] Pier B, Crellin C, Katre A, Conner MG, Novak L, Young SL, et al. Large, Non-Cavity Distorting Intramural Leiomyomas Decrease Leukemia Inhibitory Factor in the Secretory Phase Endometrium. Reprod Sci. febrero de 2020;27(2):569-574.

[30] Somigliana E, De Benedictis S, Vercellini P, Nicolosi AE, Benaglia L, Scarduelli C, et al. Fibroids not encroaching the endometrial cavity and IVF success rate: a prospective study. Hum Reprod. 1 de abril de 2011;26(4):834-839.

[31] Levy G, Hill MJ, Beall S, Zarek SM, Segars JH, Catherino WH. Leiomyoma: genetics, assisted reproduction, pregnancy and therapeutic advances. J Assist Reprod Genet. agosto de 2012;29(8):703-712.

[32] Parazzini F, Tozzi L, Bianchi S. Pregnancy outcome and uterine fibroids. Best Pract Res Clin Obstet Gynaecol. julio de 2016;34:74-84.

[33] Pritts EA, Parker WH, Olive DL. Fibroids and infertility: an updated systematic review of the evidence. Fertil Steril. abril de 2009;91(4): 1215-1223.

[34] Casini ML, Rossi F, Agostini R, Unfer V. Effects of the position of fibroids on fertility. Gynecol Endocrinol. enero de 2006;22(2):106-109.

[35] Bul C. The Role of Leiomyomas in Infertility. :5.

[36] Johnson G, MacLehose RF, Baird DD, Laughlin-Tommaso SK, Hartmann KE. Uterine leiomyomata and fecundability in the Right from the Start study. Hum Reprod. 1 de octubre de 2012;27(10):2991-2997.

[37] Sunkara SK, Khairy M, El-Toukhy T, Khalaf Y, Coomarasamy A. The effect of intramural fibroids without uterine cavity involvement on the outcome of IVF treatment: a systematic review and meta-analysis. Hum Reprod. 1 de febrero de 2010;25(2):418-429.

[38] Wang X, Chen L, Wang H, Li Q, Liu X, Qi H. The Impact of Noncavity-Distorting Intramural Fibroids on the Efficacy of In Vitro Fertilization-Embryo Transfer: An Updated Meta-Analysis. BioMed Res Int. 4 de septiembre de 2018;2018:1-13.

[39] Hart R, Khalaf Y, Yeong C-T, Seed P, Taylor A, Braude P. A prospective controlled study of the effect of intramural uterine fibroids on the outcome of assisted conception. Hum Reprod. noviembre de 2001;16(11):2411-2417.

[40] Yan L, Yu Q, Zhang Y, Guo Z, Li Z, Niu J, et al. Effect of type 3 intramural fibroids on in vitro fertilization–intracytoplasmic sperm injection outcomes: a retrospective cohort study. Fertil Steril. mayo de 2018;109(5):817-822.e2.

[41] Bai X, Lin Y, Chen Y, Ma C. The impact of FIGO type 3 fibroids on in-vitro fertilization outcomes: A nested retrospective case-control study. Eur J Obstet Gynecol Reprod Biol. abril de 2020;247:176-180.

[42] Klatsky PC, Tran ND, Caughey AB, Fujimoto VY. Fibroids and reproductive outcomes: a systematic literature review from conception to delivery. Am J Obstet Gynecol. abril de 2008;198(4):357-366.

[43] Singh SS, Belland L. Contemporary management of uterine fibroids: focus on emerging medical treatments. Curr Med Res Opin. 2 de enero de 2015;31(1):1-12.

[44] Garnock-Jones KP, Duggan ST. Ulipristal Acetate: A Review in Symptomatic Uterine Fibroids. Drugs. octubre de 2017;77(15):1665-1675.

[45] Donnez J, Donnez O, Matule D, Ahrendt H-J, Hudecek R, Zatik J, et al. Long-term medical management of uterine fibroids with ulipristal acetate. Fertil Steril. enero de 2016;105(1):165-173.e4.

[46] Powell M, Dutta D. Esmya ® and the PEARL studies: A review. Womens Health. noviembre de 2016;12(6):544-548.

[47] Luyckx M, Squifflet J-L, Jadoul P, Votino R, Dolmans M-M, Donnez J. First series of 18 pregnancies after ulipristal

acetate treatment for uterine fibroids. Fertil Steril. noviembre de 2014;102(5):1404-1409.

[48] Dolmans M, Donnez J, Fellah L. Uterine fibroid management: Today and tomorrow. J Obstet Gynaecol Res. julio de 2019;45(7):1222-1229.

[49] Donnez J, Arriagada P, Marciniak M, Larrey D. Liver safety parameters of ulipristal acetate for the treatment of uterine fibroids: a comprehensive review of the clinical development program. Expert Opin Drug Saf. 2 de diciembre de 2018;17(12):1225-1232.

[50] Donnez J, Dolmans M-M. Hormone therapy for intramural myoma-related infertility from ulipristal acetate to GnRH antagonist: a review. Reprod Biomed Online. septiembre de 2020;41(3):431-442.

[51] Lethaby A, Puscasiu L, Vollenhoven B. Preoperative medical therapy before surgery for uterine fibroids. Cochrane Gynaecology and Fertility Group, editor. Cochrane Database Syst Rev [Internet]. 15 de noviembre de 2017 [citado 18 de abril de 2021]; Disponible en: http://doi.wiley.com/10.1002/14651858.CD000547.pub2

[52] Lewis EI, Gargiulo AR. The Role of Hysteroscopic and Robot-assisted Laparoscopic Myomectomy in the Setting of Infertility. Clin Obstet Gynecol. marzo de 2016;59(1):53-65.

[53] Bosteels J, van Wessel S, Weyers S, Broekmans FJ, D'Hooghe TM, Bongers MY, et al. Hysteroscopy for treating subfertility associated with suspected major uterine cavity abnormalities. Cochrane Gynaecology and Fertility Group, editor. Cochrane Database Syst Rev [Internet]. 5 de diciembre de 2018 [citado 9 de abril de 2021]; Disponible en: http://doi.wiley.com/10.1002/14651858.CD009461.pub4

[54] Vitale SG, Sapia F, Rapisarda AMC, Valenti G, Santangelo F, Rossetti D, et al. Hysteroscopic Morcellation of Submucous Myomas: A Systematic Review. BioMed Res Int. 2017;2017:1-6.

[55] Friedman JA, Wong JMK, Chaudhari A, Tsai S, Milad MP. Hysteroscopic myomectomy: a comparison of techniques and review of current evidence in the management of abnormal uterine bleeding. 2018;30(4):9.

[56] van Dongen H, Emanuel MH, Wolterbeek R, Trimbos JB, Jansen FW. Hysteroscopic Morcellator for Removal of Intrauterine Polyps and Myomas: A Randomized Controlled Pilot Study among Residents in Training. J Minim Invasive Gynecol. julio de 2008;15(4):466-471.

[57] Osorio W. Hysteroscopic myomectomy for submucosal type 2 fibroids with cold enucleation technique and complete fibroid extraction using a double-lumen intracervical cannula. 2021;115(2):3.

[58] Mazzon I, Favilli A, Grasso M, Horvath S, Bini V, Di Renzo GC, et al. Predicting success of single step hysteroscopic myomectomy: A single centre large cohort study of single myomas. Int J Surg. octubre de 2015;22:10-14.

[59] Kotani Y, Tobiume T, Fujishima R, Shigeta M, Takaya H, Nakai H, et al. Recurrence of uterine myoma after myomectomy: Open myomectomy versus laparoscopic myomectomy: Recurrence after laparotomy vs LM. J Obstet Gynaecol Res. febrero de 2018;44(2):298-302.

[60] Oxley SG, Mallick R, Odejinmi F. Laparoscopic Myomectomy: An Alternative Approach to Tackling Submucous Myomas? J Minim Invasive Gynecol. enero de 2020;27(1): 155-159.

[61] Cela V, Freschi L, Simi G, Tana R, Russo N, Artini PG, et al. Fertility and endocrine outcome after robot-assisted laparoscopic myomectomy (RALM). Gynecol Endocrinol. enero de 2013;29(1):79-82.

[62] Fortin CN, Hur C, Radeva M, Falcone T. Effects of myomas and myomectomy on assisted reproductive technology outcomes. J Gynecol Obstet Hum Reprod. noviembre de 2019;48(9):751-755.

[63] Bulletti C, De Ziegler D, Levi Setti P, Cicinelli E, Polli V, Stefanetti M. Myomas, Pregnancy Outcome, and *In Vitro* Fertilization. Ann N Y Acad Sci. diciembre de 2004;1034(1):84-92.

[64] Oliveira FG, Abdelmassih VG, Diamond MP, Dozortsev D, Melo NR, Abdelmassih R. Impact of subserosal and intramural uterine fibroids that do not distort the endometrial cavity on the outcome of in vitro fertilization–intracytoplasmic sperm injection. Fertil Steril. marzo de 2004;81(3):582-587.

[65] Galliano D, Bellver J, Díaz-García C, Simón C, Pellicer A. ART and uterine pathology: how relevant is the maternal side for implantation? Hum Reprod Update. 1 de enero de 2015;21(1):13-38.

[66] Lee SR, Lee ES, Lee Y-J, Lee S-W, Park JY, Kim D-Y, et al. Robot-Assisted Laparoscopic Myomectomy versus Abdominal Myomectomy for Large Myomas Sized over 10 cm or Weighing 250 g. Yonsei Med J. 2020;61(12):1054.

[67] Guo XC, Segars JH. The Impact and Management of Fibroids for Fertility. Obstet Gynecol Clin North Am. diciembre de 2012;39(4):521-533.

[68] Ciavattini A, Tsiroglou D, Piccioni M, Lugnani F, Litta P, Feliciotti F, et al. Laparoscopic cryomyolysis: An alternative to myomectomy in women with symptomatic fibroids. Surg Endosc. diciembre de 2004;18(12):1785-1788.

Chapter 4

Endometrial Receptivity in Patients with Polycystic Ovary Syndrome

Alice Albu and Dragoş Albu

Abstract

Polycystic ovary syndrome (PCOS) is a frequent disorder affecting women of reproductive age characterized by infertility. Affected endometrial receptivity seems to contribute to decreased fertility of these patients as suggested by several studies. Understanding the mechanism behind this reduced endometrial receptivity could contribute to discovery of new therapeutic targets for infertility of PCOS. The aim of the paper is to review the current data regarding endometrial receptivity in PCOS patients, the potential mechanisms involved with particular focus on recent findings as the impact of gut microbiota on endometrium, the relationship between vitamin D and endometrial receptivity and the different impact of letrozole and clomiphene citrate on endometrial receptivity in infertile PCOS women.

Keywords: polycystic ovary syndrome, endometrial receptivity, endometrium, implantation, pregnancy

1. Introduction

Polycystic ovary syndrome (PCOS) is the most common endocrine disorder in women of reproductive age, having a prevalence of 8 to 13% and of 21% in high-risk groups [1]. Moreover, it is a leading cause of female infertility [2, 3] and the most common cause of anovulatory infertility [4]. A systematic review from 2020 [5] found that there is significant variation in prevalence probably according to ethnic background and design of the published studies, but also to diagnosis criteria used to identify the disease. Thus, they found that the reported prevalence of PCOS vary between 2,2% and 15–20%, with the studies using the Rotterdam criteria reporting the highest prevalence [5].

PCOS has significant consequences on the women health, being associated with infertility, menstrual irregularities, metabolic abnormalities, cardiovascular risk and psychological disturbances [6] and, therefore, impairing the quality of life. The latest guidelines [7] recommend the use of Rotterdam Consensus criteria for PCOS diagnosis, which assumes that two out of the following three features are present: oligo- or anovulation, hyperandrogenism (clinical or biochemical) and polycystic ovaries [8]. The use of these criteria generates several clinical phenotypes with variate impact on reproductive potential and metabolic profile, with some of them diagnosed with difficulty due to a scarce clinical picture. Therefore, PCOS can be a challenging disorder in the reproductive medicine practice.

Hyperandrogenism is a key feature of PCOS, being the result of increased production of both ovarian and adrenal androgens. Ovarian over-secretion of androgens is the consequence of LH stimulation and also the action of high insulin levels on insulin receptors from the ovarian theca cells. Moreover, bioavailability of androgens is increased due to insulin effect to reduce the hepatic production of sex-hormone binding globulin.

2. Fertility in patients with polycystic ovary syndrome

PCOS is considered the most common cause of anovulation, being responsible for 70% of cases of anovulatory infertility [9]. Infertility is a significant complaint among women with PCOS, being reported in 72% of women with PCOS compared with 16% in women without PCOS. However, it seems that the number of children of women with PCOS is similar with those without, suggesting that treatment for infertility is effective [10].

It was also showed that 44% of women with unexplained infertility are probable PCOS cases, underlying that the subtle clinical phenotypes in some of the patients can be the cause of misdiagnosis and, therefore, inappropriate diagnosis and treatment [11].

It seems that the criteria used for diagnosis can also impact the prevalence of infertility which is higher in women with polycystic ovary morphology in patients diagnosed according to Androgen Excess Society criteria (21,7%), while in patients diagnosed according to Rotterdam criteria infertility is present in only 6% of them [5].

Older studies report that 78% of infertile women with PCOS respond to clomiphene citrate (CC) administration [12], with only the remaining 22% requiring alternative therapies, suggesting that anovulation is not the only cause of infertility in PCOS patients. Indeed, even after restoration of ovulation, PCOS patients still have reduced cumulative pregnancy rate and higher rates of implantation failure [13]. Even in cycles with excellent embryos selected for transfer, the success of in vitro fertilization in PCOS patients remain low [14]. In animal models the transfer of blastocysts from normal mice to DHEA-induced PCOS mice resulted in a reduced implantation rate [15]. Moreover, patients with PCOS had an increased risk of miscarriage with reported rates between 30 and 50% of all conceptions [16, 17]. In addition, PCOS seems to be responsible for more than 30% of cases of recurrent miscarriages [18].

Since oocytes and embryo quality do not seems to be the cause of low implantation and pregnancy rate in PCOS patients as demonstrated by donor oocyte models [19, 20], the decreased receptivity of the endometrium seems more probable. Indeed, accumulating data support the hypothesis that endometrium of PCOS patients is affected probably as a consequence of hormonal imbalance. Thus, unopposed estrogens, hyperinsulinemia, hyperandrogenism and the members of insulin-like growth factor family were reported as possible contributors to endometrial pathology in PCOS [21]. Factors associated with unexplained recurrent pregnancy loss like high serum levels of free testosterone and LH, decreased luteal phase progesterone and delayed endometrial development [22] are also found in PCOS patients, suggesting their involvement in the high miscarriage rate in PCOS.

Several abnormalities of the endometrium were reported in PCOS women. Thus, endometrial gene expression and sex hormone receptors, co-receptors, adhesion molecules expression and endometrial markers were reported to be abnormal [23].

3. Endometrial receptivity in women with polycystic ovary syndrome

Endometrial receptivity is a complex feature of the endometrium that allow the embryo to attach and invade the endometrium, and its further development into a viable fetus. For normal implantation both embryo and endometrial quality are important. In normal women the endometrium is receptive to embryo implantation for a period of 3–6 days which starts seven to ten days after ovulation known as the window of implantation. In pathological conditions this window can be shorten or shifted, resulting in infertility or pregnancy loss.

Human endometrium is a tissue whose development depends on the level of circulating hormones. During the follicular phase of the cycle, the increasing circulating estradiol levels determine the proliferation of the endometrial cells and increased endometrial sensitivity to estrogen through increasing the estrogen receptors (ER) ER-α levels [24, 25]. The ER expression is highest in the late proliferative phase, decreasing in the luteal phase [25]. Following ovulation, the progesterone production determines inhibition of cellular proliferation, mitotic activity, DNA synthesis and stimulates the differentiation of the endometrial cells [26]. The inhibition of proliferation of the epithelial endometrial cells is the consequence of the progesterone-induced regulation of genes resulting in down regulation of estrogen receptors and the induction of the enzymes that metabolize estrogens reducing its cellular effects [26]. Moreover, progesterone reduces the expression of androgen receptor in endometrial cells and stroma [26]. As a consequence of all these changes the 'window of implantation' occur. Progesterone is also essential for decidualization, a process that allow trophoblast invasion in case the implantation occur and establish a cytokine milieu and immunomodulatory network in the stroma. The decidualization is the consequence of endometrial stromal cells modifications of the cytoskeleton and up-regulation of prolactin, insulin-like growth factors, IGF binding proteins, insulin receptor and other factors. In the case the implantation does not occur, the decreasing estrogen and progesterone levels determines a shift from the expression of the innate immune genes to inflammatory genes expression in association with cellular apoptosis, increased production of metalloproteinases and prostaglandins, followed by endometrial desquamation and menstruation [26].

In women with PCOS, in the absence of ovulation the progesterone effects on the endometrium are lacking or severely decreased, affecting the decidualization and the window of implantation. Moreover, women with PCOS may have increased exposure to estrogen levels [27] as a consequence of aromatization of increased androgens in adipose tissue and decreased sex hormone binding globulin due to hyperinsulinemia [28, 29]. Several experimental studies support the alteration of endometrium especially in the window of implantation. Thus, Avellaira et al. [30] found that the tissue homeostasis in secretory endometrium of untreated women with PCOS is affected by an imbalance between apoptosis and cell proliferation which is increased as demonstrated by a study evaluating the expression of the proteins related with the two processes [30].

It was also suggested that some endometrial alterations in PCOS are the consequence of prenatal intrauterine exposure to androgens being considered primary endometrial abnormalities [23]. Thus, the endometrium of PCOS women has a preponderance of estrogen and androgen action and decreased progesterone action as a consequence of hormone receptors expression and function.

3.1 Estrogen receptors (ER) expression and function

In PCOS patients the level of ER seems to be increased in all the cycle phases [31–35]. Moreover, some coactivators of the ER-α like TIF2 and AIB1 were also found in higher levels in the proliferative endometrium of the PCOS patients compared with controls [32–35]. Moreover, during the proliferative phase, the endometrium of PCOS women showed a higher Bcl-2/Bax ratio, indicating the predominance of anti-apoptotic factors in the estrogen receptor increased environment [31]. The higher levels of mRNA and protein for ER-α and coactivators compared with normal women were reported in the mid-secretory phase endometrium of PCOS as well [32]. Moreover, the coactivator ARA70 was increase and epithelial expression of beta3-integrin, a protein involved in cell adhesion and cell surphace mediated signaling, was decreased in endometrium of PCOS versus control [32].

Enhanced ER-α activation was associated with rare or absent apoptosis and increased in cell proliferation in the endometrium in the mid luteal phase [30, 36–38]. On the other hand, it is possible that high circulating estrogens as in patients performing ovarian stimulation to determine the apoptosis of the endometrial glandular cells, as showed by an experimental study by Chen et al. [39].

Other factors can contribute to increased exposure of endometrial cells to estrogens. Thus, the modified activity of the endometrial enzymes 17-β-hydroxysteroid dehydrogenase, which is downregulated and hydroxysteroid dehydrogenase type 1, which is upregulated, could contribute to increased local production of estradiol and androstenediol with increased estrogenic activity [40–42].

3.2 Progesterone receptor (PR) expression and function

In endometrium of PCOS women progesterone receptors (PR) alpha and beta mRNA is overexpressed and the stromal immunostaining of PR-b and Ki67 is higher compared with BMI-matched controls [43]. Moreover, an imbalance between PR-a expression and PR-b was found in proliferative endometrium of obese PCOS women, with the predominance of the later [43]. It was also reported that endometrial tissue of PCOS patients has decreased responsiveness to progesterone [44], also known as 'P resistance' [45]. This progesterone resistance might be due to reduced binding and activation of PR [46] or to an altered expression of its isoforms [46, 47]. Elevated PR isoform expression was showed to be associated with increased systemic levels of estrogen [48] and of androgen [49, 50]. Thus, hyperandrogenism modulates the expression and function of PR being associated with inactive or less active isoforms of PR [49–51], being probably responsible for progesterone resistance in PCOS women.

Mucin 1 (MUC1) is a progesterone-regulated molecule that carries selectin ligands recognized by the human blastocyst. Thus, Margarit et al. [52] showed that MUC1 expression is lower in anovulatory PCOS than in fertile patients, being a possible contributor to decreased implantation.

3.3 Androgen receptor

In the endometrium of PCOS women the androgen receptor (AR) mRNA and protein expression is increased [23] and coactivators of AR were found to be overexpressed as well [37]. Among these coactivators, Melanoma-associated antigen 11 (MAGEA11) was showed to bind to AR resulting in alteration of window of implantation [11]. Endometrial microenvironment can also contribute to over-exposure to androgen. Thus, low level of SHBG can increase the bioavailable testosteron at endometrial level [53] and increased activity of endometrial 5a-reductase generates potent androgens such as di-hydro-testosterone [37]. The uptake of intracrine precursors of testosterone [38, 54] and increased activity of hydroxi-steroid-dehydrogenase might contribute to high androgen exposure of endometrium in PCOS [55].

3.4 Hyperandrogenism

During the mid-secretory phase of the menstrual cycle and the window of implantation the level of circulating androgens reach a nadir in normal cycles [56], while in PCOS patients with hyperandrogenism the level of circulating androgens is constantly increased. There is a significant body of evidence suggesting that overexposure to androgens may affect the normal development of endometrium and, therefore the endometrial receptivity. Thus, Cermik et al. [57] studied the effect of testosterone on HOXA10 expression in endometrium, a gene well known to be involved in endometrial receptivity. They demonstrated that, in vitro testosterone exposure decreases the expression on HOXA10 and prevents the increase of this gene in response to estrogen and progesterone [57]. They also confirmed that the expression of HOXA10 is decreased in the endometrium of the hyperandrogenic PCOS patients [57]. Homebox (HOX) are genes essential for endometrial receptivity which are maximally expressed in endometrium during the window of implantation [58]. Their importance in implantation is demonstrated by experimental studies on female mice with disruption of HOXA10 which show infertility with implantation failure in spite of the presence of ovulation [59].

It was also showed that Wilms tumor suppressor (WT1) gene which is expressed in endometrium in the window of implantation, was downregulated in ovulatory women with PCOS in comparison with normal controls and that this downregulation is the consequence of androgen exposure in in vitro models [60] Since high androgen are associated with elevated PR isoforms, it was suggested that hyperandogenism could be a contributor to progesterone resistance found in PCOS women [50, 61]. High androgens can also affect the number and function of endometrial pinopodes which are associated with endometrial receptivity [62, 63]. Androgens can also influence the decidualization by their ability to modulate the oxidative stress response in decidualized endometrial cells [64] since the oxidative stress was showed to influence factors involved in embryo implantation like cytokeratin 8 (CK-8) [65]. Other androgens can also act on endometrium. Thus, DHEA seems to block glucose utilization resulting in inhibition of decidualization [66] and modulation of cell survival and apoptosis [67]. In pregnant mice treated with DHEA an impaired LIF-signal transducer and activator of transcription 3 (STAT3) pathway was observed, which was associated with implantation failure [68].

Clinical data showed that pregnant women with PCOS have lower endovascular trophoblast invasion in relation to circulating testosterone and the clinical phenotypes involving hyperandrogenism [69, 70].

3.5 Hyperinsulinemia and insulin resistance

In clinical studies, in PCOS patients undergoing in vitro maturation-in vitro fertilization embryo transfer cycle insulin resistance was associated with decreased implantation, clinical pregnancy and ongoing pregnancy rates [71]. Energy metabolism is vital for proper endometrial function taking into consideration the rapid turnover of endometrial tissue. Therefore, insulin action on endometrial tissue might be essential for endometrial receptivity. Insulin resistance and compensatory hyperinsulinemia can have detrimental effects on the implantation process as hyperinsulinemia has been shown to impair stromal cell decidualization in vitro [72–74]. In PCOS endometrium several abnormalities in insulin signaling and glucose transport have been reported. Thus, hyperinsulinemia can reduce insulin receptor substrate 1 (InRS-1) activation and glucose transport in endometrial stromal cells in PCOS women [75–76], probably via inflammatory pathways [76, 77]. Experimental studies showed that in vitro exposure to dihydrotestosterone altered the expression of insulin receptor and insulin receptor substrates and the phosphorylation of insulin receptor in endometrial stromal cells [74]. Other studies suggests that insulin action is decreased in endometrium of hyperinsulinemic women with PCOS, by showing that pAS160T642 and SLC2A4 which are substrates of insulin receptor are decreased in comparison with non-hyperinsulinemic PCOS and controls [75].

In vitro studies showed that insulin inhibits the production of IGFBP-1 in the endometrial stoma. IGFBP-1 is considered a biomarker of decidualization [73]. It is also possible that adiponectin, an insulin regulating molecule and regulator of glucose metabolism, which is decreased in PCOS patients, to be involved in endometrial receptivity of these patients. Thus, adiponectin receptors were found to be highly expressed in the human endometrium during the window of implantation [78]. Moreover, decidualized mouse endometrium is able to secrete adiponectin and adiponectin receptors were found both in decidual cells and embryo after implantation [79]. This data supports the hypothesis that adiponectin might play a role in endometrial receptivity and implantation. Studies showing that metformin reduces the miscarriage rates in PCOS patients indirectly support the hypothesis of insulin resistance involvement in endometrial receptivity [80].

3.6 Vitamin D

Vitamin D deficiency is a frequent condition among women with infertility or PCOS. Numerous studies suggested a role of vitamin D in reproductive health at variate level of reproductive system, including endometrium. However, clinical data regarding the association between serum vitamin D level and endometrial pathology are divergent. A prospective controlled study [81] analyzed factors associated with recurrent implantation failure and found higher prevalence of chronic endometritis, a lower vitamin D level and a borderline lower progesterone level in comparison with controls [81]. However, two recent systematic reviews found no association between serum vitamin D level and miscarriage rate in women who performed in vitro fertilization [82, 83], while one of these reviews reported higher pregnancy rates in vitamin D replete patients undergoing assisted reproduction treatments [82].

Experimental studies support the role of vitamin D in endometrial receptivity. Thus, Guo et al. [84] found that circulating level of vitamin D was positively associated with vitamin D receptor and HOXA10 protein level expression in the endometrium and these were substantially elevated in pregnant women compared to non-pregnant women. During the window of implantation, higher serum vitamin D levels were associated with more mature pinopodes (84). Another study showed that in patients with recurrent implantation failure vitamin D treatment increases progesterone receptor mRNA and protein level and its phosphorylation on Ser294 residues in the endometrial cells (85). These results suggest that vitamin D may play a key role in the endometrial receptivity [85].

In patients with PCOS vitamin D deficiency is frequently found [86]. However, specific data regarding the relationship between serum vitamin D and endometrium in PCOS patients are scarce. Several studies reported that vitamin D treatment can improve the features associated with endometrial receptivity like hyperandrogenism [87], hyperinsulinism and insulin resistance [88], inflammation and oxidative stress [89].

In an experimental study in a rat model of PCOS it was found that immunohistochemical staining of caspase-3 and Ki-67 were decreased with vitamin D treatment compared non-treated group [90]. Moreover, endometrial, epithelial and stromal thickness measurements were decreased in the vitamin D treatment group compared to non-treated PCOS group [90].

4. Strategies to improve endometrial function in PCOS

4.1 Ovulation induction agents

First-line treatment for ovulation induction in the treatment of infertility in PCOS are oral agents, with letrozole being superior to clomiphene citrate (CC) in terms of endometrial thickness and markers of endometrial receptivity [7, 91, 92]. Gonadotropins are the second line treatment and it seems that they have a less deleterious impact on endometrium [93]. However, no data today support the ovulation induction in infertile ovulatory PCOS for the modification of endometrial receptivity.

Several studies evaluated the different impact of ovarian stimulation with letrozole versus clomiphene citrate in patients with PCOS. Thus, Wallace et al. published in 2011 a randomized controlled study which reported that letrozole positively influenced a number of markers of endometrial receptivity like mRNA expression of leukemia inhibitory factor, dickkhopf homolog 1, fibroblast growth factor 22 compared with CC [94]. Another randomized controlled study which included 160 patients diagnosed with PCOS found that indices of endometrial receptivity like the volume, vascularization index, flow index and vascularization flow index of endometrium on the day of hCG administration and 7–9 days after ovulation were significantly increased in letrozole group compared with CC [95]. Moreover, the biochemical pregnancy rate, clinical pregnancy rate and ongoing pregnancy rate in letrozole group were significantly higher compared with CC group [95]. The same authors evaluated the indices of endometrial receptivity in treated PCOS patients (Letrozole or clomiphene citrate) and non-treated [96]. They noticed that, although the successful ovulation rate did not differ between the letrozole group and CC group, endometrial thickness, endometrial volume, vascularization index, flow index, vascularization flow index, integrin $\alpha v\beta 3$ and VEGF concentrations in uterine fluid were significantly higher in the window of implantation in the letrozole group compared with the CC group and natural cycle group [96]. Moreover, the clinical pregnancy and ongoing pregnancy rates of the letrozole group were significantly higher than in the CC group [96]. The markers of endometrial receptivity analyzed were significantly higher in pregnant patients [96]. The endometrial flow index during the implantation window had the highest predictive value for pregnancy. The integrin $\alpha v\beta 3$ in uterine fluid had better predictive value than VEGF [96].

In an experimental study on female rats it was found that the expression of integrin $\alpha v\beta 3$ in the clomiphene citrate group was lower than in the letrozole and saline solution groups [97]. The expression of HOXA10 was statistically significantly higher in the saline solution group than in the letrozole group, and the letrozole group showed a statistically significantly higher expression of HOXA10 compared with the clomiphene citrate group. The authors concluded that, in rats, letrozole affects the expression of HOXA10 in uterine epithelium but has no effect on the expression of integrin $\alpha v\beta 3$, which suggests that clomiphene suppresses endometrial receptivity more than letrozole.

4.2 Antiandrogens

Antiandrogens as flutamide, finasteride and spironolactone are used in clinical practice to improve the signs of clinical hyperandrogenism like hirsutism, acne, alopecia. Animal studies demonstrated the ability of antiandrogens to improve endometrial function [98, 99]. However, their use in patients seeking infertility treatment is prohibited by their teratogenic effects, being generally recommended to be administrated only in association with oral contraception [100]. Another way to improve hyperandrogenism is by administration of combined oral contraceptives which decrease ovarian androgen production and decrease androgen bioavailability through stimulation of sex hormone binding globulin production. Indeed, oral contraceptives, administrated in a successive or unsuccessive manner before in vitro fertilization, were showed to increase the implantation and pregnancy rate and reduce the risk of pregnancy complications along with significant decrease in circulating androgens [101]. However, in a randomized controlled trial ovulation rate and live birth rate were superior in PCOS patients receiving life style modification with or without oral contraceptive in comparison with oral contraceptive alone [102].

4.3 Freeze all strategy

Elective frozen embryo transfer after a freeze-all strategy was suggested for infertile PCOS patients undergoing IVF [103]. This approach could be particularly effective in PCOS due to exposure of the endometrium to high estrogen levels during controlled ovarian stimulation. Thus, transfer of the embryo in a subsequent cycle may avoid failure of implantation due to inadequate endometrium receptivity. This strategy was showed of particular benefit in PCOS patients and only in case of more than 16 oocytes or estradiol higher than 3000 pg./ml, resulting in higher live birth rate [104]. Regarding the preparation of endometrium, it seems that the pregnancy rate is higher in natural cycles over the hormone replacement cycles in women performing frozen embryo transfer [105]. However, specific data for PCOS women are lacking.

In women with PCOS, no difference in live birth/ongoing pregnancy and clinical pregnancy rates was detected between FET cycles stimulated with hMG and cycles artificially prepared with E2 valerate [106–108].

4.4 Gut microbiota and endometrial receptivity

There is accumulating evidence that gut microbiota might play a role in PCOS pathogenesis [109, 110]. Thus, it was showed that gut microbiota of PCOS patients is different from controls [111] and that variate profiles of gut microbiota are associated with features of PCOS such as hyperandrogenism [112], hyperinsulinemia and insulin resistance [113] and obesity [114]. In experimental studies transplantation of feces from PCOS women leads to development of PCOS features in mice [109] and oral administration of variate bacteria was associated with improvement of PCOS manifestation [110]. Thus, Qi X et al. [109] showed that Bacteroides vulgatus was markedly elevated in the gut microbiota of individuals with PCOS and that transplantation of fecal microbiota from women with PCOS or B. vulgatus-colonized recipient mice resulted in increased disruption of ovarian functions, insulin resistance, altered bile acid metabolism, reduced interleukin-22 secretion and infertility [109]. It was also showed that IL-22 improved the PCOS phenotype [109]. Guo Y et al. [110] showed that PCOS rats displayed different composition of gut microbiota that in the controls. Lactobacillus, Ruminococcus and Clostridium were lower while Prevotella was higher in PCOS rats when compared with control rats. After treating PCOS rats with Lactobacillus and fecal microbiota transplantation from healthy rats estrous cycles were improved with decreasing androgen biosynthesis [110].

However, it is possible that the relationship between gut microbiota and PCOS to be bidirectional since in androgen-induced PCOS animal models the disturbances of gut microbiota was reported [115, 116]. In turn, DHEA-shaped gut microbiota transplanted to pseudo germ-free rats recipients trigged disturbances in reproductive hormone [115]. Another study showed that both androgens and high fat diet could shift the overall gut microbial composition, being associated with the development and pathology of PCOS by shaping gut microbial communities [117]. Although direct evidence of a connection between gut microbiota and endometrial receptivity was not reported yet, we can hypothesize a connection between these two due to the recognized involvement of insulin resistance, hyperandrogenemia and obesity in endometrial receptivity which, in turn, can be shaped by intestinal bacterial community.

Regarding the mechanisms connecting gut microbiota and PCOS, Tremellen and Pearce suggest that dysbiosis of the gut microbiota brought about by a high fat-sugar diet in PCOS patients leads to an increase in intestinal permeability. Lipopolysaccharide produced by Gram-negative bacteria traverse the gut wall to enter the circulation, leading to a chronic state of low-grade inflammation. Activation of the immune system interferes with insulin receptor, driving up insulin levels, which boost testosterone production in the ovary, leading to PCOS [118].

Another way by which gut microbiota might influence the endometrial receptivity is through its recently demonstrated close connection with genital tract microbiota [119–122]. The crosstalk between gut and vaginal microbiota is highlighted by studies showing that oral administration of probiotics or bacteria can influence immunity in the vagina [120]. Thus, oral administration of Lactobacillus johnsonii was showed to inhibit the expression of inflammatory molecules in the vagina and to alleviate Gardnerella vaginalis induced vaginosis [122]. Kutteh et al. [121] demonstrated that intestinal tract immunization by oral and rectal route is followed by the induction of specific antibodies in human female genital tract secretions [Kutteh 2001]. Kim et al. [120] showed that in ovarectomized female mice, the oral administration of anti-inflammatory *Lactobacillus plantarum* NK3 and Bifidobacterium longum NK49 from kimchi and human fecal lactic acid bacteria collection was associated with alleviation of Gardnerella vaginalis induced vaginosis, inhibition of NF-κB activation and TNF-α expression in the vagina and uterus, and decreased the Gardnerella vaginalis population in the vagina [120]. In turn, Gardnerella vaginalis-induced vaginosis increased colonic myeloperoxidase activity, TNF-α expression, and fecal Proteobacteria population. NK3 and/or NK49 treatments reduced TNF-α expression and NF-κB activation in the colon and restored Gardnerella vaginalis disrupted gut microbiota composition [120].

This interplay between gut and reproductive tract microbiota may be related with endometrium function since, recently, it was showed that pathological modification of the profile of the bacterial community of the endometrial fluid might play a role in poor reproductive outcome for in vitro fertilization patients [123]. Thus, the presence of a non-Lactobacillus-dominated microbiota in a receptive endometrium was associated with significant decreases in implantation, pregnancy, ongoing pregnancy, and live birth rates [123]. Haahr et al. [124] found a decreased pregnancy rate in patients with abnormal vaginal microbiota performing IVF [124]. These studies highlight the importance of reproductive tract microbiota in fertility, possibly by modulation of endometrial receptivity.

All these data offer future therapeutic strategies to counteract decreased endometrial receptivity in PCOS women by modulating gut or reproductive tract microbiota or by administration of interleukin 22 as suggested by Qi X et al. [109].

4.5 Assessment of endometrial receptivity and therapeutical implications

The evaluation of endometrial receptivity was historically done by endometrial histology. However, recent studies find little concordance with new transcriptomic methods of endometrial receptivity assessment [125]. Endometrial receptivity array

(ERA) is a test that analyzes the gene expression of the endometrium using a panel of 238 genes that have been implicated in endometrial receptivity. The indication of this test in the clinical practice is to identify the window of implantation in patients with accelerated or delayed endometrial luteal phase development, therefore allowing the transfer of the embryo in the right moment for the embryonic-endometrial synchrony. However, data regarding the benefit of this test are limited [126]. Although in PCOS patients performing IVF ERA test has hypothetical indications, studies evaluating this aspect are lacking.

Another aspect that should be clarified further is the consistency of the ERA findings from cycle to cycle since the transfer of the embryo should be done in a non-biopsy cycle. This aspect was analyzed in seven women who performed the ERA test in separate endometrial samples obtained 29–40 months apart and found high similarity across the samples [127]. However, only five samples were from the luteal phase and only four were in the receptive phase, all the samples being normal. Therefore, the possibility to extrapolate these findings to patients with endometrium receptivity abnormalities or dyssynchrony is unknown.

The ERA test was studied in several categories of infertile patients. Tan et al. [128] found that among patients with a history of at least one euploid blastocyst implantation failure personalized frozen embryo transfer (FET) according to ERA test results was superior to standard FET in terms of implantation and ongoing pregnancy rate, although the difference was not statistically different [128]. Other studies showed a similar pregnancy rate between patients with receptive and non-receptive endometrium according to the ERA test when a personalized embryo transfer was performed in patients with recurrent implantation failure [129] or with a history of implantation failure [125]. On the other hand, Eisman et al. [130] found a similar pregnancy rate in women who had a prior failed embryo transfer and personalized frozen embryo transfer following ERA test compared with women without a prior failed embryo transfer [130]. However, the pregnancy rate was lower in patients with more than three failed embryo transfer despite personalized transfer [130].

A multicenter, open-label randomized controlled trial evaluated patients at their first appointment for IVF after exclusion of patients with recurrent miscarriage and implantation failure. They found that a personalized frozen embryo transfer guided by ERA test was superior in terms of cumulative pregnancy and live birth rate to standard frozen embryo transfers and fresh embryo transfers [131]. At the first embryo transfer cycle, although the pregnancy rate and implantation rates were significantly higher compared with the two groups without ERA guidance, the live birth rates were similar [131]. Basil et al. [132] performed a single center retrospective cohort study and found that using the ERA test in patients undergoing frozen embryo transfer, there is no benefit in terms of ongoing pregnancy rate in good prognosis patients [132].

Taken all together, these studies suggest that the ERA test might be beneficial in patients with implantation failure, although future studies are necessary to clarify this aspect. In patients at their first attempt of IVF personalized frozen embryo transfer guided by ERA test may increase the cumulative pregnancy and live birth rate, although without obvious benefits at the first transfer. Whether these results are also valid for PCOS patients remains to be established.

5. Conclusion

An increasing body of evidence suggests that endometrial receptivity in PCOS patients is decreased, being a significant contributor to infertility in these patients. However, specific strategies to overcome this barrier in infertile PCOS women should be created in order to improve fertility treatment outcome.

Author details

Alice Albu* and Dragoș Albu
'Carol Davila' University of Medicine and Pharmacy, Bucharest, Romania

*Address all correspondence to: albualice@yahoo.com

References

[1] Bozdag G, Mumusoglu S, Zengin D, Karabulut E, Yildiz BO. The prevalence and phenotypic features of polycystic ovary syndrome: a systematic review and meta-analysis. Hum Reprod 2016; 31 (12) 2841-2855

[2] Azziz, R. et al. The prevalence and features of the polycystic ovary syndrome in an unselected population. The Journal of clinical endocrinology and metabolism 89, 2745-2749, doi: 10.1210/jc.2003-032046 (2004).

[3] Norman RJ, Dewailly D, Legro RS, Hickey TE. Polycystic ovary syndrome. Lancet 370, 685-697, doi: 10.1016/S0140-6736(07)61345-2 (2007).

[4] Franks S, Stark J, Hardy K. Follicle dynamics and anovulation in polycystic ovary syndrome. Human reproduction update 14, 367-378, doi: 10.1093/humupd/dmn015 (2008)

[5] Deswal R, Narwal V, Dang A and Pundir CS. The Prevalence of Polycystic Ovary Syndrome: A Brief Systematic Review. J Hum Reprod Sci. 2020 Oct-Dec; 13(4): 261-271. Published online 2020 Dec 28. doi: 10.4103/jhrs.JHRS_95_18

[6] Cooney LG, Lee I, Sammel MD, Dokras A.Hum Reprod. High prevalence of moderate and severe depressive and anxiety symptoms in polycystic ovary syndrome: a systematic review and meta-analysis. 2017 May 1;32(5):1075-1091. doi: 10.1093/humrep/dex044.

[7] Teede HJ, Misso ML, Costello MF, Dokras A, Laven J, Moran L, Piltonen T, Norman RJ; International PCOS Network. Recommendations from the international evidence-based guideline for the assessment and management of polycystic ovary syndrome. Hum Reprod. 2018 Sep 1;33(9):1602-1618. doi: 10.1093/humrep/dey256.

[8] Rotterdam ESHRE/ASRM-Sponsored PCOS Consensus Workshop Group. Revised 2003 consensus on diagnostic criteria and long-term health risks related to polycystic ovary syndrome. Fertil Steril 2004; 81 (01) 19-25

[9] Brassard M, AinMelk Y, Baillargeon JP. Basic infertility including polycystic ovary syndrome. Med Clin North Am. 2008 Sep;92(5):1163-1192, xi. doi: 10.1016/j.mcna.2008.04.008.

[10] Joham AE, Teede HJ, Ranasinha S, Zoungas S, Boyle J. Prevalence of infertility and use of fertility treatment in women with polycystic ovary syndrome: data from a large community-based cohort study. J Womens Health (Larchmt). 2015 Apr;24(4):299-307. doi: 10.1089/jwh.2014.5000. Epub 2015 Feb 5.

[11] Younas K, Quintela M, Thomas S, Garcia-Parra J, Blake L, Whiteland H, Bunkheila A, Francis LW, Margarit L, Gonzalez D and Conlan RS. Delayed endometrial decidualisation in polycystic ovary syndrome; the role of AR-MAGEA11. J Mol Med (Berl). 2019; 97(9): 1315-1327. Published online 2019 Jun 29. doi: 10.1007/s00109-019-01809-6

[12] Hull MG. Epidemiology of infertility and polycystic ovarian disease: endocrinological and demographic studies. Gynecol Endocrinol 1987 Sep;1(3):235-245. doi: 10.3109/09513598709023610.

[13] Bellver J, et al. Endometrial gene expression in the window of implantation is altered in obese women especially in association with polycystic ovary syndrome. Fertil and Steril 95, 2335-2341, doi:10.1016/j.fertnstert.2011.03.021 (2011)

[14] Lopes IM, et al. Endometrium in women with polycystic ovary syndrome

during the window of implantation. Revista da Associacao Medica Brasileira 57,702-709 (2011)

[15] Li SY, Song Z, Song MJ et al. Impaired receptivity and decidualization in DHEA-induced PCOS mice. Sci Rep 6,38134 (2016). https://doi.org/10.1038/srep38134

[16] Balen AH, S.L. Tan, J. MacDougall, H.S.Jacobs. Miscarriage rates following in-vitro fertilization are increased in women with polycystic ovaries and reduced by pituitary desensitization with buserelin. Human Reproduction (Oxford, England), 8 (1993), pp. 959-964

[17] Sagle M, K. Bishop, N. Ridley, *et al.* Recurrent early miscarriage and polycystic ovaries. BMJ (Clinical research ed.), 297 (1988), pp. 1027-1028

[18] Nestler JE, Stovall D, Akhter N, Iuorno MJ, Jakubowicz DJ. Strategies for the use of insulin-sensitizing drugs to treat infertility in women with polycystic ovary syndrome. Fertil Steril. 2002 Feb; 77(2):209-215.

[19] Vaz GQ, Evangelista AV, Sartorio CAP, Cardoso MCA, Erthal MC, Gallo P, Oliveira MAP. Are patients with polycystic ovary syndrome ideal candidates for oocyte donation? Biomed Res Int 2016; 2016:5701609.

[20] Ashkenazi J, Farhi J, Orvieto R. Polycystic ovary syndrome patients as oocyte donors: the effect of ovarian stimulation protocol on the implantation rate of the recipient. Fertility and Sterility, 64 (1995), pp. 564-567

[21] Giudice LC. Endometrium in PCOS: Implantation and predisposition to endocrine CA. Best Practice & Research Clinical Endocrinology & Metabolism. June 2006;20(2):235-244

[22] Dosiou C, L.C. Giudice. Natural killer cells in pregnancy and recurrent pregnancy loss: endocrine and immunologic perspectives. Endocrine Reviews, 26 (2005), pp. 44-62

[23] Palomba S, Piltonen TT, Giudice LC. Endometrial function in women with polycystic ovary syndrome: a comprehensive review. Human Reproduction Update, Vol.27, No.3, pp. 584-618, 2021

[24] Giudice LC. Elucidating endometrial function in the post-genomic era. Human Reproduction Update, 9 (2003), pp. 223-235

[25] Xu XL, Deng SL, Lian ZX, Yu K. Estrogen Receptors in Polycystic Ovary Syndrome. Cells 2021 Feb; 10(2): 459. Published online 2021 Feb 21. doi: 10.3390/cells10020459

[26] Giudice LC. Endometrium in PCOS: implantation and predisposition to endocrine CA. Best Pract Res Clin Endocrinol Metab 2006;20: 235-244

[27] Venturoli S, E. Porcu, R. Fabbri, *et al.* Episodic pulsatile secretion of FSH, LH, prolactin, oestradiol, oestrone, and LH circadian variations in polycystic ovary syndrome. Clinical Endocrinology, 28 (1988), pp. 93-107

[28] Nestler JE, L.P. Powers, D.W. Matt, *et al.* A direct effect of hyperinsulinemia on serum sex hormone-binding globulin levels in obese women with the polycystic ovary syndrome. The Journal of Clinical Endocrinology and Metabolism, 72 (1991), pp. 83-89

[29] S. Robinson, D. Kiddy, S.V. Gelding, *et al.* The relationship of insulin insensitivity to menstrual pattern in women with hyperandrogenism and polycystic ovaries. Clinical Endocrinology, 39 (1993), pp. 351-355

[30] Avellaira C, Villavicencio A, Bacallao K, Gabler F, Wells P, Romero C, Vega M. Expression of molecules associated with tissue homeostasis in

secretory endometria from untreated women with polycystic ovary syndrome. Hum Reprod 2006;21:3116-3121.

[31] Maliqueo M, Clementi M, Gabler F, Johnson C, Palomino A, Sir Peterman T, Vega M. Expression of steroid receptors and proteins related to apoptosis in endometria of women with **polycystic** ovary syndrome. Fertil Steril 2003, 812-819

[32] Quezada S, Avellaira C, Johnson MC, Gabler F, Fuentes A, Vega M. Evaluation of steroid receptors, coregulators, and molecules associated with uterine receptivity in secretory endometria from untreated women with polycystic ovary syndrome. Fertil Steril 2006;85:1017-1026.

[33] Gregory CW, Wilson EM, Apparao EKB, Lininger RA, Meyer WR, Kowalik A, Fritz MA, Lessey BA. Steroid receptor coactivator expression throughout the menstrual cycle in normal and abnormal endometrium. J Clin Endocrinol Metab 2002;87: 2960-2966,

[34] Villavicencio A, Bacallao K, Avellaira C, Gabler F, Fuentes A, Vega M. Androgen and estrogen receptors and co-regulators levels in endometria from patients with polycystic ovarian syndrome with and without endometrial hyperplasia. Gynecol Oncol 2006;103: 307-314

[35] Wang A, Ji L, Shang W, Li M, Chen L, White RE, Han G. Expression of GPR30, ERalpha and ERbeta in endometrium during window of implantation in patients with polycystic ovary syndrome: a pilot study. Gynecol Endocrinol 2011;27:251-255

[36] Plaza-Parrochia F, Bacallao K, Poblete C, Gabler F, Carvajal R, Romero C, Valladares L, Vega M. The role of androst-5-ene3b,17b-diol (androstenediol) in cell proliferation in endometrium of women with polycystic ovary syndrome. Steroids 2014;89: 11-19.

[37] Plaza-Parrochia F, Oro´ stica L, Garcı´a P, Vera C, Romero C, Valladares L, Vega M. Molecular mechanisms of androstenediol in the regulation of the proliferative process of human endometrial cells. Reprod Sci 2017a;24:1079-1087.

[38] Plaza-Parrochia F, Romero C, Valladares L, Vega M. Endometrium and steroids, a pathologic overview. Steroids 2017b;126:85-91.

[39] Chen SU, Chou CH, Chen MJ, Chen TH, Yang YS, Yang JH. Apoptotic effects of high estradiol concentrations on endometrial glandular cells. J Clin Endocrinol Metab 2014;99:E971–E980.

[40] Ito K, Utsunomiya H, Suzuki T, Saitou S, Akahira J, Okamura K, Yaegashi N, Sasano H. 17b-hydroxysteroid dehydrogenases in human endometrium and its disorders. Mol Cell Endocrinol 2006;248: 136-140

[41] Leon L, Bacallao K, Gabler F, Romero C, Valladares L, Vega M. Activities of steroid metabolic enzymes in secretory endometria from untreated women with polycystic ovary syndrome. Steroids 2008;73:88-95.

[42] Plaza F, Gabler F, Romero C, Vantman D, Valladares L, Vega M. The conversion of dehydroepiandrosterone into androst-5-ene-3b, 17b-diol (androstenediol) is increased in endometria from untreated women with polycystic ovarian syndrome. Steroids 2010; 75:810-817.

[43] Paulson M, Norstedt G, Sahlin L, Hirschberg AL. Association between prolactin receptor expression and proliferation in the endometrium of obese women with polycystic ovary syndrome. Gynecol Endocrinol 2020a;36:226-232.

[44] Chrousos GP, MacLusky NJ, Brandon DD, Tomita M, Renquist DM, Loriaux DL, Lipsett MB. Progesterone resistance. Adv Exp Med Biol 1986;196:317-328.45. Graham and Clarke, 1997

[45] Graham JD, Clarke CL. Physiological action of progesterone in target tissues. Endocr Rev 1997;18:502-519.

[46] Mote PA, Balleine RL, McGowan EM, Clarke CL. Heterogeneity of progesterone receptors A and B expression in human endometrial glands and stroma. Hum Reprod 2000:15 Suppl 3:48-56.

[47] Patel B, Elguero S, Thakore S, Dahoud W, Bedaiwy M, Mesiano S. Role of nuclear progesterone receptor isoforms in uterine pathophysiology. Hum Reprod Update 2015;21: 155-173.

[48] Hu M, Li J, Zhang Y, Li X, Bra¨nnstro¨m M, Shao LR, Billig H. Endometrial progesterone receptor isoforms in women with polycystic ovary syndrome. Am J Transl Res 2018;10:2696-2705.

[49] Babayev SN, Park CW, Keller PW, Carr BR, Word RA, Bukulmez O. Androgens upregulate endometrial epithelial progesterone receptor expression: potential implications for endometriosis. Reprod Sci 2017;24:1454-1461.

[50] Young SL. Androgens and endometrium: new lessons from the corpus luteum via the adrenal cortex? Fertil Steril 2018;109:623-624.

[51] Su S, Blackwelder AJ, Grossman G, Minges JT, Yuan L, Young SL, Wilson EM. Primate-specific melanoma antigen-A11 regulates isoform-specific human progesterone receptor-B transactivation. J Biol Chem 2012;287:34809-34824.

[52] Margarit L, A. Taylor, M. H. Roberts, L. Hopkins, C. Davies, A. G. Brenton, R. S. Conlan, A. Bunkheila, L. Joels, J. O. White ... Show more. MUC1 as a Discriminator between Endometrium from Fertile and Infertile Patients with PCOS and Endometriosis. The Journal of Clinical Endocrinology & Metabolism, Volume 95, Issue 12, 1 December 2010, Pages 5320-5329

[53] Maliqueo M, Bacallao K, Quezada S, Clementi M, Gabler F, Johnson MC, Vega M. Sex hormone-binding globulin expression in the endometria of women with polycystic ovary syndrome. Fertil Steril 2007;87:321-328

[54] Plaza-Parrochia F, Poblete C, Gabler F, Carvajal R, Romero C, Valladares L, Vega M. Expression of steroid sulfated transporters and 3b-HSD activity in endometrium of women having polycystic ovary syndrome. Steroids 2015;104:189-195.

[55] Bacallao K, Leon L, Gabler F, Soto E, Romero C, Valladares L, Vega M. In situ estrogen metabolism in proliferative endometria from untreated women with polycystic ovarian syndrome with and without endometrial hyperplasia. J Steroid Biochem Mol Biol 2008;110: 163-169.

[56] Schulte MMB, J, KH. The Effect of Metabolic Derangements on Endometrial Receptivity at the Time of Implantation. Reprod Sci. 2015 Jan; 22(1): 6-14.

[57] Cermik D, Selam B, Taylor HS. Regulation of HOXA-10 expression by testosterone in vitro and in the endometrium of patients with polycystic ovary syndrome. J Clin Endocrinol Metab. 2003 Jan; 88(1):238-243. doi: 10.1210/jc.2002-021072.

[58] Du H, Sarno J, Taylor HS. HOXA10 inhibits Kruppel-like factor 9 expression in the human endometrial epithelium. Biol Reprod. 2010;83 (2):205-211.

[59] Satokata I, Benson G, Maas R. Sexually dimorphic sterility phenotypes in Hoxa10-deficient mice. Nature. 1995;374 (6521):460-463.

[60] Gonzalez D, Thackeray H, Lewis PD, et al. Loss of WT1 expression in the endometrium of infertile PCOS patients: a hyperandrogenic effect? J Clin Endocrinol Metab. 2012;97 (3):957-966

[61] Babayev SN, Park CW, Keller PW, Carr BR, Word RA, Bukulmez O. Androgens upregulate endometrial epithelial progesterone receptor expression: potential implications for endometriosis. Reprod Sci 2017;24: 1454-1461.

[62] Bentin-Ley U. Relevance of endometrial pinopodes for human blastocyst implantation. Hum Reprod 2000;15:67-73.

[63] Mokhtar HM, Giribabu N, Muniandy S, Salleh N. Testosterone decreases the expression of endometrial pinopode and L-selectin ligand (MECA-79) in adult female rats during uterine receptivity period. Int J Clin Exp Pathol 2014;7:1967-1976

[64] Kajihara T, Tochigi H, Prechapanich J, Uchino S, Itakura A, Brosens JJ, Ishihara O. Androgen signaling in decidualizing human endometrial stromal cells enhances resistance to oxidative stress. Fertil Steril 2012;97:185-191.

[65] Hu M, Zhang Y, Li X, Cui P, Li J, Bra¨nnstro¨m M, Shao LR, Billig H. Alterations of endometrial epithelial-mesenchymal transition and MAPK signaling components in women with PCOS are partially modulated by metformin in vitro. Mol Hum Reprod 2020c;26: 312-326

[66] Frolova AI, O'Neill K, Moley KH. Dehydroepiandrosterone inhibits glucose flux through the pentose phosphate pathway in human and mouse endometrial stromal cells, preventing decidualization and implantation. Mol Endocrinol. 2011;25 (8):1444-1455

[67] Maliqueo MA, Quezada S, Clementi M, Bacallao K, Anido M, Johnson C, Vega M. Potential action of androstenedione on the proliferation and apoptosis of stromal endometrial cells. Reprod Biol Endocrinol 2004;2:81

[68] Li SY, Song Z, Song MJ, Qin JW, Zhao ML, Yang ZM. Impaired receptivity and decidualization in DHEA-induced PCOS mice. Sci Rep 2016;6:6

[69] Palomba S, Russo T, Falbo A, Di Cello A, Amendola G, Mazza R, Tolino A, Zullo F, Tucci L, La Sala GB. Decidual endovascular trophoblast invasion in women with polycystic ovary syndrome: an experimental case-control study. J Clin Endocrinol Metab 2012;97: 2441-2449

[70] Palomba S, Falbo A, La Sala GB. Metformin and gonadotropins for ovulation induction in patients with polycystic ovary syndrome: a systematic review with meta-analysis of randomized controlled trials. Reprod Biol Endocrinol 2014b;12:3.

[71] Chang EM, Han JE, Seok HH, Lee DR, Yoon TK, Lee WS. Insulin resistance does not affect early embryo development but lowers implantation rate in in vitro maturation-in vitro fertilization-embryo transfer cycle. Clin Endocrinol (Oxf). 2013;79 (1):93-99.

[72] Irwin JC, de las Fuentes L, Dsupin BA, Giudice LC. Insulin-like growth factor regulation of human endometrial stromal cell function: coordinate effects on insulin-like growth factor binding protein-1, cell proliferation and prolactin secretion. Regul Pept 1993;48:165-177

[73] Ujvari D, Jakson I, Babayeva S, Salamon D, Rethi B, Gidlöf S, Hirschberg AL. Dysregulation of In Vitro Decidualization of Human Endometrial Stromal Cells by Insulin via Transcriptional Inhibition of Forkhead Box Protein O1. PLoS One. 2017 Jan 30;12(1):e0171004. doi: 10.1371/journal.pone.0171004. eCollection 2017.

[74] Lee MH, Yoon JA, Kim HR, Kim YS, Lyu SW, Lee BS, Song H, Choi DH. Hyperandrogenic milieu dysregulates the expression of insulin signaling factors and glucose transporters in the endometrium of patients with polycystic ovary syndrome. Reprod Sci 2020;27: 1637-1647

[75] Fornes R, Ormazabal P, Rosas C, et al. Changes in the expression of insulin signaling pathway molecules in endometria from polycystic ovary syndrome women with or without hyperinsulinemia. Mol Med. 2010;16 (3-4):129-136.

[76] Oro´ stica L, Poblete C, Romero C, Vega M. Pro-inflammatory markers negatively regulate IRS1 in endometrial cells and endometrium from women with obesity and PCOS. Reprod Sci 2020;27: 290-300.

[77] Piltonen TT, Chen JC, Khatun M, Kangasniemi M, Liakka A, Spitzer T, Tran N, Huddleston H, Irwin JC, Giudice LC. Endometrial stromal fibroblasts from women with polycystic ovary syndrome have impaired progesterone-mediated decidualization, aberrant cytokine profiles and promote enhanced immune cell migration in vitro. Hum Reprod 2015;30:1203-1215.

[78] Takemura Y, Osuga Y, Yamauchi T, et al. Expression of adiponectin receptors and its possible implication in the human endometrium. Endocrinology. 2006;147 (7):3203-3210

[79] Dunaif A, Graf M. Insulin administration alters gonadal steroid metabolism independent of changes in gonadotropin secretion in insulin-resistant women with the polycystic ovary syndrome. J Clin Invest. 1989;83 (1):23-29.

[80] Nestler JE. Should patients with polycystic ovarian syndrome be treated with metformin?: an enthusiastic endorsement. Hum Reprod. 2002 Aug;17(8):1950-1953. doi: 10.1093/humrep/17.8.1950.

[81] Saxtorph MH, Hallager T, Persson G, Petersen KB, Eriksen JO, Larsen LG, Hviid TV, Macklon N. Assessing endometrial receptivity after recurrent implantation failure: a prospective controlled cohort study. Reprod Biomed Online. 2020 Dec;41(6):998-1006. doi: 10.1016/j.rbmo.2020.08.015.

[82] Chu J, Gallos I, Tobias A, Tan B, Eapen A, Coomarasamy A. Vitamin D and assisted reproductive treatment outcome: a systematic review and meta-analysis. Hum Reprod 2018 Jan 1;33(1):65-80. doi: 10.1093/humrep/dex326

[83] Cozzolino M, Busnelli A, Pellegrini L, Riviello E, Vitagliano A. How vitamin D level influences in vitro fertilization outcomes: results of a systematic review and meta-analysis. Fertil Steril 2020 Nov;114(5):1014-1025. doi: 10.1016/j.fertnstert.2020.05.040. Epub 2020 Oct 1.

[84] Guo J, Liu S, Wang P, Ren H, Li Y. Characterization of VDR and CYP27B1 expression in the endometrium during the menstrual cycle before embryo transfer: implications for endometrial receptivity. Reprod Biol Endocrinol 2020 Mar 17;18(1):24. doi: 10.1186/s12958-020-00579-y.

[85] Hosseinirad H, Novin MG, Hosseini S, Nazarian H, Amidi F, Paktinat S, Azizi E, Mofarahe ZS. Effect of 1,25(OH)2-vitamin D3 on expression

and phosphorylation of progesterone receptor in cultured endometrial stromal cells of patients with repeated implantation failure. Acta Histochem. 2020 Feb;122(2):151489. doi: 10.1016/j.acthis.2019.151489. Epub 2019 Dec 24

[86] Li HWR, Brereton RE, Anderson RA, Wallace AM, Ho CKM. Vitamin D deficiency is common and associated with metabolic risk factors in patients with polycystic ovary syndrome. Metabolism 2011 Oct;60(10):1475-1481. doi: 10.1016/j.metabol.2011.03.002. Epub 2011 May 6.

[87] Al-Bayyari N, Al-Domi H, Zayed F, Hailat R, Eaton A. Androgens and hirsutism score of overweight women with polycystic ovary syndrome improved after vitamin D treatment: A randomized placebo controlled clinical trial. Clin Nutr 2021 Mar;40(3):870-878. doi: 10.1016/j.clnu.2020.09.024. Epub 2020 Sep 24.

[88] Wang L, Wen X, Lv S, Tian S, Jiang Y, Yang X. Effects of vitamin D supplementation on metabolic parameters of women with polycystic ovary syndrome: a meta-analysis of randomized controlled trials. Gynecol Endocrinol 2021 May;37(5):446-455. doi: 10.1080/09513590.2020.1813272. Epub 2020 Sep 10.

[89] Foroozanfard F, Jamilian M, Bahmani F, Talaee R, Talaee N, Hashemi T, Nasri K, Asemi Z, Esmaillzadeh A. Calcium plus vitamin D supplementation influences biomarkers of inflammation and oxidative stress in overweight and vitamin D-deficient women with polycystic ovary syndrome: a randomized double-blind placebo-controlled clinical trial. Clin Endocrinol (Oxf) 2015 Dec;83(6):888-894. doi: 10.1111/cen.12840. Epub 2015 Jul 23.

[90] Kuyucu Y, Çelik LS, Kendirlinan O, Tap O, Mete UO. Investigation of the uterine structural changes in the experimental model with polycystic ovary syndrome and effects of vitamin D treatment: An ultrastructural and immunohistochemical study. Reprod Biol 2018 Mar;18(1):53-59. doi: 10.1016/j.repbio.2018.01.002. Epub 2018 Jan 8.

[91] Gadalla MA, Huang S, Wang R, Norman RJ, Abdullah SA, El Saman AM, Ismail AM, van Wely M, Mol BW. Effect of clomiphene citrate on endometrial thickness, ovulation, pregnancy and live birth in anovulatory women: systematic review and meta-analysis. Ultrasound Obstet Gynecol 2018;51:64-76

[92] Mehdinejadiani S, Amidi F, Mehdizadeh M, Barati M, Safdarian L, Aflatoonian R, Alyasin A, Aghahosseini M, Pazhohan A, Hayat P et al. The effects of letrozole and clomiphene citrate on ligands expression of Wnt3, Wnt7a, and Wnt8b in proliferative endometrium of women with polycystic ovarian syndrome. Gynecol Endocrinol 2018;34:775-780

[93] Weiss NS, Kostova E, Nahuis M, Mol BWJ, van der Veen F, van Wely M. Gonadotrophins for ovulation induction in women with polycystic ovary syndrome. Cochrane Database Syst Rev 2019;1: CD010290

[94] Wallace KL, Venessia Johnson, Victoria Sopelak, Randall Hines. Clomiphene citrate versus letrozole: molecular analysis of the endometrium in women with polycystic ovary syndrome. Fertil Steril. 2011 Oct;96(4):1051-1056. doi: 10.1016/j.fertnstert.2011.07.1092.

[95] Wang L, Xinqiang Wen, Shulan Lv, Juan Zhao, Ting Yang, Xiaofeng Yang. Comparison of endometrial receptivity of clomiphene citrate versus letrozole in women with polycystic ovary syndrome: a randomized controlled study. Gynecol Endocrinol 2019 Oct;35(10):862-865. doi: 10.1080/09513590.2019.1612358. Epub 2019 May 12.

[96] Wang L, Shulan Lv, Fen Li, E Bai, Xiaofeng Yang. Letrozole Versus

Clomiphene Citrate and Natural Cycle: Endometrial Receptivity During Implantation Window in Women With Polycystic Ovary Syndrome. Front Endocrinol (Lausanne). 2021 Jan 18;11:532692. doi: 10.3389/fendo. 2020.532692. eCollection 2020.

[97] Bao SH, Shi Le Sheng, Yi Feng Peng, Qi De Lin. Effects of letrozole and clomiphene citrate on the expression of HOXA10 and integrin alpha v beta 3 in uterine epithelium of rats. Fertil Steril 2009 Jan;91(1):244-248. doi: 10.1016/j. fertnstert.2007.11.024. Epub 2008 Feb 4.

[98] Gong H, Wu W, Xu J, Yu D, Qiao B, Liu H, Yang B, Li Y, Ling Y, Kuang H. Flutamide ameliorates uterine decidualization and angiogenesis in the mouse hyperandrogenemia model during mid-pregnancy. PLoS One 2019;14:e0217095.

[99] Slayden OD, Brenner RM. Flutamide counteracts the antiproliferative effects of antiprogestins in the primate endometrium. J Clin Endocrinol Metab 2003;88:946-949.

[100] ACOG. ACOG Practice Bulletin N. 194. Polycystic ovary syndrome. Obstet Gynecol 2018;131:e157–e171.

[101] Pan JX, Liu Y, Ke ZH, Zhou CL, Meng Q, Ding GL, Xu GF, Sheng JZ, Huang HF. Successive and cyclic oral contraceptive pill pretreatment improves IVF/ICSI outcomes of PCOS patients and ameliorates hyperandrogenism and antral follicle excess. Gynecol Endocrinol 2015;31:332-336.

[102] Legro RS, Dodson WC, Kris-Etherton PM, Kunselman AR, Stetter CM, Williams NI, Gnatuk CL, Estes SJ, Fleming J, Allison KC et al. Randomized controlled trial of preconception interventions in infertile women with polycystic ovary syndrome. J Clin Endocrinol Metab 2015;100:4048-4058

[103] Wei D, Shi Y, Li J, Wang Z, Zhang L, Sun Y, Zhou H, Xu Y, Wu C, Liu L et al. Effect of pretreatment with oral contraceptives and progestins on IVF outcomes in women with polycystic ovary syndrome. Hum Reprod 2017;32:354-361.

[104] Wei D, Yu Y, Sun M, Shi Y, Sun Y, Deng X, Li J, Wang Z, Zhao S, Zhang H et al. The effect of supraphysiological estradiol on pregnancy outcomes differs between women with PCOS and ovulatory women. J Clin Endocrinol Metab 2018;103:2735-2742.

[105] Levi Setti PE, Cirillo F, De Cesare R, Morenghi E, Canevisio V, Ronchetti C, Baggiani A, Smeraldi A, Albani E, Patrizio P. Seven years of vitrified blastocyst transfers: comparison of 3 preparation protocols at a single ART center. Front Endocrinol (Lausanne) 2020; 11:346

[106] Muasher SJ, Kruithoff C, Simonetti S, Oehninger S, Acosta AA, Jones GS. Controlled preparation of the endometrium with exogenous steroids for the transfer of frozen-thawed pre-embryos in patients with anovulatory or irregular cycles. Hum Reprod 1991;6:443-445.

[107] Yu J, Ma Y, Wu Z, Li Y, Tang L, Li Y, Deng B. Endometrial preparation protocol of the frozen-thawed embryo transfer in patients with polycystic ovary syndrome. Arch Gynecol Obstet 2015;291: 201-211.

[108] Kollmann M, Martins WP, Lima ML, Craciunas L, Nastri CO, Richardson A, Raine-Fenning N. Strategies for improving outcome of assisted reproduction in women with polycystic ovary syndrome: systematic review and meta-analysis. Ultrasound Obstet Gynecol 2016;48:709-718.

[109] Qi X, Chuyu Yun, Lulu Sun, Jialin Xia, Qing Wu, Ying Wang, Lina Wang, Yangming Zhang, Xianyi Liang, Liying Wang, Frank J Gonzalez, Andrew D Patterson, Huiying Liu, Liangshan Mu, Zehong Zhou, Yue Zhao, Rong Li, Ping Liu, Chao Zhong, Yanli Pang, Changtao Jiang, Jie Qiao. Gut microbiota-bile acid-interleukin-22 axis orchestrates polycystic ovary syndrome. Nat Med. 2019 Aug;25(8):1225-1233. doi: 10.1038/s41591-019-0509-0. Epub 2019 Jul 22.

[110] Guo Y, Yane Qi, Xuefei Yang, Lihui Zhao, Shu Wen, Yinhui Liu, Li Tang. Association between Polycystic Ovary Syndrome and Gut Microbiota. PLoS One. 2016 Apr 19;11(4):e0153196. doi: 10.1371/journal.pone.0153196. eCollection 2016.

[111] Lindheim L, Bashir M, Münzker J, Trummer C, Zachhuber V, Leber B, Horvath A, Pieber TR, Gorkiewicz G, Stadlbauer V, Obermayer-Pietsch B. Alterations in Gut Microbiome Composition and Barrier Function Are Associated with Reproductive and Metabolic Defects in Women with Polycystic Ovary Syndrome (PCOS): A Pilot Study. PLoS One. 2017 Jan 3;12(1):e0168390. doi: 10.1371/journal.pone.0168390. eCollection 2017.

[112] Torres PJ, Martyna Siakowska M, Banaszewska B, Pawelczyk L, Duleba AJ, Kelley ST, Thackray VG. Gut Microbial Diversity in Women With Polycystic Ovary Syndrome Correlates With Hyperandrogenism. J Clin Endocrinol Metab. 2018 Apr 1;103(4):1502-1511. doi: 10.1210/jc.2017-02153.

[113] He F, Li Y. The gut microbial composition in polycystic ovary syndrome with insulin resistance: findings from a normal-weight population. J Ovarian Res. 2021 Mar 27;14(1):50. doi: 10.1186/s13048-021-00799-9.

[114] Zhou L, NI Z, Yu J, Cheng W, Cai Z, You C. Correlation Between Fecal Metabolomics and Gut Microbiota in Obesity and Polycystic Ovary Syndrome. Front Endocrinol (Lausanne). 2020 Sep 8;11:628. doi: 10.3389/fendo.2020.00628. eCollection 2020.

[115] Han Q, Wang J, Weiping Li, Zi-Jiang Chen, Yanzhi Du. Androgen-induced gut dysbiosis disrupts glucolipid metabolism and endocrinal functions in polycystic ovary syndrome. Microbiome. 2021 May 6;9(1):101. doi: 10.1186/s40168-021-01046-5.

[116] Kelley ST, Danalea V Skarra, Alissa J Rivera , Varykina G Thackray. The Gut Microbiome Is Altered in a Letrozole-Induced Mouse Model of Polycystic Ovary Syndrome. PLoS One. 2016 Jan 5;11(1):e0146509. doi: 10.1371/journal.pone.0146509. eCollection 2016.

[117] Yanhua Zheng, Jingwei Yu, Chengjie Liang, Shuna Li, Xiaohui Wen, Yanmei Li. Characterization on gut microbiome of PCOS rats and its further design by shifts in high-fat diet and dihydrotestosterone induction in PCOS rats. Bioprocess Biosyst Eng. 2021 May;44(5):953-964. doi: 10.1007/s00449-020-02320-w. Epub 2020 Mar 10.

[118] Tremellen K, Pearce K. Dysbiosis of Gut Microbiota (DOGMA)--a novel theory for the development of Polycystic Ovarian Syndrome. Med Hypotheses. 2012 Jul;79(1):104-112. doi: 10.1016/j.mehy.2012.04.016. Epub 2012 Apr 27.

[119] Quaranta G, Sanguinetti M, Masucci L. Fecal Microbiota Transplantation: A Potential Tool for Treatment of Human Female Reproductive Tract Diseases. Front Immunol. 2019; 10: 2653. Published online 2019 Nov 26. doi: 10.3389/fimmu.2019.02653

[120] Kim DE, Kim JK, Han SK, Jang SE, Han MJ, Kim DH. Lactobacillus plantarum NK3 and Bifidobacterium

longum NK49 Alleviate Bacterial Vaginosis and Osteoporosis in Mice by Suppressing NF-κB-Linked TNF-α Expression. J Med Food. (2019) 22:1022-1031. 10.1089/jmf.2019.4419

[121] Kutteh WH, Kantele A, Moldoveanu Z, Crowley-Nowick PA, Mestecky J. Induction of specific immune responses in the genital tract of women after oral or rectal immunization and rectal boosting with Salmonella typhi Ty 21a vaccine. J Reprod Immunol. (2001) 52:61-75. 10.1016/S0165-0378(01)00109-7

[122] Joo HM, Hyun YJ, Myoung KS, Ahn YT, Lee JH, Huh CS, et al. Lactobacillus johnsonii HY7042 ameliorates Gardnerella vaginalis-induced vaginosis by killing Gardnerella vaginalis and inhibiting NF-κB activation. Int Immunopharmacol. (2011) 11:1758-65. 10.1016/j.intimp.2011.07.002

[123] Moreno I, Codoner FM, Vilella F, Valbuena D, Martinez-Blanch JF, Jimenez-Almazab J, Alonso R, Alama P, Remohi J, Pellicer A, Ramon D, Simon C. Evidence that the endometrial microbiota has an effect on implantation success or failure. Am J Obstet Gynecol. 2016 Dec;215(6):684-703. doi: 10.1016/j.ajog.2016.09.075. Epub 2016 Oct 4.

[124] Haahr T, Jensen JS, Thomsen L, Duus L, Rygaard K, Humaidan P. Abnormal vaginal microbiota may be associated with poor reproductive outcomes: a prospective study in IVF patients. Hum Reprod. 2016 Apr;31(4):795-803. doi: 10.1093/humrep/dew026. Epub 2016 Feb 23.

[125] Cohen AM, Ye XY, Colgan TJ, Greenblatt EM, Chan C. Comparing endometrial receptivity array to histologic dating of the endometrium in women with a history of implantation failure. Syst Biol Reprod Med. 2020 Dec;66(6):347-354. doi: 10.1080/19396368.2020.1824032.Epub 2020 Sep 30.

[126] Lessey BA, Young SL. What exactly is endometrial receptivity? Fertil Steril 2019;111(4):611-617

[127] Ruiz-Alonso M, Blesa D, Bosch N, Martínez-Conejero J.A, Alamá P. The accuracy and reproducibility of the endometrial receptivity array is superior to histology as a diagnostic method for endometrial receptivity. Fertil Steril. 2013; 99: 508-517

[128] Tan J, Kan A, Hitkari J, Taylor B, Tallon N, Warraich G, Yuzpe A, Nakhuda G. The role of the endometrial receptivity array (ERA) in patients who have failed euploid embryo transfers. J Assist Reprod Genet. 2018 Apr;35(4):683-692. doi: 10.1007/s10815-017-1112-2.Epub 2018 Jan 11

[129] Hashimoto T, Koizumi M, Doshida M, Toya M, Sagara E, Oka N, Nakajo Y, Aono N, Igarashi H, Kiono K. Efficacy of the endometrial receptivity array for repeated implantation failure in Japan: A retrospective, two-centers study. Reprod Med Biol. 2017 Jul; 16(3): 290-296. doi: 10.1002/rmb2.12041

[130] Eisman LE, Pisarska MD, Wertheimer S, Chan JL, Akopians AL, Surrey MW, Danzer HC, Ghadir S, Chang WY, Alexander CJ, Wang ET. Clinical utility of the endometrial receptivity analysis in women with prior failed transfers. J Assist Reprod Genet. 2021 Mar;38(3):645-650. doi: 10.1007/s10815-020-02041-9. Epub 2021 Jan 17.

[131] Simon C, Gomez C, Cabanillas S, Vladimirov I, Castillon G, Giles J, Boynukalin K, Findikli N, Bahceci M, Ortega I, Vidal C, Funabiki M, Izquierdo A, Lopez L, Portela S, Frantz N, Kulmann M, Taguchi S, Labarta E, Colucci F, Mackens S, Santamaria X, Munoz E, Barrera S, Garcia-Velasco A, Fernandez M, Ferrando M, Ruiz M, Mol BW, Valbuena

D for the ERA-RCT Study Consortium Group. A 5-year multicentre randomized controlled trial comparing personalized, frozen and fresh blastocyst transfer in IVF. Reprod BioMed Online 2020;41(3):402-415

[132] Bassil R, Casper R, Samara N, Hsieh T, Barzilay E, Orvieto R, Haas J. Does the endometrial receptivity array really provide personalized embryo transfer? J Assist Reprod Genet. 2018 Jul;35(7):1301-1305. doi: 10.1007/s10815-018-1190-9.Epub 2018 May 8.

Chapter 5

Non-Invasive Chromosome Screening for Embryo Preimplantation Using Cell-Free DNA

Jin Huang, Yaxin Yao, Yan Zhou, Jialin Jia, Jing Wang, Jun Ren, Ping Liu and Sijia Lu

Abstract

Preimplantation genetic testing (PGT) is widely adopted to select embryos with normal ploidy but requires invasive embryo biopsy procedures. Therefore, non-invasive PGT (niPGT) detection of cell-free DNA (cfDNA) in blastocyst culture medium has gradually become a hot area in the field of assisted reproduction. This chapter will systematically summarize how researchers use embryonic cfDNA to conduct niPGT detection worldwide. It will also thoroughly review the factors that affect the accuracy of the test and its underlying issues, as well as prospective applications. We hope to provide a useful reference for the standardized operation of non-invasive PGT that can be widely applied in clinical practice.

Keywords: niPGT, Spent Culture Media, cfDNA, Aneuploid

1. Introduction

In vitro fertilization and embryo transfer (IVF-ET) is an effective method for the treatment of infertility, yet it still has a relatively low success rate [1]. Furthermore, the multiple pregnancy rate remains high as a result of multiple embryos being transferred, which can increase the chances of adverse pregnancy outcomes and affect the health of both the mother and children [2]. Elective single embryo transfer (eSET) is the most effective way to reduce the rate of multiple pregnancies and is increasingly used worldwide [3]. Nonetheless, the success rate of single embryo transplantation is not satisfactory, mainly due to the lack of a systematic approach for evaluating the conceivability of embryonic development. Presently, embryonic morphological assessment is still the most commonly used method, but this method has many problems due to the lack of quantifiable indicators and its susceptibility to subjective factors of laboratory embryologist [4–6].

Studies have shown that there is an approximately 40%–60% risk of chromosomal aneuploidy even before embryo implantation [7–9]. PGT-A can be used to identify embryos with chromosomal aneuploidy, thereby improving clinical outcomes in IVF patients [10–13]. Nonetheless, PGT-A relies on embryo biopsy, and its invasive biopsy approaches may increase its technical limitations for the following reasons: (1) it may have an influence on the quality and the level of development of the embryo [14]; (2) it may increase the chance of abnormal epigenetic modifications [15, 16]; (3) it has high requirements on the environment and operating instruments, and there is a potential risk of sampling failure; and (4) the accuracy of test results may be affected by mosaicism. Consequently, it is necessary to establish an optimal selection procedure in line with the morphological assessment for embryos that truly reflects the chromosome ploidy status of the embryo, avoids invasive operations, and does not require expensive equipment. Recently, several studies have found the presence of cfDNA in the culture medium and blastocyst fluid of embryos [17–21]. Noninvasive PGT-A detection through cfDNA has become a growing niche in the field of assisted reproduction. In this chapter, we will comprehensively review the advancements and attempts at noninvasive PGT-A using foetal cfDNA and discuss the pros and cons as well as insights into its clinical applications in IVF-ET.

2. cfDNA research based on Spent culture media (SCM)

2.1 The discovery of cfDNA in SCM

Stigliani et al. [18] first demonstrated the presence of cfDNA in SCM in 2013, where genomic DNA (gDNA) was found in 63% (205/326) of the 326 SCMs collected, ranging from 41 pg to 1.8 ng. Subsequently, Hammond et al. [19] also detected mitochondrial DNA (mtDNA) and gDNA in SCMs. In addition, Stigliani et al. [22] reported that the ratio of mtDNA to gDNA in the SCM of D3 was positively correlated with the formation rate of blastocysts. These results suggest that SCM can serve as a sampling source for early embryonic DNA, laying the foundation for the development of the non-invasive method of PGT-A.

2.2 Application of SCM in PGT-A

In recent years, an increasing number of studies have been conducted to evaluate the feasibility of SCM-based non-invasive PGT-A approaches, and some of the results are encouraging. Many studies have found that PGT-A by trophectoderm (TE) biopsy or whole embryo of SCM has a high consistency rate (as shown in **Table 1**. Pro). Nevertheless, other research groups have reported relatively low consistency rates when compared with TE or whole embryo results (see **Table 1**. Con). These contradictory results may be related to factors such as the difference in SCM sampling methods and sampling time used in the studies, embryo treatment, and the definition of consistency. By improving the detection method, non-invasive PGT-A using SCM is expected to meet the requirements of clinical diagnosis.

2.3 Factors affecting the accuracy of non-invasive PGT-A

When comparing the ploidy consistency of cfDNA in SCM, all studies have reported a high success rate of cfDNA amplification and detection, ranging from 77.3% to 100% (as shown in **Figure 1**). However, its consistency to the conventional PGT-A results fluctuated widely, ranging from 33% to 100% [23, 26, 27, 39] (as shown in **Figure 2**). Hence, it is critical to recognise the factors influencing accuracy.

Study	Fertilization method	Media system	Frozen: yes or no	Timing of collection and embryo manipulation	Volume for WGA	Amplification method	WGA products detection %(n)	DNA analysis	Concordance rate, %(n)
PRO									
Kuznyetsov et al. [23]	ICSI	Single medium	Yes	D5/D6 embryo (**freeze-thaw**): The thawed blastocysts were cultured in 25μL medium for 24h; Laser collapse to mix BF and SCM	-	SurePlex	100%(28/28)	NGS	96.4% vs WB (27/28) 87.5% vs TE (21/24)
Huang et al. [24]	ICSI	Single medium	Yes	D5/D6 embryo (**freeze-thaw**): The thawed blastocysts were cultured for 24h in 15μL medium, then the medium was collected	3.5μL	MALBAC	92.3%(48/52)	NGS	93.8% vs WB (45/48)
Jiao et al. [25]	ICSI	-	Yes	D5/D6 embryo (**freeze-thaw**): The thawed blastocysts were cultured in 12μL medium for 15h; Laser collapse to mix BF and SCM	10 μL	Improved MALBAC (MICS-Inst)	100%(41/41)	NGS	90.48% vs WB (19/21)
Li et al. [26]	ICSI	-	Yes	D5/D6 embryo (**freeze-thaw**): The thawed blastocysts were cultured in 15μL medium for 14~18h; Laser collapse to mix BF and SCM	10 μL	Improved MALBAC (MICS-Inst)	97.6% (40/41)	NGS	87.2% vs WB (34/39)
Chen et al. [27]	ICSI	Sequential medium	No	D3-D5/D6 (Fresh): On day 3, each embryo was washed and moved to an individual 30-μL drop and cultured to blastocyst stage	20~25 μL	MALBAC	100% (256/256)	NGS	78.1% vs WB (200/256)
Kuznyetsov et al. [23]	ICSI	Sequential medium	No	D4 ~ D5/D6 (**Fresh**): On day 4, each embryo was washed and moved to an individual 10-μL drop and cultured to blastocyst stage, followed by laser collapse to mix BF and SCM	-	SurePlex	100%(19/19)	NGS	100% vs TE (19/19)

Study	Fertilization method	Media system	Frozen: yes or no	Timing of collection and embryo manipulation	Volume for WGA	Amplification method	WGA products detection%(n)	DNA analysis	Concordance rate, %(n)
Rubio et al. [28]	ICSI	Single medium	No	D4~ D6/D7 (**Fresh**): On day 4, each embryo was washed and moved to an individual 10-μL drop and cultured to blastocyst stage(D6/7)	8-10μL	IonReproseq PGS Kit	94.8%(109/115)	NGS	84% VS TE (68/81)
				D4 ~ D5 (**Fresh**): On day 4, each embryo was washed and moved to an individual 10-μL drop and cultured to blastocyst stage(D5)					63% VS TE (17/27)
Rubio et al. [29]	ICSI or IVF	Sequential medium or Single medium	No	D4 ~ D6/D7 (**Fresh**): On day 4, each embryo was washed and moved to an individual 10-μL drop for at least 40 hours in culture.	10 μL	IonReproseq PGS Kit	92%(1197/ 1301)	NGS	78.2%(866/ 1108)
Lledo et al. [30]	ICSI	Single medium	No	D3-D5 (**Fresh**): On day 3, each embryo was washed and moved to an individual 20-μL drop and cultured to blastocyst stage(D5)	7.5μL	NICS-Inst	92.4%(85/92)	NGS	60.9% vs TE (28/46)
				D3-D6 (**Fresh**): On day 3, each embryo was washed and moved to an individual 20-μL drop and cultured to blastocyst stage(D6)					92.0% vs TE (34/37)
				D3-D5 (**Fresh**): On day 3, each embryo was washed and moved to an individual 20-μL drop and cultured to blastocyst stage(D5)	7.5μL	Sureplex	92.4%(85/92)	NGS	60.9% vs TE (28/46)
				D3-D6 (**Fresh**): On day 3, each embryo was washed and moved to an individual 20-μL drop and cultured to blastocyst stage(D6)					86.5%vsTE (32/37)

Study	Fertilization method	Media system	Frozen: yes or no	Timing of collection and embryo manipulation	Volume for WGA	Amplification method	WGA products detection %(n)	DNA analysis	Concordance rate, %(n)
Xu et al. [31]	ICSI	Sequential medium	Yes	D3 (**freeze-thaw**) ~D5: Warmed D3 embryos were placed in 30-μL droplets and cultured to blastocyst stage(D5)	5 to 20 μL	MALBAC	100%(42/42)	NGS	85.7% vs TE (36/42)
CON									
Hanson et al. [32]	ICSI	Sequential medium	No	D3/4-D5/6/7 (**Fresh**): On day 3, each embryo was washed and moved to an individual 30-μL drop and cultured to blastocyst stage, an additional media changeover occurred on day 4 for some samples.	-	NICS-Inst	62.7% (104/166)	NGS	59.6% vs TE (62/104)
Yin et al. [33]	ICSI	Sequential medium	No	D5/D6 embryo (**freeze-thaw**): The thawed blastocysts were cultured in 25μL medium for 24h;	- (Collected 20-25 μL)	NICS-Inst	78.7% (59/75)	NGS	32.2% vs WB (19/59)
Yeung et al. [34]	ICSI	Sequential medium	No	D3-D5/D6 (**Fresh**): On day 3, each embryo was washed and moved to an individual 30-μL drop and cultured to blastocyst stage	3μL (Collected 20 μL)	SurePLEX	77.3%(116/168)	NGS	62.1% VS TE (72/116)
Li et al. [35]	ICSI	Sequential medium	No	D3-D5(**Fresh**): On day 3, each embryo was washed and moved to an individual 30-μL drop and cultured to blastocyst stage, followed by laser collapse to mix BF and SCM	NA (Collected 25 μL)	MALBAC	97.5%(39/40)	NGS	50% VS WB (19/38)
									44.7% vs TE (17/38)
Vera-Rodriguez et al. [41]	ICSI	Sequential medium	No	D3-D5(**Fresh**): On day 3, each embryo was washed and moved to an individual 25-μL drop and cultured to blastocyst stage	20μL	SurePLEX	91.1%(51/56)	NGS	33.0% vs TE (17/51)
Feichtinger et al. [36]	ICSI	Single medium	No	D1-D5/6(**Fresh**): Embryos were cultured in single 25-μL droplets using a single step medium from fertilization until day 5/6.	5 μL	Sureplex	81.8%(18/22)	aCGH	72.2% vs PB (13/18)

Study	Fertilization method	Media system	Frozen: yes or no	Timing of collection and embryo manipulation	Volume for WGA	Amplification method	WGA products detection %(n)	DNA analysis	Concordance rate, %(n)
Ho et al. [37]	ICSI	Single medium	Yes	D1 (**freeze-thaw**) ~D3: Warmed 2PNs embryos were cultured in 25-μL medium until D3	5 μL	Picoplex	39%(16/41)	NGS	56.3% vs WB (9/16)
				D1 (**freeze-thaw**) ~D5: Warmed 2PNs embryos were cultured in 25-μL medium until D5	5 μL		80.4%(33/41)		65% vs TE (26/40)
Liu et al. [38]	ICSI	Single medium	No	D1-D5(**Fresh**): Embryos were cultured in single 30-μL droplets using a single step medium from fertilization until day 5/6.	30 μL	MALBAC	90.90% (80/88)	NGS	64.5% VS TE (20/31)
Shamonki et al. [39]	ICSI	Sequential medium	No	D3-D5/D6(**Fresh**): On day 3, each embryo was washed and moved to an individual 15-μL drop and cultured to blastocyst stage	-	Repli-G	96.5%(55/57)	-	-
Galluzi et al. [40]	ICSI	Sequential medium	No	D1-D3(**Fresh**): Embryos were cultured in single 10-μL droplets from fertilization until day D3.	2.5μL	PicoPLEX	93.7%(30/32)	qPCR	
				D3-D5/6(**Fresh**): On day 3, each embryo was washed and moved to an individual 10-μL drop and cultured to blastocyst stage	2.5μL		94.4%(51/54)		
Stigliani et al. [18]	ICSI	Sequential medium	No	D1-D2/D3(**Fresh**): SCM were collected after embryo transferor cryopreservation on Day 2 or Day 3	-	GenomePlex	63%(205/326)	qPCR	

Table 1.
Concordance rates between niPGT-A based on SCM and TE or WB.

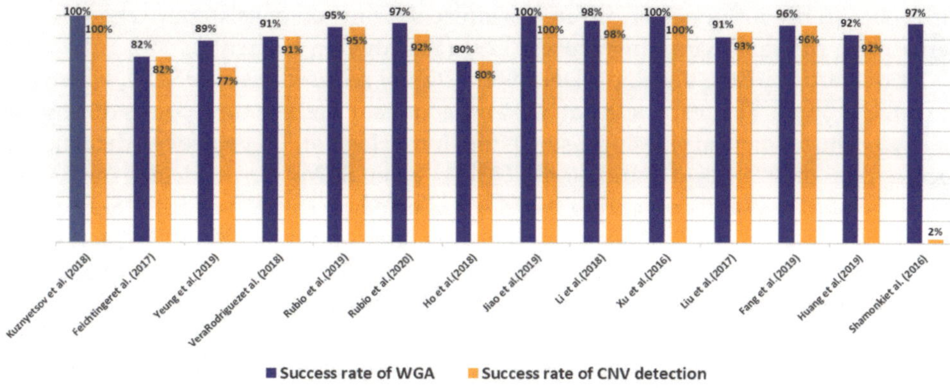

Figure 1.
Success rates of WGA amplification and CNV detection reported in different niPGT studies.

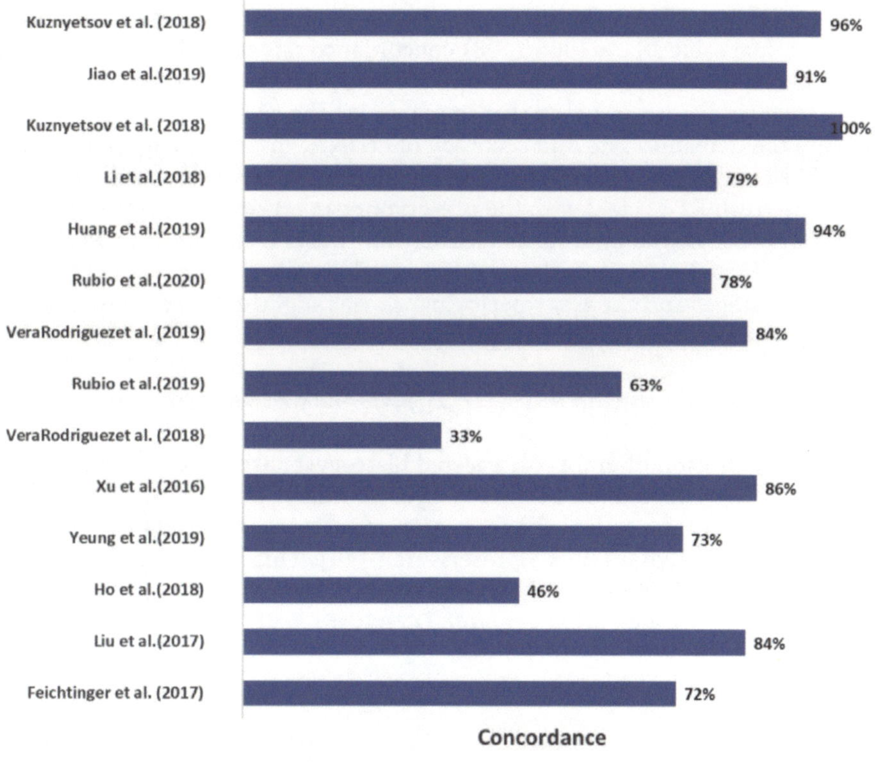

Figure 2.
CNV concordance rate reported in studies comparing SCM with TE or whole embryo samples.

2.3.1 Influence of sampling time on accuracy

At present, there are two common types of commercial embryo culture systems: sequential culture and single culture systems. However, the quality of DNA in SCM degrades as a result of cfDNA degradation over time. Therefore, the time and opportunity for cfDNA degradation could be minimized via media changes. Additionally, the maternal DNA contamination introduced by residual cumulus cells could be reduced or eliminated by media change to a certain extent. The results of a few studies using a single culture system [36–38] and sequential culture medium [31, 39, 41] are listed in **Table 1**. Importantly, Rubio et al. showed no significant difference in the influence of different culture systems on consistency when performing the same sampling process [29] (as shown in **Figure 3**).

As the fertilized egg develops, DNA is constantly released into the SCM, which is a dynamic process. The test results of SCM collected at different time points during embryo culture may vary. Using a single medium, Ho et al. [37] achieved detection success rates of 39% (16/41) and 80.4% (33/41) when SCMs were collected on D3 and D5, respectively. When comparing the SCM collected on D3-D5 and D4-D5, Lane et al. [43] found that the accuracy was higher in later samples, with >95% ploidy consistency and 100% consistency of the sex chromosome. The primary explanation for these observations may be that the number of embryonic cells increases exponentially with in line with embryonic development and that the concentration of cfDNA surges dramatically at later stages of the development. Rubio et al. [28] transferred embryos into new culture drops onD4 and collected SCM on D5 to D7. The SCM consistency of D4-D6/7 was significantly higher than that of D4-D5 (84.0% vs. 63.0%), and the level of maternal contamination was also reduced. A multicentre clinical study which supports the above assumption. conducted by the same team that compared SCM and TE samples using a large sample size of 1,301 embryos, also achieved a remarkable 78.2% (866/1108) concordance rate using D4-D6/7 SCM samples [29]. While the consistency rate jumped to 92.0% if the culture were last until D6.

The above studies have shown that to maximize the collection of cfDNA content and ensure the detection rate and accuracy of cfDNA, there is an optimal collection time for SCM on the premise of ensuring the blastocyst rate and excellent embryo rate. For the fresh ET cycle, D4 to the pre-cryopreservation blastocyst stage (D5/D6/D7) could be the optimal collection time. Several studies of ni-PGTA have also been conducted on frozen-thaw embryos, where the culture media were collected at later stages and the assay performance was slightly better compared to that of the fresh embryos (as shown in **Figure 4**).

2.3.2 Fresh-frozen embryos yield better niPGT performance than fresh embryos

In cryopreservation of embryos, assisted blastocyst shrinkage is usually performed during vitrification of the embryo. Shrinkage of the blastocyst cavity before vitrification can prevent the formation of ice crystals and improve the survival rate of embryos after cryopreservation [44]. This process leads to lysis of cell membrane, which increases the likelihood of that embryonic cells releasing cytoplasmic materials, including genomic DNA, into the SCM, thereby increasing

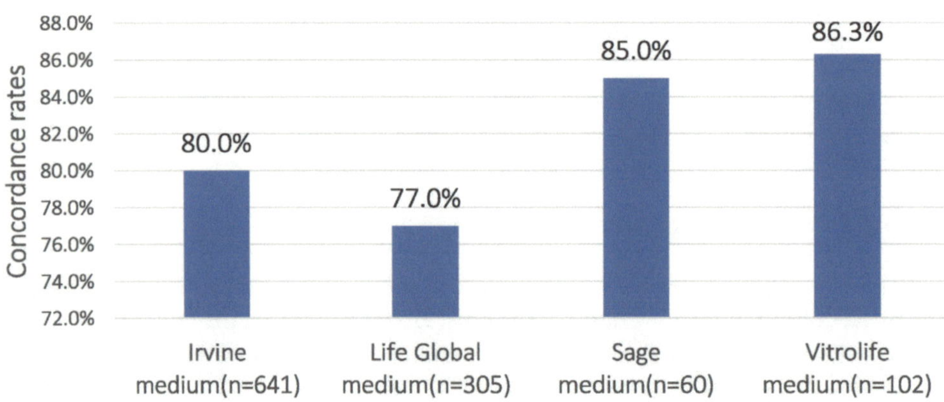

Figure 3.
CNV concordance rates of SCM versus TE biopsies in using different brands of culture media. No statistical differences were observed in four major brands of media. Data from Rubio et al. [42] (Ref). Data from Rubio et al. Embryonic cell-free DNA released to the spent blastocyst media. Am J Obstet Gynecol 2020.

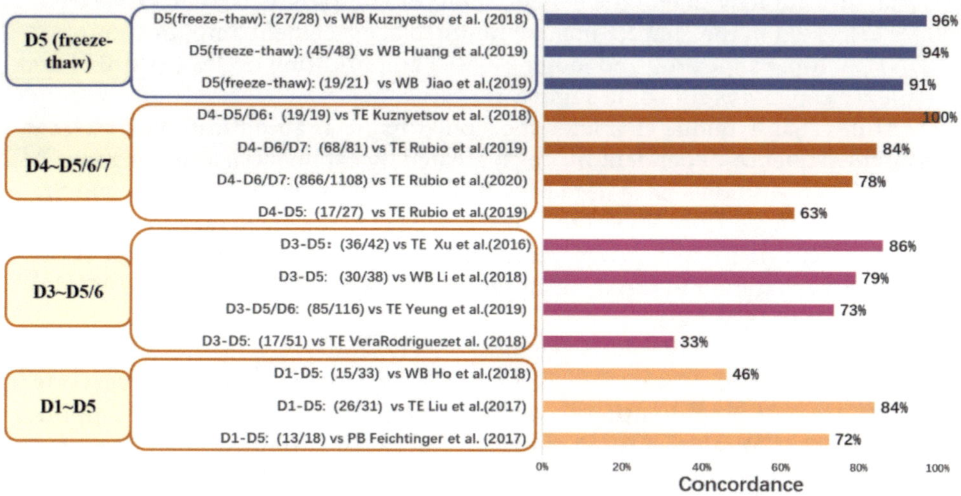

Figure 4.
Comparing SCM collection strategies and its impact on CNV concordance rate.

the concentration of DNA templates available for the downstream whole genome amplification (WGA) of niPGT-A. Furthermore, the vitrification process may lead to a higher rate of cell apoptosis, which also potentially increases the amount of cfDNA in the media after thawing and recovery. Kuznyetsov et al. [23] compared the amplification outcomes of a mixture of SCM and blastocyst fluid collected before vitrification (19) and after vitrification (30). The average amount of DNA obtained from fresh embryo culture amplification (6.3 ng/μL ~36.0 ng/μL) was lower than that obtained from vitrification-revival blastocysts (10.5 ng/μL ~44.0 ng/μL). After thawing 52 donated frozen blastocysts with TE biopsy results, Huang et al. [24] found that 48 of them (92.3%) were successfully amplified, and the data could be used for the analysis, with a consistency of 93.8% (45/48) to the whole embryo results. Jiao et al. [25] assessed 41 frozen blastocysts donated by 22 couples with known chromosomal rearrangements and 21 frozen blastocysts donated by 8 couples with normal karyotypes for PGT-SR and PGT-A analysis, respectively. All BCM (a mixture of SCM and BF) samples (62/62, 100%) were amplified successfully, and the clinical consistency between the niPGT-A results and the whole embryo was 90.48% (19/21). For PGT-SR results, the clinical consistency of BCM in chromosomal rearrangement and its corresponding whole embryo sample was 100% (41/41). Li et al. [26], using similar sampling methods, assessed 41 embryos and 97.6% were successfully amplified, and the clinical consistency between the niPGT-A results and the whole embryo was 87.2%. In summary, the SCM of cryopreserved-and-thawed embryos may contain more cfDNA than fresh embryos, which would minimize amplification failures and improve the reliability of the test results. This finding may be beneficial for patients who have had miscarriages due to embryo chromosomal abnormalities in the previous ART cycle. Providing that patients have sufficient cryopreserved embryos, they may take advantage of niPGT-A to screen euploid embryos for transplantation prior to the next transplantation cycle with resuscitated media (as shown in **Figure 4**).

2.3.3 Methods of whole-genome amplification

Given the challenge of low-concentration cfDNA in SCM, a WGA method with high uniformity and fidelity is required to amplify a small amount of genetic material to accurately detect the genetic status of embryos. Different WGA techniques discussed in the chapter include multiple displacement amplification (MDA), multiple annealing and looping-based amplification cycles (MALBA) and Sureplex/Picoplex (as shown in **Figure 5**).

MALBAC has a unique characteristic similar to linear amplification, which can reduce the sequence-dependent bias exacerbated by exponential amplification [34]. Several niPGT-A studies have used MALBAC to amplify cfDNA in SCM, and the success rates ranged from 90.9% to 100% [24, 31, 35, 38]. In 2019, Jiao et al. developed NICS-INST technology based on MALBAC, which incorporated WGA and library preparation in the same amplification step, achieving a 100% (41/41) detection rate in SCM [25].

Picoplex/Sureplex is currently the most widely used WGA methods for conventional PGT-A. One study used Picoplex for SCM amplification with a success rate of 97% [37]. In another study using the Sureplex amplification method, the amplification rate of 22 SCM samples reached 81.8%, and all the amplified samples produced PGT-A results by aCGH [36]. A study using Sureplex WGA in combination with blastocyst fluid (BF) and SCM found amplification rates of 100% in 28 samples, all of which produced PGT-A results [23]. In one SCM study with a large sample size of 168, 89.3% of the samples were successfully amplified by Sureplex, and 77.3% of the sequenced samples yielded PGT-A results [34]. Lledo et al. compared Veriseq (Illumina®) and NICS (Yikon®), which both achieved 92.4% amplification success rates. The consistency of the culture medium collected on D6 and TE biopsy was 92.0% and 86.5%, respectively [30].

MDA is an isothermal amplification reaction using Phi29 DNA polymerase [45]. Amplification bias due to nonlinear amplification remains a significant fault in the technique. Studies using MDA on SCM have shown an amplification success rate of 97%; however, only 2% of the amplified samples produced reliable PGT-A results [39]. Since the cfDNA of SCM is dominated by short fragments with a length of 160–220 bp [46], this would especially affect the MDA-based method, which requires longer DNA fragments to achieve optimal amplification.

The Phi29DNA polymerase used in MDA technology has high fidelity but is restricted by the starting amount of the DNA template. When the starting amount is very low, the coverage rate and accuracy of the amplified products can decrease

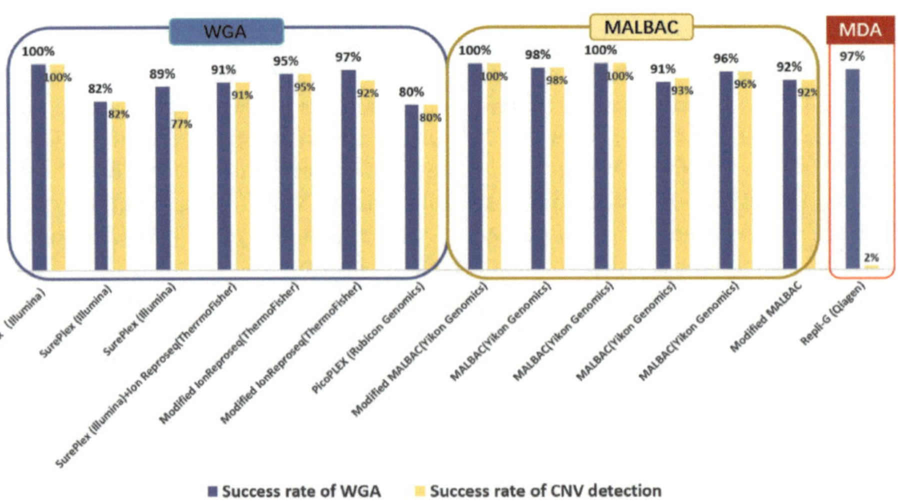

Figure 5.
Comparing SCM amplification methods and the concordance of CNV in different study MALBAC and SurePlex, PicoPLEX and IonReproseq are the main methods, MDA is not applicable.

dramatically. Malbac and Sureplex have the advantages of high genome coverage, low ADO rate, and a low number of starting DNA templates required. However, DNA polymerase has lower fidelity than Phi29 polymerase, which leads to an increased false positive rate compared to MDA.

2.3.4 Standard of the mosaic threshold of embryo

Embryonic mosaicism refers to the existence of two or more cell lines with different genotypes in the same embryo. Some studies suggest that abnormal cells in a mosaic embryo are gradually diminished, i.e., a certain degree of self-repair occurs during embryonic development [47–49]. Mosaic embryos, especially those with a low proportion, still have a decent success rate of pregnancy after being implanted [50, 51]. Therefore, there is a trend of accepting low-frequency mosaic embryos in clinical practice.

Chromosome ploidy of mosaic embryos can be quantified by the proportion of mosaics (M), and samples with results above a certain threshold of M are identified as aneuploidy embryos. Therefore, the proportion of false positives and false negatives in embryo chromosome detection relies on the threshold setting of M. We observed that different studies had different criteria for reporting mosaicism, ranging from 30% to 60%. Yeung et al. [34] set the minimum threshold as 30% and recommend against the implantation of mosaic embryos >30%. Bolton et al. [47] found that the elimination of aneuploidy cells in the ICM through apoptosis may result in an increase in aneuploidy fragments in the SCM. Thus, increasing the chimaerism threshold of SCM samples may reduce the false positive rate and improve the consistency rate. In the study of Jiao et al., samples with a mosaic ratio of less than 40% were defined as euploid, while samples with ≥40% were defined as aneuploid [25]. Rubio et al.'s study directly defined samples with a chimaerism ratio of <50% as euploidy and ≥ 50% as aneuploidy, and no mosaic embryos were reported [28]. Huang et al. observed that using 60% as the threshold for distinguishing aneuploidy from euploid embryos achieved a false negative rate of zero, significantly improving the results of non-invasive PGT-A [24]. This study suggests that appropriately increasing the aneuploidy threshold can minimize the mosaic false positives caused by NGS results to a certain extent; however, these adjustments would require validation on a much larger scale.

2.3.5 Whole embryo samples are more suitable as the gold standard for niPGT evaluation

Individual research groups may use different gold standards when evaluating the accuracy of SCM or BF detection results. At present, TE biopsy is the standard clinical practice for PGT-A; thus, TE biopsy is often used as the gold standard. However, due to the presence of chimaeric embryos, studies have questioned whether a couple of TE biopsy cells is able to accurately represent the ploidy of the inner cell masses. There was also a study performed to compare the ploidy results from cfDNA and polar body biopsy [36]. Although the polar body is naturally released from oocytes, which are minimally invasive, it only examines aneuploidy of maternal meiosis origin and is limited by its inability to directly evaluate the genetic status of the entire embryo [52].

Consequently, the D5 whole embryo for comparison with cfDNA as the gold standard may be the most appropriate when considering the accuracy of the given selected comparison criteria. Several studies have reported the use of the whole embryo as the gold standard. SCM collected from thawed blastocysts was assessed, which achieved overall consistency with the WB samples, ranging from 90.48% to 96.4% in all these studies [23–25]. Nevertheless, it can be challenging to obtain donated WB, even though it may be the best representation of the genetic status of the entire embryonic genome.

2.3.6 The determination for concordance

The concordance between the SCM and the selected gold standard, e.g., conventional TE biopsy or whole embryo, can be analysed from several aspects, as shown in **Table 2**.

First, the statistics of the consistency rate can be grouped into the following three situations: (1) the negative consistency rate (euploidy vs. euploidy), that is, both SCM and gold standard are negative results reported as euploidy, which is also the most critical indicator in clinical practice. Generally, clinicians choose euploid embryos for transplantation, and the accuracy of this indicator often directly impacts the clinical outcome. (2) The positive consistency rate (aneuploidy vs. aneuploidy), that is, both SCM and gold standard are positive results reported as aneuploidy. Usually, clinicians would not choose such embryos for transplantation. Hence, the accuracy will directly affect the availability of embryos for transplantation and the cycle cancellation rate. (3) The overall consistency, which is a comprehensive evaluation including both euploidy and aneuploidy.

Second, the researchers likewise have different ways to calculate consistency. (1) Clinical consistency refers to the test results for the impact on the clinical decision, as some researchers suppose that only euploid embryos would be considered for implantation, which means clinical consistency is the foundation, which agrees with the transplant decision (as shown in **Figure 6**). (2) Full consistency: it can only be considered consistent when the test result is absolutely in line with the karyotype, especially for patients with known chromosomal abnormalities (as shown in **Figure 6**). (3) Partial consistency: Some researchers consider SCM and the gold standard to be two different types of samples. Thus, they should be considered as consistent if there is partial consistency with the karyotypes.

Third, the criteria for the reporting of aneuploidy are not uniform. Researchers usually consider whether to report fragmentation abnormalities or whole chromosome abnormalities and whether to report mosaic results and their reporting criteria.

Through the analysis of a series of related studies (see **Table 2**), we observed that although different investigators used different methods to calculate consistency, the consistency results were superior to other methods when only clinical consistency rates were considered.

In the studies of Huang et al. [24], Jiao et al. [25], Li et al. [35], Liu et al. [38], and Yeung et al. [34], when the karyotype was completely consistent or partially consistent, the results' coincidence rates to the gold standard were 83.3%, 76.2%, 50%, 64.5% and 62.1%, respectively. However, the consistency rates increased to 93.8%, 90.5%, 78.9%, 83.9% and 73.3%, respectively, when only clinical consistency was considered.

In addition, in the analysis of Kuznyetsov et al., if only chromosomal aneuploidy was considered, the clinical consistency rate was often better than the results of fragment abnormalities and consistent karyotypes. The clinical concordance of frozen embryos and fresh embryos was 96.4% and 100% without considering chimaerism and fragment abnormalities, respectively, but decreased to 78.5% and 73.7% when considering chimaerism and fragment abnormalities, respectively. In addition, only euploidy and aneuploidy were distinguished according to the chromosomal test results given, and the positive and negative consistency rates in each study were calculated.

Study	Concordance rate			Definition of concordance			Definition of aneuploidy			
	Concordance	PPV	NPV	Clinical concordance	Karyotype complete concordance	Karyotype partial concordance	Chromosomal level(mosaic)	Chromosomal level (No mosaic)	Chromosomal segment level (mosaic)	Chromosomal segment level (No mosaic)
Huang et al. [24]	93.8%(45/48) vs WB	91.7% (33/36)	100% (12/12)	√					√	
	83.3%(40/48) vs WB	91.7% (33/36)	100% (12/12)		√				√	
Jiao et al. [25]	90.5%(19/21) vs WB	75%(6/8)	100% (13/13)	√					√	
	76.2%(16/21)	75%(6/8)	100% (13/13)		√					
Xu et al. [31]	85.7%(36/42) vs TE	78.9% (15/19)	91.3% (21/23)	√					√	
Li et al. [35]	78.9%(30/38) vs WB	73.9% (17/23)	86.7% (13/15)	√					√	
	50%(19/38) vs WB	73.9% (17/23)	86.7% (13/15)		√				√	
Liu et al. [38]	83.9%(26/31) vs WB	80%(8/10)	90% (18/20)	√					√	
	64.5%(20/31) vs WB	80%(8/10)	90% (18/20)		√				√	
Rubio et al. [28]	78.7%(85/108) vs TE	77.6% (52/67)	91.7% (33/36)	√						√
Yeung et al. [34]	73.3%(85/116)	82.6% (71/86)	46.7% (14/30)	√					√	
	62.1%(72/116) vs TE	82.6% (71/86)	46.7% (14/30)			√			√	
Vera-Rodriguez et al. [41]	33.3% (17/51) vs TE	90.9% (20/22)	20.7% (6/29)	√					√	

Study	Concordance rate			Definition of concordance			Definition of aneuploidy			
	Concordance	PPV	NPV	Clinical concordance	Karyotype complete concordance	Karyotype partial concordance	Chromosomal level(mosaic)	Chromosomal level (No mosaic)	Chromosomal segment level (mosaic)	Chromosomal segment level (No mosaic)
Kuznyetsov et al. [23]	96.4% (27/ 28)vs WB	100% (21/21)	85.7% (6/7)	√			√			
	92.8%(26/28) vs WB	100% (21/ 21))	85.7% (6/7)		√		√			
	78.5%(22/28) vs WB	79.2% (19/24)	75%(3/ 4)		√				√	
	100% (19/19) vs TE	100% (8/8)	100% (11/11)	√			√			
	100%(19/19) vs TE	100% (8/8)	100% (11/11)		√		√			
	73.7%(14/19) vs TE	72.7% (8/11)	75%(6/ 8)		√				√	

Table 2.
The different definitions of concordance and the aneuploidy affect the concordance rate.

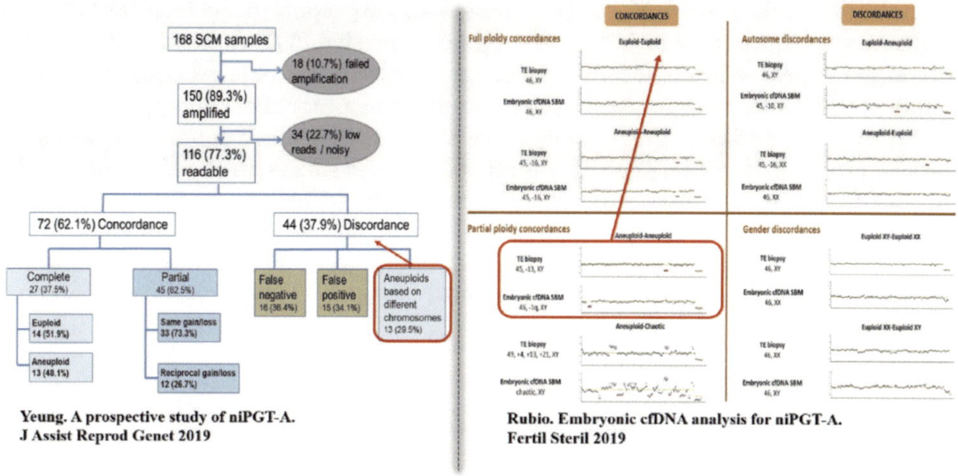

Figure 6.
Definition of concordance between SCM and the gold standard are at different levels in studies. Yeung et al. defines concordance at chromosome level, while Rubio et al. defines at the level of clinical concordance.

In general, the negative consistency rate is better than the positive consistency rate in SCM, which may indicate high false positives in the niPGT-A test. On the other hand, it also shows that the negative result of this approach is more reliable. In summary, the definition of consistency has a direct impact on the final results of the assessment method. Considering the speciality of cfDNA presented in SCM, it seems insufficient to define consistency purely based on the perfect match of the CNV patterns. Chen et al. [27] proposed the embryos can be categorized or scored by the obtained niPGT-A results into three groups: (A) chromosomal normal, (B) chromosomal abnormal, and (C) multiple abnormal chromosomes or uncertain. The results showed group A predicts a normal embryo with 90.0% probability, while groups B and C predict 27.8% and 72.2% normal probability, respectively. Thus, it may be necessary to fully consider the conditions, such as mosaicism, ploidy status and test resolution, when establishing the analytical model.

It seems more appropriate to use whole blastocysts as the gold standard for evaluation of the accuracy of niPGTA. Apparently, the establishment of the model would require large embryos of SCM and WB paired samples, with standardized sample collection and data analysis procedures. Furthermore, the model can evaluate SCM according to the euploidy probability of embryos to obtain the priority or exclusion order of embryos for implantation to avoid the waste of embryos due to false-positive decisions led by conventional PGT-A.

2.4 Clinical application of non-invasive PGT-A

At present, several studies have applied non-invasive PGT-A to diverse patient groups to preliminarily evaluate the clinical manifestations of the technique. Xu et al. [31] used non-invasive PGT-A for the first time in balanced translocation patients and obtained five live births from seven couples. Rubio et al. [28] compared the clinical outcomes of two groups of patients, one with both TE biopsy and SCM results of euploidy and the other with TE biopsy negative and SCM results of aneuploidy. The transplant success rate of patients with both euploidy TE and SCM results was twofold (52.9% vs. 16.7%) higher than that of the latter group. Zero miscarriages were observed (0/9) when both the TE and SCM results indicated that the embryos were euploid. Moreover, Fang et al. [53] reported the results of a single-centre clinical trial in 2019 applying non-invasive PGT-A on patient groups with either repeated implant failures (≥3) or repeated miscarriages (≥3). The trial included 45 couples with 50 ART cycles, resulting in a biochemical pregnancy rate of 72% (36/50), a clinical pregnancy rate of 58% (29/50), and a spontaneous miscarriage rate of ~10% (3/29), with a total of 27 babies successfully delivered. While the clinical trial scale of the above studies was small, the cfDNA-based niPGT-A proved in principle that it could reduce miscarriage and improve the ongoing pregnancy rate. Conversely, large-scale randomized controlled clinical trials are needed to conclude whether non-invasive PGT-A can be an effective way to evaluate embryo implantation potential.

3. Studies of cfDNA in blastocyst fluid (BF)

3.1 Presence of cfDNA in in blastocyst fluid (BF)

The presence of cfDNA in blastocyst fluid (BF) was revealed as early as 2013. For the first time, Palini et al. [17] reported that genomic DNA has identified in 90% (26/29) BF by qPCR, with an average amount of gDNA at 9.9 pg. TBC1D3 on chr17 and TSPY1Y on the Y chromosome were successfully amplified, which confirmed that the sex of embryos could be determined by qPCR using BF. In addition, genome-wide amplification (WGA) was demonstrated for blastocyst fluid amplification, and aneuploidy detection of WGA products was performed using microarray comparative genomic hybridization (aCGH). The aCGH results revealed the presence of the Y chromosome in two BF samples, which was consistent with previous data obtained by PCR analysis. It also showed multiple chromosomal abnormalities that agreed with the karyotype, suggesting that the WGA product DNA was indeed of embryonic origin. Subsequently, Zhang et al. [46] performed next-generation sequencing on WGA-amplified BF DNAs and compared the data with paired blastomere biopsy samples. The results showed decent concordance in genomic coverage and pattern regions between the two DNA sources. Further analysis of the gene annotation results suggested that cfDNA in the BF contained the sequences of the majority of genes, indicating that cfDNA in the BF could be used for solving monogenic diseases.

3.2 Sampling method of blastocyst fluid

BF can be isolated from embryos for downstream analysis using blastocyst puncture, which is a microscopy-assisted puncture made with an ICSI injection pipette on the trophoblast side, opposite of the inner cell mass. The fluid is then taken until the blastocyst completely collapses around the pipette [54]. This method can only isolate minute amounts (~0.01 μL) of BF for analysis [55, 56].

3.3 Study of PGT-A using blastocyst fluid

Recently, BF has been studied as a source for minimally invasive PGT-A. In 2014, Gianaroli et al. [57] isolated BF from 51 blastocysts, and the average concentration of WGA-amplified DNA detected in 39 BF samples (76.5%) was 900.38 ng/μL (ranging between 876.3–939.5 ng/μL). The results of BF detected in 38 cases (38/39, 97.4%) were consistent with the ploidy of TE biopsy results, and 9 cases (9/9, 100%) were consistent with the ploidy of the blastomere biopsy, and the coincidence rate of PB ploidy was 93.3% (28/30). Magli et al. [55] of the same group improved the sampling and amplification of BF samples to a success rate of 82% (95/116). aCGH was performed on 87 of these samples, of which 82 samples (94%) were used for subsequent analysis. The ploidy consistency of BF and TE samples was 97.1% (67/69), 94.4% (34/36) with blastomere biopsy and 94.1% (32/34) with polar body biopsy. In 2019, Magli et al. [12] used the same approach to amplify blastocyst fluid extracted from 256 blastocysts with a 71% (182/256) WGA amplification rate. Compared with the results of the corresponding TE cells, the overall ploidy consistency was 93.6% (161/172). The above results suggested that the cfDNA of the BF was highly predictive of embryo ploidy; however, the results from other research groups have been less satisfactory.

Tobler et al. [58] obtained a WGA amplification success rate of 63% (60/96) after thawing and culturing donated embryos to extract BF. The concordance between the BF karyotype and the whole embryo was 48.3% (29/60) by aCGH analysis, suggesting that BF may not be suitable for the PGT test. In 2018, Tsuiko performed chromosome analysis using NGS on 16 donated blastocysts, and the success rate of BF amplification was 87.5% (14/16). However, only 10 samples (10/16, 62.5%) passed sequencing and quality control for the subsequent analysis. The results showed that only 40% (4/10) of the BF samples completely agreed with the TE or ICM results. In addition, significantly more mosaicisms were found in BF samples than in TE and ICM samples. These results together suggest that although BF-DNA can be successfully amplified for NGS, one would not recommend using BF as a single DNA source for preimplantation genetic screening due to its low concordance with ICM and TE results. Capalbo et al. [59] (2018) performed PGT-A on 23 BF samples and compared the results with TE. Only 8 cases (34.8%) were successfully amplified, and only 3 cases (37.5%) were consistent with the ploidy of TE detection results.

In summary, studies assessing the reliability of BF DNA as a template for PGT-A have yielded conflicting conclusions, with 37.5%–97.4% concordance with TE samples (**Table 3**). Differences in consistency levels between studies may be related to differences in embryo handling. Tsuiko and Tobler used frozen embryos donated by patients after treatment, and BF was absorbed after blastocyst resuscitation and expansion; Tobler's study [58] specifically suggests that they are not suitable for clinical use. In contrast, the BF samples of Gianaroli, Magli and colleagues were obtained from fresh culture cycles and underwent many procedures (PB biopsies, assisted incubation and blastomere biopsies) that were not performed or relatively few procedures were performed in other studies. Thus, the observed increased rates of amplification and concordance may be due to the superior quality of BF obtained from freshly cultured embryos over frozen embryos or to an increase in the amount of DNA in the blastocyst cavity resulting from unintentional cell lysis or death during the procedure. It is also important to point out that the sample size in the Capalbo and Tsuiko studies was much smaller than that of Gianaroli, Magli and colleagues, so different results might have been obtained if a larger sample size had been studied.

According to the results of available studies collectively, BF DNA presented a high percentage of DNA amplification failure. The percentage of blastocyst fluid samples that successfully underwent whole genome amplification and produced detectable levels of DNA ranged from 34.8% to 82% [46, 58–60]. The difficulty in the successful amplification of BF-DNA lies in the small amount of fluid obtained from the cystic cavity, and the BF volume reported in various studies ranged from 0.3 nl to 1 μl. The volume difference would significantly impact the concentration of BF-DNA and may impose a negative effect on the efficiency of subsequent amplification. Another major reason for failure in BF-DNA amplification would be degradation. The success rate of whole genome amplification was generally much higher (≥98%) [58, 61] in TE biopsy, which makes BF DNA less suitable as an alternative source for clinical application [19].

Study	Fresh/frozen embryos	Method of BF collection	Day of BF isolation	Volume used of WGA	WGA method	WGA products detection%(n)	DNA analysis	Concordance, %(n)
PRO								
Gianaroli et al. [57]	Fresh	Blastocentesis	D5	1 μL	Sureplex	76.5%(39/51)	aCGH	100% vs BM(9/9) 97.4% vs TE (38/39) 93.3% vs PB(28/30)
Magli et al. [55]	Fresh	Blastocentesis	D5	0.01 μL	SurePlex	82%(95/116)	aCGH	94.4% vs BM(34/36) 97.1% vs TE (67/69) 94.1% vs PB(32/34)
Magli et al. [60]	Fresh	Blastocentesis	D5	The aspirated fluid was transferred into a 1-μL droplet of PBS	SurePlex	71%(182/256)	aCGH	93.6% vs TE (161/172)
CON								
Tsuiko et al. [56]	Cryopreserved blastocysts	Blastocentesis	D5	0.01 μL	Picoplex	62.5% (10/16)	NGS	40% vs ICM 或TE(4/10)
Tobler et al. [58]	Cryopreserved blastocysts	Blastocentesis	D5	1 μL	SurePlex	63%(60/96)	aCGH	48.3% vs EB(29/60)
Capalbo et al. [59]	Fresh	Blastocentesis	D5	The aspirated fluid was transferred into a 5-μL droplet of medium	SurePlex	34.8%(8/23)	NGS	37.5% vs TE(3/8)

Table 3.
Summary of BF cfDNA study.

In addition, blastocyst puncture is still a minimally invasive procedure, as an ICSI needle is inserted into the blastocyst cavity to extract the fluid. However, with the presence of amplifiable cfDNA in the BF, the low consistency of the test results to TE or other gold standards suggests that technical variability may still exist. The process may accidentally acquire loose cells trapped in the lumen or shed cell material, resulting in inconsistent test outcomes. Thus, further optimization is required before using BF DNA for PGT.

3.4 Correlation between BF test results and clinical outcomes

The DNA concentration in the BF was very low, and the total amount varied greatly between samples, implying that the BF DNA amount could be related to the developmental status of embryos. In 2019, Magli et al. [60] showed a significantly higher WGA amplification success rate of BF in aneuploid blastocysts (n = 150, 81%) versus euploid blastocysts (n = 32, 45%), suggesting differences in the quality or total amount of DNA in the BF of euploidy and aneuploidy embryos. Moreover, the clinical pregnancy rate was 77% in the group with failed BF amplification and 37% in the group with successful BF amplification when following the clinical outcome of 53 TE euploid blastocysts. The same trend was found in the rate of persistent pregnancies in failed and successful amplified BF samples, which were 68% and 31.5%, respectively. These clinical results suggest that the success of BF amplification may have predictive value for the viability of the corresponding blastocyst; nevertheless, further validation is required to draw conclude. Given that the total amount of DNA in the BF is relatively low, combining blastocyst fluid and culture medium may increase the amount of cfDNA, therefore improving the amplification success rate and consistency of detection.

4. Problems in the application of cfDNA to PGT-A

Before the large-scale use of SCM in PGT-A, further investigations are needed to trace the origin of cfDNA and confirm whether cfDNA represents the euploidy of embryos.

4.1 The origin of cfDNA

At present, there are several opinions about the origin of cfDNA. It is believed that during embryonic development, cfDNA may be released into the culture media through cell lysis, apoptosis, cell debris or other mechanisms [19]. In apoptotic cells, DNA is cleaved to form fragments. These fragment sizes are multiples of approximately 180-bp oligomers [62]. Zhang's [46] research shows that the fragments have two peaks. The first peak had a range of 160–220 bp, whereas the second peak was broader, ranging from 300 to 400 bp. Bolton et al. [63] found that apoptosis was frequently observed within the ICM and TE between euploid cells and aneuploid cells in a mouse model. The results also showed that in aneuploid embryos, the percentages of apoptotic cells in the ICM and TE were 41.4% and 3.3%, respectively. In euploid embryos, the percentage of apoptotic cells in euploid cells was 19.5% and 0.6%, respectively. If cfDNA mainly comes from apoptotic cells, Bolton's and other studies demonstrate that cfDNA mainly originates from the ICM.

Moreover, Victor et al. [51] tracked the development of embryos dynamically using immunofluorescence technology, especially cell proliferation and apoptosis in euploid embryos, aneuploid embryos and mosaic embryos. The TE and ICM in euploid cells showed lower level of activities in both not only in cell proliferation but also in apoptosis. Nevertheless, in mosaic and aneuploid embryos, the levels of the two processes were both higher.

4.2 Maternal contamination

The discordant results in SCM and control embryos were mainly attributable to a high percentage of maternal DNA in the spent culture media. The Vera Rodriguez team [41] analysed the SCM and TE results from 56 samples. Among them, 17 embryos were detected as aneuploid or aneuploid males (XY) by TE, while all of them were detected as aneuploid females (XX) by SCM. When Feichtinger et al. compared the consistency between the SCM and polar body, the negative control (SCM of fertilization failure oocytes) was also effectively amplified. Oocytes are unlikely to abandon their DNA to the culture media. Therefore, this maternal contamination may come from cumulus cells or other exogenous DNA [36]. However, contamination may be minimized with the degradation of DNA in vitro by changing the solution in the sequential culture at D3 and delaying the sampling time. In sequential culture, if the granular cells before ICSI are not removed entirely, it is recommended to remove them again during the culture medium change on Day 3.

To reduce the interference of human judgement, we should develop a calculation method to eliminate maternal DNA for the purpose of internal quality control. To confirm whether there was maternal DNA contamination in the embryo medium, Hammond et al. carried out a short tandem repeat (STR) analysis on abandoned spent culture media (n = 10), media controls (n = 2) and the corresponding cumulus cells [64]. Maternal DNA from cumulus cells successfully amplified all gene loci, but the amount of DNA in the SCM was too small to identify DNA. STR analysis is a long-range amplification, and highly fragmented SCM DNA seems unsuitable for this detection. Vera Rodriguez et al. conducted SNP sequencing of three groups of samples (TE/follicular fluid DNA/embryonic SCM DNA) from 35 embryos and successfully quantified the proportion of maternal DNA contamination in SCM [41]. This suggests that SNP detection can be used to evaluate maternal contamination in SCM.

In addition, considering that the fragment size of cfDNA may be different from that of maternal contamination DNA, or according to the cleavage characteristics of cfDNA at the restriction site, it can be considered to identify the target fragment size and restriction site characteristics, and only analyse the DNA that conforms to the embryonic DNA. The hypothesis is that there is a DNA amplification and database construction method that can maintain the characteristics of DNA fragments or restriction sites, and the original cfDNA template can be amplified with high fidelity.

4.3 Background cfDNA contamination of SCM

Some studies have suggested that another source of exogenous DNA contamination is the low level of background DNA in SCM. In 2017, Hammond et al. [64] detected low baseline levels of DNA in the base media and protein supplement components of three commercial culture media. They also detected a copy of nuclear DNA in the culture media with no previous contact with embryos. Vera Rodriguez et al. [41] detected DNA quantification using qPCR in 53 spent culture media and 17 control samples (culture media with no previous contact with embryos). Then, PGT-A analysis was performed in 56 spent culture media and 11 control samples. The SCM was amplified successfully, and 11 controls generated an amplification-failure pattern, causing downstream analysis failure. In addition, Li et al. [35] found that the background DNA of the control culture did not interfere with the detection results, and all samples from the same embryo had the same sex chromosome diagnosis. The results testified that although there was a low baseline of exogenous DNA in the control SCM, the effect could be ignored due to the small amount of exogenous DNA. In addition, some commercial media use human serum albumin (HSA) to improve embryo development. Because HSA can adsorb DNA, the amount that is added should be controlled within a reasonable range. We suggest that the blank culture medium should be set as the parallel culture at the same time as recovering blastocyst culture media for quality control of SCM samples.

5. Prospects

Using SCM cfDNA for PGT-A has become a hot topic in the assisted reproductive field. The current research focuses on the aneuploidy consistency between cfDNA and embryos. However, the consistency comparison needs to consider many influencing factors, such as the definition of consistency, sampling methods, analysis methods, etc. We need to reach a certain consensus and standard before making an objective evaluation. Through the summary and introduction of this review, we found that a suitable sampling time, WB as the gold standard, suitable amplification methods and NGS platforms may provide the basis for the standardization of non-invasive PGT-A.

In the future, we should develop a standardized and automatic embryo culture and sample collection system based on the operating habits and culture process of the embryo laboratory. Meanwhile, we need to combine the sample downstream detection technology with corresponding software analysis to select the best embryos, which are those with the lowest probability of chromosomal abnormalities, for transplantation to improve the success rate of the whole IVF-ET cycle. It is believed that with the development of technology, the realization of automatic collection and detection platforms, the accumulation of detectable sample sizes, and the average cost of PGT-A detection on each embryo will be greatly reduced, and it is encouraging that SCM sample collection and detection will be developed into the routine process of embryo laboratories.

With the accumulation of data, SCM can be used to develop detection content for different populations. For the low-risk population with chromosomal abnormalities, we can give the risk value of chromosomal abnormalities on chromosome 16, which easily causes abortion, and on chromosomes 13, 15, 18, 21 and X, which easily cause birth defects. Referring to the NIPT method, the influence, caused by a proportion of false positive cfDNA, will be reduced. For high-risk populations with chromosomal abnormalities, such as elderly individuals, the consistency between SCM test results and embryos is high, and the interference of false-positives is relatively low. For this group of people, it is recommended to conduct whole chromosome screening, determine the risk value of chromosomal abnormalities of each embryo and determine the order of embryo transfer according to the risk value. For people with clear indications of PGT-A, we suggest that SCM samples be stored while biopsy samples are collected, especially for the laboratory or biopsy operator who has just performed biopsy. If there is no result or the result of biopsy cannot be used, SCM test results could provide remedial measures for the failure of detection due to sample loss or operation. In addition, for IVF cycles with poor quality or a small number of embryos, we should minimize the damage of biopsy operations to embryos and consider the detection of chromosome aneuploidy by SCM under the premise of full knowledge.

Exogenous contamination of embryos has been a more concerning issue at present. To improve the accuracy of detection, DNA fragments from embryos should be identified by differentiated DNA fragment length or linkage analysis in a bioinformatics platform. In addition, due to the different fertilization methods of IVF embryos, researchers have been worried that sperm will interfere with SCM. If we find a way to eliminate maternal or paternal contamination, it will be supplied to IVF embryos. We can use this technology to eliminate the problem of chromosome aneuploidy through non-invasive PGT-A to achieve ideal clinical outcomes for a wider population.

At the same time, non-invasive PGT detection can try not only for aneuploidy detection but expand to the comprehensive evaluation on the based on morphology and take into account the DNA concentration, chimaeric ratio, resolution, consistency with the gold standard and other factors of embryonic SCM. With the accumulation of clinical outcomes, it can also be combined with the clinical data of patients as an index to predict the clinical outcomes of embryos.

A noninvasive artificial intelligence embryo evaluation model could be established, which not only provides suggestions for clinicians on the order of embryo implantation but also provides patients with the most suitable and economical detection scheme, ultimately saving time for pregnancy and improving the overall success rate of IVF-ET.

6. Conclusions

As the findings of non-invasive PGT-A (NIPGT-A) research have been discussed, and researchers have noticed that the success rate and accuracy of the test are closely related to the types of culture medium, culturing and methods, sampling method, detection platform s and gold-standard reference used of detection. This chapter systematically expounds on how researchers use foetal free DNA for non-invasive PGT-A detection and thoroughly analyses the factors affecting its accuracy, possible problems and future application prospects. We hope that it serves as a good reference for non-invasive PGT-A being widely used in standardized operations before clinical application.

Acknowledgements

This work was supported by the National Key Research and Development Program (Grant No. 2018YFC1003100).

Conflict of interest

The authors declare that the research was conducted in the absence of any commercial or financial relationships that could be construed as potential conflicts of interest.

Acronyms and abbreviations

PGT-A	Preimplantation Genetic Testing For Aneuploidy
cfDNA	Cell-free DNA
niPGT-A	non-invasive PGT-A
IVF-ET	In vitro fertilization and embryo transfer
eSET	elective single embryo transfer
BCM	blastocoel fluid and spent culture medium
SCM	spent culture media

BF	blastocoel fluid
gDNA	genomic DNA
mtDNA	mitochondrial DNA
TE	trophectoderm
NICS-INST	Non-invasive chromosome screening: an improved MALBAC whole genome amplification (WGA) strategy
PGT-SR	Preimplantation Genetic Testing for Structural Rearrangement
WGA	whole genome amplification
MDA	multiple displacement amplification
MALBAC	multiple annealing and looping-based amplification cycles
NICS	Non-Invasive Chromosome Screening
ADO	allele dropout
NGS	next-generation sequencing
WB	whole blastocyst
CNV	copy number variations
aCGH	array-based comparative genomic hybridization
ICSI	Intracytoplasmic sperm injection
PB	Polar body
STR	short tandem repeat
SNP	single nucleotide polymorphism
HSA	Human serum albumin

Author details

Jin Huang[1,2,3,4†], Yaxin Yao[5†], Yan Zhou[5], Jialin Jia[1,2,3,4], Jing Wang[5], Jun Ren[5], Ping Liu[1,2,3,4*] and Sijia Lu[5*]

1 Centre for Reproductive Medicine, Department of Obstetrics and Gynecology, Peking University Third Hospital, Beijing, China

2 National Clinical Research Center for Obstetrics and Gynecology (Peking University Third Hospital), Beijing, China

3 Key Laboratory of Assisted Reproduction (Peking University), Ministry of Education, Beijing, China

4 Beijing Key Laboratory of Reproductive Endocrinology and Assisted Reproductive Technology, Beijing, China

5 Department of Clinical Research, Yikon Genomics Co. Ltd., Suzhou, China

*Address all correspondence to: pingliu7703@sina.com; lusijia@yikongenomics.com

† These authors contribute equally to the manuscript.

References

[1] Kupka M S, Ferraretti A P, De Mouzon J, et al. Assisted reproductive technology in Europe, 2010: results generated from European registers by ESHREdagger Hum Reprod, 2014, 29 (10): 2099-2113.doi:10.1093/humrep/deu175

[2] Elster N. Less is more the risks of multiple births Fertility and Sterility, 2000, 74(4): 617-623.doi:

[3] Maheshwari A, Griffiths S, Bhattacharya S. Global variations in the uptake of single embryo transfer Hum Reprod Update, 2011, 17(1): 107-120. doi:10.1093/humupd/dmq028

[4] Kirkegaard K, Agerholm I E, Ingerslev H J. Time-lapse monitoring as a tool for clinical embryo assessment Hum Reprod, 2012, 27(5): 1277-1285.doi: 10.1093/humrep/des079

[5] Basile N, Vime P, Florensa M, et al. The use of morphokinetics as a predictor of implantation: a multicentric study to define and validate an algorithm for embryo selection Hum Reprod, 2015, 30 (2): 276-283.doi:10.1093/humrep/deu331

[6] Rubio I, Galan A, Larreategui Z, et al. Clinical validation of embryo culture and selection by morphokinetic analysis: a randomized, controlled trial of the EmbryoScope Fertil Steril, 2014, 102(5): 1287-1294 e 1285.doi:10.1016/j.fertnstert.2014.07.738

[7] Rabinowitz M, Ryan A, Gemelos G, et al. Origins and rates of aneuploidy in human blastomeres Fertil Steril, 2012, 97(2): 395-401.doi:10.1016/j.fertnstert.2011.11.034

[8] Fragouli E, Alfarawati S, Spath K, et al. O-1 The origin and impact of embryonic aneuploidy Reproductive BioMedicine Online, 2013, 26(10.1016/s1472-6483(13)60034-6

[9] Franasiak J M, Forman E J, Hong K H, et al. The nature of aneuploidy with increasing age of the female partner: a review of 15,169 consecutive trophectoderm biopsies evaluated with comprehensive chromosomal screening Fertil Steril, 2014, 101(3): 656-663 e651. doi:10.1016/j.fertnstert.2013.11.004

[10] Chen M, Wei S, Hu J, et al. Can Comprehensive Chromosome Screening Technology Improve IVF/ICSI Outcomes? A Meta-Analysis PLoS One, 2015, 10(10): e0140779.doi:10.1371/journal.pone.0140779

[11] Scott R T, Jr., Upham K M, Forman E J, et al. Blastocyst biopsy with comprehensive chromosome screening and fresh embryo transfer significantly increases in vitro fertilization implantation and delivery rates: a randomized controlled trial Fertil Steril, 2013, 100(3): 697-703.doi:10.1016/j.fertnstert.2013.04.035

[12] Forman E J, Hong K H, Ferry K M, et al. In vitro fertilization with single euploid blastocyst transfer: a randomized controlled trial Fertil Steril, 2013, 100(1): 100-107 e101.doi:10.1016/j.fertnstert.2013.02.056

[13] Rubio C, Bellver J, Rodrigo L, et al. In vitro fertilization with preimplantation genetic diagnosis for aneuploidies in advanced maternal age: a randomized, controlled study Fertil Steril, 2017, 107(5): 1122-1129.doi: 10.1016/j.fertnstert.2017.03.011

[14] Wu Y, Lv Z, Yang Y, et al. Blastomere biopsy influences epigenetic reprogramming during early embryo development, which impacts neural development and function in resulting mice Cell Mol Life Sci, 2014, 71(9): 1761-1774.doi:10.1007/s00018-013-1466-2

[15] Zhao H C, Zhao Y, Li M, et al. Aberrant epigenetic modification in

murine brain tissues of offspring from preimplantation genetic diagnosis blastomere biopsies Biol Reprod, 2013, 89(5): 117.doi:10.1095/biolreprod.113.109926

[16] Zeng Y, Lv Z, Gu L, et al. Preimplantation genetic diagnosis (PGD) influences adrenal development and response to cold stress in resulting mice Cell Tissue Res, 2013, 354(3): 729-741.doi:10.1007/s00441-013-1728-1

[17] Palini S, Galluzzi L, De Stefani S, et al. Genomic DNA in human blastocoele fluid Reprod Biomed Online, 2013, 26(6): 603-610.doi:10.1016/j.rbmo.2013.02.012

[18] Stigliani S, Anserini P, Venturini P L, et al. Mitochondrial DNA content in embryo culture medium is significantly associated with human embryo fragmentation Hum Reprod, 2013, 28 (10): 2652-2660.doi:10.1093/humrep/det314

[19] Hammond E R, Shelling A N, Cree L M. Nuclear and mitochondrial DNA in blastocoele fluid and embryo culture medium: evidence and potential clinical use Hum Reprod, 2016, 31(8): 1653-1661.doi:10.1093/humrep/dew132

[20] Farra C, Choucair F, Awwad J. Non-invasive pre-implantation genetic testing of human embryos: an emerging concept Hum Reprod, 2018, 33(12): 2162-2167.doi:10.1093/humrep/dey314

[21] Leaver M, Wells D. Non-invasive preimplantation genetic testing (niPGT): the next revolution in reproductive genetics? Hum Reprod Update, 2020, 26(1): 16-42.doi:10.1093/humupd/dmz033

[22] Stigliani S, Persico L, Lagazio C, et al. Mitochondrial DNA in Day 3 embryo culture medium is a novel, non-invasive biomarker of blastocyst potential and implantation outcome Mol Hum Reprod, 2014, 20(12): 1238-1246. doi:10.1093/molehr/gau086

[23] Kuznyetsov V, Madjunkova S, Antes R, et al. Evaluation of a novel non-invasive preimplantation genetic screening approach PLoS One, 2018, 13 (5): e0197262.doi:10.1371/journal.pone.0197262

[24] Huang L, Bogale B, Tang Y, et al. Noninvasive preimplantation genetic testing for aneuploidy in spent medium may be more reliable than trophectoderm biopsy Proc Natl Acad Sci U S A, 2019, 116(28): 14105-14112. doi:10.1073/pnas.1907472116

[25] Jiao J, Shi B, Sagnelli M, et al. Minimally invasive preimplantation genetic testing using blastocyst culture medium Hum Reprod, 2019, 34(7): 1369-1379.doi:10.1093/humrep/dez075

[26] Li X, Hao Y, Chen D, et al. Non-invasive preimplantation genetic testing for putative mosaic blastocysts: a pilot study Human reproduction, 2021, 36(7): 2020-34. doi:10.1093/humrep/deab080.

[27] Chen L, Sun Q, Xu J, et al. A Non-invasive Chromosome Screening Strategy for Prioritizing in vitro Fertilization Embryos for Implantation Frontiers in Cell and Developmental Biology. 2021, 9. doi: 10.3389/fcell.2021.708322

[28] Rubio C, Rienzi L, Navarro-Sanchez L, et al. Embryonic cell-free DNA versus trophectoderm biopsy for aneuploidy testing: concordance rate and clinical implications Fertil Steril, 2019, 112(3): 510-519.doi:10.1016/j.fertnstert.2019.04.038

[29] Rubio C, Navarro-Sanchez L, Garcia-Pascual C M, et al. Multicenter prospective study of concordance between embryonic cell-free DNA and trophectoderm biopsies from 1301 human blastocysts Am J Obstet Gynecol, 2020, 223(5): 751 e751-751 e713.doi:10.1016/j.ajog.2020.04.035

[30] Lledo B, Morales R, Ortiz J A, et al. Consistent results of non-invasive PGT-A of human embryos using two different techniques for chromosomal analysis Reprod Biomed Online, 2021, 42(3): 555-563.doi:10.1016/j.rbmo.2020.10.021

[31] Xu J, Fang R, Chen L, et al. Noninvasive chromosome screening of human embryos by genome sequencing of embryo culture medium for in vitro fertilization Proc Natl Acad Sci U S A, 2016, 113(42): 11907-11912.doi:10.1073/pnas.1613294113

[32] Hanson B M, X Tao, K H Hong, et al. Noninvasive preimplantation genetic testing for aneuploidy exhibits high rates of deoxyribonucleic acid amplification failure and poor correlation with results obtained using trophectoderm biopsy Fertility and sterility, 2021, 115, 1461-1470, doi: 10.1016/j.fertnstert.2021.01.028.

[33] Yin B, Zhang H, Xie J, et al. Validation of preimplantation genetic tests for aneuploidy (PGT-A) with DNA from spent culture media (SCM): concordance assessment and implication Reproductive biology and endocrinology: RB&E, 2021, 19, 41, doi: 10.1186/s12958-021-00714-3.

[34] Yeung Q S Y, Zhang Y X, Chung J P W, et al. A prospective study of non-invasive preimplantation genetic testing for aneuploidies (NiPGT-A) using next-generation sequencing (NGS) on spent culture media (SCM) J Assist Reprod Genet, 2019, 36(8): 1609-1621.doi: 10.1007/s10815-019-01517-7

[35] Li P, Song Z, Yao Y, et al. Preimplantation Genetic Screening with Spent Culture Medium/Blastocoel Fluid for in Vitro Fertilization Sci Rep, 2018, 8 (1): 9275.doi:10.1038/s41598-018-27367-4

[36] Feichtinger M, Vaccari E, Carli L, et al. Non-invasive preimplantation genetic screening using array comparative genomic hybridization on spent culture media: a proof-of-concept pilot study Reprod Biomed Online, 2017, 34(6): 583-589.doi:10.1016/j.rbmo.2017.03.015

[37] Ho J R, Arrach N, Rhodes-Long K, et al. Pushing the limits of detection: investigation of cell-free DNA for aneuploidy screening in embryos Fertil Steril, 2018, 110(3): 467-475 e462.doi: 10.1016/j.fertnstert.2018.03.036

[38] Liu W, Liu J, Du H, et al. Non-invasive pre-implantation aneuploidy screening and diagnosis of beta thalassemia IVSII654 mutation using spent embryo culture medium Ann Med, 2017, 49(4): 319-328.doi:10.1080/07853890.2016.1254816

[39] Shamonki M I, Jin H, Haimowitz Z, et al. Proof of concept: preimplantation genetic screening without embryo biopsy through analysis of cell-free DNA in spent embryo culture media Fertil Steril, 2016, 106(6): 1312-1318.doi: 10.1016/j.fertnstert.2016.07.1112

[40] Galluzzi L, S Palini, S Stefani, et al. Extracellular embryo genomic DNA and its potential for genotyping applications Future science OA, 2015, 1, Fso62, doi: 10.4155/fso.15.62

[41] Vera-Rodriguez M, Diez-Juan A, Jimenez-Almazan J, et al. Origin and composition of cell-free DNA in spent medium from human embryo culture during preimplantation development Hum Reprod, 2018, 33(4): 745-756.doi: 10.1093/humrep/dey028

[42] Rubio et al. Embryonic cell-free Rubio et al. Embryonic cell-free Rubio et al. Embryonic cell-free

[43] Lane M, Zander-Fox D L, Hamilton H, et al. Ability to detect aneuploidy from cell free DNA collected from media is dependent on the stage of development of the embryo Fertility and Sterility, 2017, 108(3): 10.1016/j.fertnstert.2017.07.192

[44] Wong K M, Mastenbroek S, Repping S. Cryopreservation of human embryos and its contribution to in vitro fertilization success rates Fertil Steril, 2014, 102(1): 19-26.doi:10.1016/j.fertnstert.2014.05.027

[45] Mai M, Hoyer J D, Mcclure R F. Use of multiple displacement amplification to amplify genomic DNA before sequencing of the alpha and beta haemoglobin genes J Clin Pathol, 2004, 57(6): 637-640.doi:10.1136/jcp.2003.014704

[46] Zhang Y, Li N, Wang L, et al. Molecular analysis of DNA in blastocoele fluid using next-generation sequencing J Assist Reprod Genet, 2016, 33(5): 637-645.doi:10.1007/s10815-016-0667-7

[47] Bolton H, Graham S J L, Van Der Aa N, et al. Mouse model of chromosome mosaicism reveals lineage-specific depletion of aneuploid cells and normal developmental potential Nat Commun, 2016, 7(11165.doi:10.1038/ncomms11165

[48] Mccoy R C. Mosaicism in Preimplantation Human Embryos: When Chromosomal Abnormalities Are the Norm Trends Genet, 2017, 33 (7): 448-463.doi:10.1016/j.tig.2017.04.001

[49] Babariya D, Fragouli E, Alfarawati S, et al. The incidence and origin of segmental aneuploidy in human oocytes and preimplantation embryos Hum Reprod, 2017, 32(12): 2549-2560.doi:10.1093/humrep/dex324

[50] Zore T, Kroener L L, Wang C, et al. Transfer of embryos with segmental mosaicism is associated with a significant reduction in live-birth rate Fertil Steril, 2019, 111(1): 69-76.doi:10.1016/j.fertnstert.2018.08.057

[51] Victor A R, Tyndall J C, Brake A J, et al. One hundred mosaic embryos transferred prospectively in a single clinic: exploring when and why they result in healthy pregnancies Fertil Steril, 2019, 111(2): 280-293.doi:10.1016/j.fertnstert.2018.10.019

[52] Salvaggio C N, Forman E J, Garnsey H M, et al. Polar body based aneuploidy screening is poorly predictive of embryo ploidy and reproductive potential J Assist Reprod Genet, 2014, 31(9): 1221-1226.doi:10.1007/s10815-014-0293-1

[53] Fang R, Yang W, Zhao X, et al. Chromosome screening using culture medium of embryos fertilised in vitro: a pilot clinical study J Transl Med, 2019, 17(1): 73.doi:10.1186/s12967-019-1827-1

[54] D'alessandro A, Federica G, Palini S, et al. A mass spectrometry-based targeted metabolomics strategy of human blastocoele fluid: a promising tool in fertility research Mol Biosyst, 2012, 8(4): 953-958.doi:10.1039/c1mb05358b

[55] Magli M C, Pomante A, Cafueri G, et al. Preimplantation genetic testing: polar bodies, blastomeres, trophectoderm cells, or blastocoelic fluid? Fertil Steril, 2016, 105(3): 676-683 e675.doi:10.1016/j.fertnstert.2015.11.018

[56] Tsuiko O, Zhigalina D I, Jatsenko T, et al. Karyotype of the blastocoel fluid demonstrates low concordance with both trophectoderm and inner cell mass Fertil Steril, 2018, 109(6): 1127-1134 e1121.doi:10.1016/j.fertnstert.2018.02.008

[57] Gianaroli L, Magli M C, Pomante A, et al. Blastocentesis: a source of DNA for preimplantation genetic testing. Results from a pilot study Fertil Steril, 2014, 102 (6): 1692-1699 e1696.doi:10.1016/j.fertnstert.2014.08.021

[58] Tobler K J, Zhao Y, Ross R, et al. Blastocoel fluid from differentiated blastocysts harbors embryonic genomic material capable of a whole-genome

deoxyribonucleic acid amplification and comprehensive chromosome microarray analysis Fertil Steril, 2015, 104(2): 418-425.doi:10.1016/j.fertnstert.2015.04.028

[59] Capalbo A, Romanelli V, Patassini C, et al. Diagnostic efficacy of blastocoel fluid and spent media as sources of DNA for preimplantation genetic testing in standard clinical conditions Fertil Steril, 2018, 110(5): 870-879 e875.doi:10.1016/j.fertnstert.2018.05.031

[60] Magli M C, Albanese C, Crippa A, et al. Deoxyribonucleic acid detection in blastocoelic fluid: a new predictor of embryo ploidy and viable pregnancy Fertil Steril, 2019, 111(1): 77-85.doi:10.1016/j.fertnstert.2018.09.016

[61] Handyside A H. Noninvasive preimplantation genetic testing: dream or reality? Fertil Steril, 2016, 106(6): 1324-1325.doi:10.1016/j.fertnstert.2016.08.046

[62] Matassov D, Kagan T, Leblanc J, et al. Measurement of apoptosis by DNA fragmentation Methods Mol Biol, 2004, 282(1-17.doi:10.1385/1-59259-812-9:001

[63] Bolton H, Graham S J L, Van Der Aa N, et al. Mouse model of chromosome mosaicism reveals lineage-specific depletion of aneuploid cells and normal developmental potential Nature Communications, 2016, 7(1): 10.1038/ncomms11165

[64] Hammond E R, Mcgillivray B C, Wicker S M, et al. Characterizing nuclear and mitochondrial DNA in spent embryo culture media: genetic contamination identified Fertil Steril, 2017, 107(1): 220-228 e225.doi:10.1016/j.fertnstert.2016.10.015

Chapter 6

You Have a New Super Power: Ethics of Oocyte Cryopreservation

Leila Mohammadi, Silvia Martinez and Daniel Aranda

Abstract

This chapter will be an ethical analysis on challenging situations surrounding oocyte cryopreservation treatment in young healthy women. There has been always a complicated interaction between technology and changing societal values. This ethical discussion is not on whether or not oocyte cryopreservation in itself is ethically justifiable. Through a comprehensive literature review, this chapter discusses some ethical aspects that have emerged since oocyte cryopreservation was applied for the first time. Through a practical approach, this chapter address ethical uncertainties presenting case studies, ethical questions and terms, existing arguments in favor and against oocyte cryopreservation; and examine the individual patient's beliefs, perception and opinions.

Keywords: Egg freezing, Oocyte cryopreservation, Non-medical reason, Reproductive technology, Ethics

1. Introduction

Fertility preservation is a recent technology that provides the possibility to maintain reproductive ability to women who either face the risk of infertility for medical treatments or want to postpone childbearing for possible age-related fertility. The majority of users of Fertility Preservation technology are women who for cancer therapies receive chemo and radiotherapy that can cause infertility [1–3]. However, there are more conditions that required medical treatment can damage reproductive cells such as autoimmune diseases and myelodysplastic syndromes. Women affected by X trisomy, X-fragile, premature ovarian failure (POF) based on genetic origin as in Turner syndrome mosaicism, and syndrome, are another group that fertility preservation could help them [4]. Finally, the last group of women who can benefit from fertility preservation are those who wish to preserve and store oocytes for non-medical purposes. This procedure is called with various names such as elective egg freezing; social egg freezing, and planned oocyte cryopreservation also known as OC.

The first successful result of OC technique was a baby has born from a previously frozen oocyte in 1896, in the US [5]. Until 2012 OC has been classified as experimental by the ASRM but after a review of the scientific literature the Committee announced that the success rate of in vitro fertilization (IVF) using fresh eggs and frozen eggs are positively similar, so that they removed the experimental label from OC treatment. In addition, the existent studies about the health of babies born from frozen eggs did not prove a remarkable congenital anomalies raise when compared with other IVF babies [5]. However, while the ESHRE, ASRM and Ethics Committee approved the use of OC for Medical reasons (mostly patients affected by cancer therapies) [5, 6]. they declined the use of OC for healthy women who wish to avoid age related fertility decline for postpone the maternity (for social reasons). In spite of not being recommended OC for non-medical reasons because of insufficient data on "safety, efficacy, ethics, emotional risks, and cost-effectiveness" the number of women seeking OC for social reason as well as the numbers of clinics offering OC technique have been increasing [7–9].

One year after removing the experimental label from OC, ASRM published an article in their website in which they explained about how healthy women can benefit from OC technique to postpone childbearing [10]. This article declared that although this new medical technique is improving, it raises "ethical issues involving evaluation of evidence, balancing benefits and harms, supporting patient autonomy, avoiding conflict of interest, and promoting advances in health care" [10].

This chapter addresses the ethical issues that arise when OC is used by women whose goal is to protect their ability to have children in the future apart from an immediate threat from gonadotoxic therapy. This ethical discussion is not on whether or not oocyte cryopreservation in itself is ethically justifiable. Through a comprehensive literature review, this chapter argues some ethical uncertainties, ethical questions and terms, existing arguments in favor and against oocyte cryopreservation; and examine the individual patient's beliefs, perception and opinions.

2. Ethical uncertainties

The OC technology improvement itself was not the only reason for women's interest to postpone childbearing. In many countries, the number of women who defer childbearing to their thirties has been rising [11]. For decades, women have been having children at older ages due to substantial lifestyle changes worldwide. By 1970, the average age of the first childbirth increased to around thirty years old, which at that time was the last chance to try for motherhood. With increasing knowledge about women's reproduction and fertility, since 1980 more women started to have children at 40–45 years old [12, 13]. Among all the reasons that affected this social change, access to education and increasing participation at workplace were the most significant. Since for women the age range (20s and 30s) in which they can peruse their education and improve their social position is also the same period of being optimal fertile (20s and early 30s) and starting to weakening at late 30s [14].

Terms such as "postponing the maternity" or "delay childbearing" are often used, which refers to the idea that the most important women's duty "motherhood" is at risk and if they do not accomplish this responsibility they are blamed to be selfish and irresponsible [15]. While studies show that, many women face conflicts in their life because the optimal moment for educational and professional improvement coincides exactly with when their reproductive system is in its best condition. Other issues such as partnership and economic situation has been also reported as other barriers on women's path for childbearing at younger age. Many women who wanted to have children find themselves in an inacceptable economic condition or not having an adequate partner [16–19]. Finally, what seems like a delay might be a consequence of the extensive and continuous overestimation of female reproductive potential with age and the capacity of reproductive treatments to recover the potential [20].

Given these societal and personal reasons for late reproduction, a biological treatment emerges because the older women are the higher risk of failure to conceive as both the quantity and quality of the oocytes decreases, while chromosomal abnormalities causing fetal abnormalities increases. Men's age also affects fertility and offspring health, although not until men are older, age 40 or 50. For both men and women, the more time passes before they reproduce, the risk of some disorders, life circumstance, or accident may affect their fertility or abnormality in offspring.

Traditionally women, who wish to become a mother at younger ages, had the possibility to undergo IVF with donor oocytes, when they face oocyte quality problem or other diseases. Planned OC offers a further option for women in this condition, if they have previously stored their own oocytes, might help them to become mother. Compared with using donor oocytes, planned OC provides benefits such as genetically related with the off spring. Although planned OC ultimately will be ineffective in some percentage of cases, it will allow some women and couples who otherwise would have had to forego biological parenthood the chance to have genetically related children.

With this background, let us consider some of the ethical arguments in favor and against oocyte cryopreservation. A wide range of viewpoints on planned OC have been presented by researchers and commentators [21–27], while several commentators raise questions and concerns about planned OC, most conclude it should be available to women who are fully informed and wish to use it [24, 26].

2.1 Arguments supporting oocyte cryopreservation by healthy women

In 2012, the European Culture of Human Multiplication and Embryology (ESHRE) validated a plan to safeguard the richness of arranged OC [28]. The main advantage of planned OC is that it provides reproductive autonomy, by giving women greater number of reproductive options. There are several contributors to this argument. First, by giving women time to flourish in their education and careers, planned OC reduces the pressure of the 'ticking biological clock' and the pressure of having a child when the woman is not yet financially, emotionally, or situationally ready [17, 29–31]. Although all these factors are obvious benefits, recent research suggests that the lack of a partner is one of the main reasons a woman preserves her oocytes compared to other reasons [27, 32]. While oocyte freezing at a younger age gives the best chance to preserve oocyte quality, critics argue that an overreliance on genetic parenthood using this method might negatively impact and even stigmatize parents from pursuing other, more traditional options [15, 33].

The second strong argument for promoting planned OC is to give more control to women with regards to their preserved gametes compared to frozen embryos. In the case of embryos, which already has genes from the egg and the sperm, a divorce or separation could result in a partner retracting consent. This leads to additional difficulties on the clinical, emotional and legal front, which can be avoided by freezing individual gametes.

Thirdly, oocyte freezing is a more acceptable option for those who are not comfortable with preserving embryos due to moral and religious reasons [27, 34]. Indeed, some theologists trust ovarian cryopreservation and subsequent autologous transplantation later in life as morally acceptable because it does not rely on IVF for procreation [35]. Furthermore, women are allowed a possibility of having a genetically related child even if they do not have a partner when the oocytes are preserved. Hence, even though embryo cryopreservation is the more established procedure, women prefer oocyte preservation because of the independence it gives them from their partner [36].

It is to be noted that oocyte cryopreservation in this context is not performed in response to the onset of disease; rather, it is meant as protection against future infertility. The benefits of oocyte conservation by women are comparable to the cryopreservation of sperm by men, however, the costs, physical demands and the risks of the two procedures are completely different. Nevertheless, men face far less criticism when trying to preserve their future fertility compared to women [19].

A few authors note that planned OC may increase social justice by removing the obstacles that women face when planning for a family due to their shorter reproductive windows. Planned OC can minimize the burden of career and education that women face in their most fertile period and can extend their reproductive timeframe. Although this could significantly contribute to equality between men and women, this is currently not the case because of low uptake of the process in certain populations [19, 21, 28]. It is possible to postulate that women would feel and act equal to men if given the choice to extend their reproductive age. This could eventually mean women becoming mothers at 50 or 60 years of age, while currently they face biological constraints around the age of 40 [37].

Critics argue that advanced maternal age could be detrimental to children as older parents could have lesser energy to look after young children and might die before the children grow into young adults [31, 38]. However, preliminary data shows that most women actually plan on using their frozen oocytes in their 40s, and would rarely consider becoming parents in their 50s or 60s, mainly because of the higher risks to health that women face in advanced maternal age [30].

Interestingly, women who do become parents at an advanced age report that they have less pressures of establishing a career and more financial freedom, which gives them more time to focus on their family and enjoy parenthood [39]. Indeed, there is no conclusive evidence to show that younger mothers are better mothers, and more empirical data collected through longitudinal studies on children will help answer this. Nevertheless, a strong argument against older mothers is that women play important roles as grandmothers, and advanced maternal age would prevent children from enjoying social contact with their grandparents [38].

2.2 Arguments opposing oocyte cryopreservation by healthy women

A major hurdle in the advancement of routine oocyte cryopreservation is its safety [40], in addition to potential repercussions for future children and for mothers who choose pregnancy at older age. Several precautions should be taken, as there is a high level of uncertainty, with extra discretion applied when cryopreserving oocytes. There is currently not much data surrounding the harm to the health of children born from frozen oocytes, however; early reports suggest that these children do not have adverse health outcomes compared to children born without these interventions [41, 42].

Indeed, the Ethics Committee of the American Society for Reproductive Medicine lays out several arguments that planned OC is potentially safer than OC before gonadotoxic therapy in response to disease, because the patient is not already suffering from a serious disease nor are they delaying treatment due to fertility concerns [19]. Interestingly, ovarian hyperstimulation syndrome, the most common risk of OC, is actually decreased when the OC is planned because there is no embryo transfer once the stimulation cycle is finished. Additionally, it has been shown that the use of gonadotropin-releasing hormone agonist triggers can lead to a further reduction in the risk of ovarian hyperstimulation when they are used with gonadotropin releasing hormone antagonist cycles [43].

The committee hypothesizes that data on the long-term safety and efficacy of planned OC is not widely available because of the time involved in patients returning to use their cryopreserved oocytes and in the time it takes for the children derived from those oocytes to grow up. Additionally, the process of vitrification for easy cryopreservation was only recently adopted.

Another strong argument against the use of OC is the 'false hope' that the procedure might offer to women who are planning their future children [40]. Although the technique is undergoing significant advancements, live birth rates with cryopreserved oocytes are still low and this is difficult to predict before a pregnancy progresses. This, in addition to the fact that OC does not guarantee success for a future pregnancy, poses a significant risk for waste of resources both in terms of time and money [27, 44]. The emotional wellbeing of a woman is also under threat when she relies on this technique for her reproductive goals.

In all, the committee strongly believes that a woman must make an individual choice when it comes to using planned OC after assessing the risks involved and the benefits derived from the procedure. This 'false security blanket' issue is especially relevant when planned OC is thought of as an 'insurance policy' for women who want to bear children in the future, which can pose problems when women develop an overreliance on this technique for their reproductive goals. However, the concern of overreliance assumes without prior evidence that women will dismiss other available options such as reproduction or immediate marriage, just because of cryopreserving oocytes [15].

Education and informed consent are the best ways to address patient misunderstanding of the success rates of planned oocyte cryopreservation. Towards this, physicians and other healthcare professionals involved in the process must observe restraint when describing the technique to avoid giving false hope. However, when there is a risk of overreliance on any one method of conception, it is common for patients to struggle in their decision-making process. It is important to present appropriate medical counseling to these patients and it is imperative for the healthcare provider to place trust in the patients' capability to make an informed decision when all information is duly presented. Essentially, patient choice should not be removed because of physician bias in underestimating their capabilities. More research into this topic will be crucial to address these biases.

Current research is looking to address questions about the number of oocytes, classified by age and hormone levels, that are needed to have a higher chance of a successful pregnancy using those oocytes [45–47]. It is important that this data is relayed to patients. For instance, if a woman knows that when is 38 years old she needs to store 25–30 oocytes in order to stand a chance of having one child, she is better informed and not falsely over reliant on the procedure [47–49].

Another downside of planned OC are its costs, which are usually paid out-of-pocket by women, with multiple cycles adding to the expense even more [45]. As discussed previously, OC is sometimes the only option for women who undergo social freezing, and for couples who cannot undergo embryo freezing due to ethical and/or religious beliefs. There are also countries where embryo freezing is prohibited through legislation. Even though embryo freezing is typically covered by insurance providers, this is not the case for elective oocyte freezing. This is partly fuelled by the position of the ASRM, which still does not encourage oocyte cryopreservation for personal elective reasons but promotes OC for cancer and other medical indications by removing the term 'experimental procedure' from its recommendations [50].

In most of the western world, especially in Europe and the United States, the cost of a single cycle of egg freezing is between $10 000–15 000. Understandably, the procedure has faced a lot of criticism regarding the cost-effectiveness of the technique. Indeed, the costs are not only limited to the retrieval and storage of oocytes. After the patient decides to use the frozen oocytes, IVF needs to be used to promote embryo formation. Recent research suggests that direct IVF conception at the age of 40 years is more-cost effective when compared to cryopreserving oocytes at 35 years followed by IVF at 40 years [51, 52]. In contrast, another study that developed a cost-effectiveness algorithm shows that the highest cost–benefit is obtained when the oocytes are cryopreserved when women are 37 years of age [53].

Recent findings also suggest that only 10% of women who opted for planned OC for social reasons came back to use them for a pregnancy [54]. This indicates that the associated costs are not being realized in most cases. Elective oocyte banking does not come with the financial advantages of oocyte freezing for medical purposes, which are often discounted through compassionate donations from specialized pharmacies or are supported through organizations raising funds for cancer patients. Additionally, many countries do not recognize the right of a woman to reproduce through this method and view OC as an elective procedure similar to plastic surgery for cosmetic purposes rather than a medical necessity. The high costs associated with OC and IVF and these social restrictions contribute to women missing chances to safeguard their future fertility.

Although some large companies have started offering planned OC as a health benefit [55], they are still very few to make a difference in a majority of women's lives. Planned OC is likely an option only for a small percentage of women, which would result in the benefits of education, career and life-stability available only to these privileged women. Indeed, there are concerns raised about the inequitable societal consequences of planned OC.

The committee also discusses a related issue in its opinion on OC before gonadotoxic therapy – and suggested that a person cannot be denied having an offspring because of their potentially shortened lifespan because of disease. However, this does not mean women can carry pregnancies without concerns about maternal age. Several studies show that the mother and baby are at increased risk with an increase in the age of the pregnant woman [56–58].

Moreover, children may undergo psycho-social trauma as a result of having an older mother compared to traditional reproductive options [38, 44]. Women should be made aware of these risks when they consider cryopreserving their oocytes [59].

Next, it is important to hypothesize the social implications of planned OC if it were to become mainstream. Although generally thought of as increasing women's choices and giving reproductive freedom, it could reduce their reproductive autonomy by not giving importance to the social structures surrounding female biology [33, 38, 40]. Moreover, there is a risk of social expectations shifting to pressure women into freezing their eggs if they want to have biologically or genetically related children while pursuing a successful career [34]. Taken these into account, what first appeared as a way of empowering women to take control of their reproductive choices by giving them the freedom to pursue their dreams without the constraints of a biological clock could turn into a tool that unknowingly oppresses them [33]. This future would see women having less of a choice in their reproductive journeys, and would be socially compelled to become a parent later in life because they have the choice to do so, and in the worst case, would be expected to refrain from parenthood completely [34]. Although this seems extreme, societal structures have evolved around oppressing women before and this can happen again. For planned OC to work successfully, measures need to be in place to ensure that the reproductive autonomy of women is maintained while achieving equality, without relying on "medicalization", which is a tendency to seek medical answers to social problems [28].

Therefore, as noted by several ethicists, an important question to answer is 'who should be qualified to offer these services'? [60]. The amount of time, money, expectations and emotions that social freezing patients involved in the cryopreservation of gametes go through must be taken into consideration. Achievable standards need to be in place to guide organizations offering cryopreservation and those advertising such services. Indeed, OC has been marketed to healthy women for a few years, even though there are safety and efficacy concerns surrounding it [61].

Studies from Spain and USA report that many clinics fail to sufficiently educate clients for them to make a well-informed decision [61, 62].

Another concern raised with respect to planned OS is the uncertain ownership of the gamete. Human eggs have become widely sought-after in the assisted reproduction of infertile women, which has led to a market of women selling their own eggs to egg banks for money [63]. This system could exploit young women who are looking for ways to make money.

A related concern with planned OC and ownership relates to the disposition of gametes in the case of an accidental death or when the donor succumbs to a disease. An important question that should be addressed with patients is how the oocytes should be disposed of in case the biological owner dies. Although this issue is raised with patients that are undergoing fertility preservation for medical reasons such as cancer therapy, this should also be an important topic of discussion with patients that are preserving their oocytes for reasons that are not medical.

Additionally, ownership must also be made clear in cases where donors become ill or impaired cognitively that raises concerns over assisting them in their reproductive goals. Moreover, some women may not agree to policies that govern their ability to give their cryopreserved eggs to third parties or to donate it to research and teaching. Another point of interest is that ASRM does not support the use of frozen gametes for the donor's relatives if the donor dies, even if biological owner specially requests it [46]. This is, however, possible in some countries. Details of cryopreservation such as how long the frozen eggs can be used, and who uses these eggs need to be discussed at the time of consent; this also requires specific policies adopted by clinics and legislation.

Finally, a major hurdle facing OC, especially for patients cured by cancer is the morality of a child born to a mother who has a deadly disease. This can be categorized into four major concerns: shorter lifespan of the mother, a recurrence of the cancer or other medical conditions that will be detrimental to the mother's health, the health of children born to women who froze their oocytes after starting gonadotoxic treatment, and a genetic disposition of cancer from the mother carrying over to the child. Eventually, provisions must be made for parenting and financial responsibilities in case a single woman uses her cryopreserved oocytes at an older age or after treatment for a fatal disease.

3. Individual patient's beliefs, perception and opinions

The concept of freezing eggs as a potential method of preserving fertility has been analyzed from various viewpoints and social science disciplines. The profile of patients who would use this technology and their reasoning behind using it are all being explored [64–67], As shown previously, most women who want to freeze their eggs are single and already have a decline in their fertility and the amount of eggs [67]. They choose to freeze their eggs because of a variety of reasons, important among them the physical, economical, structural, and personal factors. Indeed, it was found that women chose to freeze eggs because of the absence of conditions crucial for pursuing motherhood, and not because of the presence of any dominant reasons [68]. Interestingly, there have been investigations into fertility preservation and the attitudes surrounding it in several countries [69–74]. The majority of studies point towards an increasing acceptance of these technology which correlates with an increase in knowledge about them [70, 72].

These studies indeed provide necessary insights into the attitudes of women towards specific aspects of the freezing process especially from medical and social viewpoints. Three major viewpoints of women regarding egg freezing is detailed below.

Owner of their life: This group of people identify women as being responsible for their own reproductive life, and is often associated with being a viewpoint that emphasizes an individual's choice without disturbances from outside factors. Although the right to reproduction is of utmost importance to these women, they are generally indifferent towards policies that intervene to facilitate being children at a younger age. This viewpoint assumes that egg freezing is a potential option for claiming their right to having a child.

Policy change requester: In this group of people, the predominant viewpoint is that assistant reproduction with technology is often unwarranted, especially for reasons that are not medical. It emphasizes on policies being enacted to ensure the wok-life balance of women. This viewpoint perceives policy chance as the only successful way of improving the conditions necessary to facilitate having a child and bringing them up.

Need for social information: This group of people need a debate on a societal scale. This point of view approves the use of egg freezing for both medical and non-medical purposes. The viewpoint encourages social debate to understand these questions in more detail and do not support the idea of a 'right' to have a child in this context. This viewpoint hence associates OC as a legitimate and responsible option to support socio-cultural changes and is not supportive of unnecessary regulatory intervention.

This final section details the challenges that assistive reproductive technologies face in the context of what is the traditional path to pursuing life and parenthood. For instance, women do not have access to infertility care or options for assistive reproductive technologies in several European countries [75].

Certainly, another important example is the utilization of parental leave. It is well established that men generally under-utilize parental leave while women take longer leaves of absence from work to care for young children. This also translates into more women with children switching to part-time work in order to facilitate the careers of men [76]. Although these balances and imbalances in family and career are acknowledged in all the viewpoints discussed above, it is perceived differently in all of them.

Viewpoint one focused on individual and autonomous choices with regards to fertility and did not care to venture into understanding policy interventions. Alternatively, viewpoint two was strongly in favor of restrictions placed on reproductive technologies with a preference for changing policies to facilitate good work-life balance. Finally, viewpoint three promoted social debate with respect to egg freezing, while disapproving regulatory interventions regarding the same. These varying viewpoints on who is responsible for their choices and how it should be regulated reflects on ideas of autonomy and maternalistic tendencies.

Indeed, the current standing of the authorities on the subject through a literature review suggests that it is important for a physician to prioritize autonomous choices compared to maternalistic tendencies [28]. However, it is important to note that viewpoints that favor these maternalistic attitudes often prevail.

Interestingly, there are several different perspectives on how egg freezing and gender equality are related. These different viewpoints suggest that freezing of eggs can be used a tool to eradicate gender inequality and the discrimination that women face. In fact, viewpoint three perceives egg freezing as a responsible choice keeping in line with changes in the socio-cultural landscape. This correlates well with the thoughts of Carroll [66], who framed this as "enacting responsible reproductive citizenship". However, despite these positive changes that egg freezing can be responsible for, it is imperative to not view it is as the solution for social injustices to women [31]. Understandably, it is important to not restrict access to egg freezing based on these debates; however, it is imperative that legislation and employers attempt to address the real reasons behind the need for delayed childbearing for working mothers [28].

Certainly, the literature suggests that it is the diversity of viewpoints surrounding egg freezing that is responsible for controversies compared to the technology of egg freezing itself. Women who decide to freeze their eggs not only deal with all the ethical issues surrounding this technology, but also have to deal with changing opinions and viewpoints on this practice in their daily life. Some of these include being pressured to freeze their eggs to be a "responsible citizen", an unrealistic understanding of the success rates of such procedures, and the stigma they face when faced with stereotypes in their environment [15, 77].

Therefore, it is important to understand that while egg freezing certainly holds benefits for women by relieving them from the pressure of the biological clock, it could be harmful in other ways by psychologically impacting their experience based on societal expectations [78]. These points need to be considered together when discussing egg freezing. It is also crucial to understand not only the opinion of women but also that of men and other groups of people who might contribute to further controversies in the decision-making process of a woman.

4. Discussion and conclusion

Several challenges that assistive reproductive technologies face stems from certain misconceptions regarding their use and a lack of understanding the power and limitation of these technologies. Adding to these challenges are dishonest marketing campaigns overestimating the success of these procedures, a difference in success rates in different clinics and a misunderstanding of the process involved in the procedures. There is an imminent need for oversight and regulation of this technology and marketing because enthusiastic entrepreneurs target women at cocktail parties and other informal events to convince them to "freeze their eggs" before it's too late, suggesting that "smart women freeze" and the others miss out. These statements and marketing strategies are ethically and morally unacceptable, especially when women are not provided the complete picture with regards to the costs, time and risks involved and the low success rates of the procedure which is typically not covered by insurance. Information such as the number of cycles to freeze enough eggs, the cost involved in each cycle of cryopreservation, including the medications and time involved, the cost of storage of eggs per year, the age-related decrease in success rates of the procedure, the cost of the use of future eggs with intracytoplasmic injection of the sperm, the risk to the women of ovarian hyperstimulation syndrome occurring as a result of ovarian stimulation and the side effects, and more importantly the chance that there will be no baby at the end of the risky procedure should all be communicated to the patient in clear terms to facilitate them making an informed decision. These discussions should also involve the fate of the gametes in case of death, disease, disability or if the donor decides to not personally use the gametes. Patients that are already confused with the options available to them will need to be guided into the system by developing trust and by portraying transparency through standardization of care. Otherwise, there is a risk that they will be further confused by the deluge of information available and might withdraw from options available to them. Finally, there is an urgent need for a change in the curriculum when training OB/GYN residents and primary care physicians to include information about fertility decline and the options available to couples and women. To eventually promote successful reproductive decision making in patients and to respect the rights of autonomous choices of women, it is important that OB/GYNs can provide the necessary knowledge for them to make an informed decision.

Conflict of interest

The authors declare no conflict of interest.

Author details

Leila Mohammadi*, Silvia Martinez and Daniel Aranda
Open University of Catalonia, Barcelona, Spain

*Address all correspondence to: limohammadi@uoc.edu

References

[1] Gidoni Y, Holzer H, Tulandi T, Tan SL. Fertility preservation in patients with non-oncological conditions. Reproductive biomedicine online. 2008 Jan 1;16(6):792-800. DOI: 10.1016/S1472-6483(10)60144-7

[2] Noyes N, Melzer K, Druckenmiller S, Fino ME, Smith M, Knopman JM. Experiences in fertility preservation: lessons learned to ensure that fertility and reproductive autonomy remain options for cancer survivors. Journal of assisted reproduction and genetics. 2013 Oct;30(10):1263-1270. DOI: 10.1007/s10815-013-0066-2

[3] Dolmans MM, Manavella DD. Recent advances in fertility preservation. Journal of Obstetrics and Gynaecology Research. 2019 Feb;45(2):266-279. DOI: 10.1111/jog.13818

[4] Gidoni Y, Holzer H, Tulandi T, Tan SL. Fertility preservation in patients with non-oncological conditions. Reproductive biomedicine online. 2008 Jan 1;16(6):792-800. DOI: 10.1016/S1472-6483(10)60144-7

[5] of the American TP. Mature oocyte cryopreservation: a guideline. Fertility and Sterility. 2013 Jan 1;99(1):37-43. 10.1016/j.fertnstert.2012.09.028

[6] Practice Committee of the American Society for Reproductive Medicine. Fertility preservation in patients undergoing gonadotoxic therapy or gonadectomy: a committee opinion. Fertility and Sterility. 2013 Nov 1;100(5):1214-1223. DOI: 10.1016/j.fertnstert.2013.08.012

[7] Goldman KN, Labella PA, Grifo JA, McCulloh D, Noyes N. The evolution of oocyte cryopreservation (OC): longitudinal trends at a single center. Fertility and Sterility. 2014 Sep 1;102(3):e164-e165. DOI: 10.1016/j.fertnstert.2014.07.563

[8] Mucowski SJ, Bendikson K, Paulson R, Chung K. Current utilization status of cryopreserved oocytes in the United States. Fertility and Sterility. 2014 Feb 1; DOI: 101(2):e31-2. 10.1016/j.fertnstert.2013.11.116

[9] Argyle CE, Harper JC, Davies MC. Oocyte cryopreservation: where are we now?. Human reproduction update. 2016 Jun 1;22(4):440-449. DOI: 10.1093/humupd/dmw007

[10] Ethics Committee of the American Society for Reproductive Medicine. Planned oocyte cryopreservation for women seeking to preserve future reproductive potential: an Ethics Committee opinion. Fertility and sterility. 2018 Nov 1;110(6):1022-1028. DOI: 10.1016/j.fertnstert.2018.08.027

[11] Jones B. Lord Winston labels egg freezing an 'expensive confidence trick'. BioNews. 2009 Jul;515.

[12] Mathews TJ, Hamilton BE. First births to older women continue to rise. US Department of Health and Human Services, Centers for Disease Control and Prevention, National Center for Health Statistics; 2014.

[13] Cedars MI. Introduction: childhood implications of parental aging. Fertility and sterility. 2015 Jun 1;103(6):1379-1380. DOI: 10.1016/j.fertnstert.2015.04.011

[14] CECOS Fédération, Schwartz D, Mayaux MJ. Female fecundity as a function of age: results of artificial insemination in 2193 nulliparous women with azoospermic husbands. New England Journal of Medicine. 1982 Feb 18;306(7):404-406. DOI: 10.1056/NEJM198202183060706

[15] Mertes H. The portrayal of healthy women requesting oocyte cryopreservation. Facts, views & vision

in ObGyn. 2013;5(2):141. https://www.ncbi.nlm.nih.gov/pmc/articles/PMC3987355/

[16] Barclay E. More women are freezing their eggs, but will they ever use them? NPR, November 25, 2015.

[17] Barritt J, Luna M, Sandler B, Duke M, Copperman AB. Elective oocyte freezing for the preservation of fertility. DOI: 10.4236/ojog.2012.21005

[18] Lemoine ME, Ravitsky V. Sleepwalking into infertility: the need for a public health approach toward advanced maternal age. The American journal of bioethics. 2015 Nov 2;15(11):37-48. DOI: 10.1080/15265161.2015.1088973

[19] Petropanagos A. Reproductive 'choice'and egg freezing. Oncofertility. 2010:223-235. DOI: 10.1007/978-1-4419-6518-9_17

[20] Goldman KN, Grifo JA. Elective oocyte cryopreservation for deferred childbearing. Current Opinion in Endocrinology, Diabetes and Obesity. 2016 Dec 1;23(6):458-464. DOI: 10.1097/MED.0000000000000291

[21] Goold I, Savulescu J. In favour of freezing eggs for non-medical reasons. Bioethics. 2009 Jan;23(1):47-58. DOI: 10.1111/j.1467-8519.2008.00679.x

[22] Cobo A, García-Velasco JA. Why all women should freeze their eggs. Current Opinion in Obstetrics and Gynecology. 2016 Jun 1;28(3):206-210. DOI: 10.1097/GCO.0000000000000269

[23] Petropanagos A, Cattapan A, Baylis F, Leader A. Social egg freezing: risk, benefits and other considerations. CMAJ. 2015 Jun 16;187(9):666-669. DOI: 10.1503/cmaj.141605

[24] Rabinowitz A. Why egg freezing is an impossible choice. Nautilus. 2015 Mar;22.

[25] Schattman GL. Cryopreservation of oocytes. New England Journal of Medicine. 2015 Oct 29;373(18):1755-1760. DOI: 10.1056/NEJMcp1307341

[26] Spar D. Should you freeze your eggs? Marie Claire 2015.

[27] Robertson JA. Egg freezing and egg banking: empowerment and alienation in assisted reproduction. Journal of Law and the Biosciences. 2014 Jun 1;1(2):113-136. DOI: 10.1093/jlb/lsu002

[28] Pennings G, ESHRE Task Force on Ethics and Law including, de Wert G, Shenfield F, Cohen J, Tarlatzis B, Devroey P. ESHRE Task Force on Ethics and Law 12: oocyte donation for non-reproductive purposes. Human Reproduction. 2007 May 1;22(5):1210-1213. DOI: 10.1093/humrep/dem025

[29] Bernstein S, Wiesemann C. Should postponing motherhood via "social freezing" be legally banned? An ethical analysis. Laws. 2014 Jun;3(2):282-300. DOI: 10.3390/laws3020282

[30] Gold E, Copperman K, Witkin G, Jones C, Copperman AB. P-187: a motivational assessment of women undergoing elective egg freezing for fertility preservation. Fertility and Sterility. 2006 Sep 1;86(3):S201. DOI: 10.1016/j.fertnstert.2006.07.537

[31] Harwood K. Egg freezing: a breakthrough for reproductive autonomy?. Bioethics. 2009 Jan;23(1):39-46. DOI: 10.1111/j.1467-8519.2008.00680.x

[32] Donnez J. Introduction: fertility preservation, from cancer to benign disease to social reasons: the challenge of the present decade. Fertility and sterility. 2013 May 1;99(6):1467-1468. DOI: 10.1016/j.fertnstert.2013.03.040

[33] Stoop D, van der Veen F, Deneyer M, Nekkebroeck J, Tournaye H. Oocyte banking for anticipated gamete

exhaustion (AGE) is a preventive intervention, neither social nor nonmedical. Reproductive biomedicine online. 2014 May 1;28(5):548-551. DOI: 10.1016/j.rbmo.2014.01.007

[34] Wunder D. Social freezing in Switzerland and worldwide--a blessing for women today?. Swiss medical weekly. 2013;143. https://serval.unil.ch/resource/serval:BIB_5CC0C719FF00.P001/REF.pdf

[35] ESHRE Task Force on Ethics and Law, including, Dondorp W, de Wert G, Pennings G, Shenfield F, Devroey P, Tarlatzis B, Barri P, Diedrich K. Oocyte cryopreservation for age-related fertility loss. Human reproduction. 2012 May 1;27(5):1231-1237. DOI: 10.1093/humrep/des029

[36] Peccatori FA, Azim HA, Orecchia R, Hoekstra HJ, Pavlidis N, Kesic V, Pentheroudakis G. Cancer, pregnancy and fertility: ESMO Clinical Practice Guidelines for diagnosis, treatment and follow-up. Annals of oncology. 2013 Oct 1;24:vi160-70. DOI: 10.1093/annonc/mdt199

[37] Sparrow R. Reproductive technologies, risk, enhancement and the value of genetic relatedness. Journal of medical ethics. 2014 Nov 1;40(11):741-743. DOI: 10.1136/medethics-2013-101807

[38] Pennings G, Mertes H. Ethical issues in infertility treatment. Best Practice & Research Clinical Obstetrics & Gynaecology. 2012 Dec 1;26(6):853-863. DOI: 10.1016/j.bpobgyn.2012.04.002

[39] Kennedy J. Yes, I froze my eggs, but am I a victim of a new fertility racket. The Guardian.[Cited 2015 Feb 18]. Available: http://www. theguardian.com/commentisfree/2014/oct/19/why-i-froze-my-eggs-at-such-a-cost. 2015.

[40] McDougall R. Systematic reviews in bioethics: types, challenges, and value. Journal of Medicine and Philosophy. 2014 Feb 1;39(1):89-97. DOI: 10.1093/jmp/jht059

[41] Lahdenperä M, Lummaa V, Helle S, Tremblay M, Russell AF. Fitness benefits of prolonged post-reproductive lifespan in women. Nature. 2004 Mar;428(6979):178-181. https://www.nature.com/articles/nature02367

[42] Johnston J, Zoll M. Is freezing your eggs dangerous. A primer. New Republic. 2014 Nov 1:1-5.

[43] Practice Committee of the American Society for Reproductive Medicine. Prevention and treatment of moderate and severe ovarian hyperstimulation syndrome: a guideline. Fertility and sterility. 2016 Dec 1;106(7):1634-1647. DOI: 10.1016/j.fertnstert.2016.08.048

[44] Noyes N, Porcu E, Borini A. Over 900 oocyte cryopreservation babies born with no apparent increase in congenital anomalies. Reproductive biomedicine online. 2009 Jan 1;18(6):769-776. DOI: 10.1016/S1472-6483(10)60025-9

[45] Devine K, Mumford SL, Goldman KN, Hodes-Wertz B, Druckenmiller S, Propst AM, Noyes N. Baby budgeting: oocyte cryopreservation in women delaying reproduction can reduce cost per live birth. Fertility and sterility. 2015 Jun 1;103(6):1446-1453. DOI: 10.1016/j.fertnstert.2015.02.029

[46] Mesen TB, Mersereau JE, Kane JB, Steiner AZ. Optimal timing for elective egg freezing. Fertility and sterility. 2015 Jun 1;103(6):1551-1556. DOI: 10.1016/j.fertnstert.2015.03.002

[47] Goldman RH, Racowsky C, Farland LV, Munné S, Ribustello L, Fox JH. Predicting the likelihood of live birth for elective oocyte cryopreservation: a counseling tool for physicians and patients. Human

reproduction. 2017 Apr 1;32(4):853-859. DOI: 10.1093/humrep/dex008

[48] Doyle JO, Richter KS, Lim J, Stillman RJ, Graham JR, Tucker MJ. Successful elective and medically indicated oocyte vitrification and warming for autologous in vitro fertilization, with predicted birth probabilities for fertility preservation according to number of cryopreserved oocytes and age at retrieval. Fertility and sterility. 2016 Feb 1;105(2):459-466. DOI: 10.1016/j.fertnstert.2015.10.026

[49] Allen R. Is egg freezing only for white women. New York Times. 2016 May;21.

[50] Hodes-Wertz B, Druckenmiller S, Smith M, Noyes N. What do reproductive-age women who undergo oocyte cryopreservation think about the process as a means to preserve fertility?. Fertility and sterility. 2013 Nov 1;100(5):1343-1349. DOI: 10.1016/j.fertnstert.2013.07.201

[51] Rebar RW. Social and ethical implications of fertility preservation. Fertility and sterility. 2016 Jun 1;105(6):1449-1451. DOI: 10.1016/j.fertnstert.2016.02.002

[52] Pfeifer S, Gldberg J, McClure R, Lobo R, Thomas M, Widra E. Practice committees of American Society for Reproductive Medicine; society for assisted reproductive technology. Mature oocyte cryopreservation: a guideline. Fertil Steril. 2013;99(1):37-43.

[53] van Loendersloot LL, Moolenaar LM, Mol BW, Repping S, van der Veen F, Goddijn M. Expanding reproductive lifespan: a cost-effectiveness study on oocyte freezing. Human reproduction. 2011 Nov 1;26(11):3054-3060. DOI: 10.1093/humrep/der284

[54] Linkeviciute A, Peccatori FA, Sanchini V, Boniolo G. Oocyte cryopreservation beyond cancer: tools for ethical reflection. Journal of assisted reproduction and genetics. 2015 Aug;32(8):1211-1220. DOI: 10.1007/s10815-015-0524-0

[55] Mertes H. Does company-sponsored egg freezing promote or confine women's reproductive autonomy?. Journal of assisted reproduction and genetics. 2015 Aug;32(8):1205-1209. DOI: 10.1007/s10815-015-0500-8

[56] Sauer MV. Reproduction at an advanced maternal age and maternal health. Fertility and sterility. 2015 May 1;103(5):1136-1143. DOI: 10.1016/j.fertnstert.2015.03.004

[57] Nekkebroeck J, Stoop D, Devroey P. O-036 A preliminary profile of women opting for oocyte cryopreservation for non-medical reasons. Human Reproduction. 2010 Jun;25 (20100600). https://oce.ovid.com/article/00004683-201006001-00043/HTML

[58] von Wolff M, Germeyer A, Nawroth F. Fertility preservation for non-medical reasons: controversial, but increasingly common. Deutsches ärzteblatt international. 2015 Jan;112(3):27. https://www.ncbi.nlm.nih.gov/pmc/articles/PMC4321210/

[59] Ethics Committee of the American Society for Reproductive Medicine. Oocyte or embryo donation to women of advanced reproductive age: an Ethics Committee opinion. Fertility and sterility. 2016 Oct 1;106(5):e3-e7. DOI: 10.1016/j.fertnstert.2016.07.002

[60] Stoop D, Maes E, Polyzos NP, Verheyen G, Tournaye H, Nekkebroeck J. Does oocyte banking for anticipated gamete exhaustion influence future relational and reproductive choices? A follow-up of bankers and non-bankers. Human reproduction. 2015 Feb 1;30(2):338-344. DOI: 10.1093/humrep/deu317

[61] Provoost V, Tilleman K, D'Angelo A, De Sutter P, de Wert G, Nelen W, Pennings G, Shenfield F, Dondorp W. Beyond the dichotomy: a tool for distinguishing between experimental, innovative and established treatment. Human Reproduction. 2014 Mar 1;29(3):413-417. DOI: 10.1093/humrep/det463

[62] Jackson S, Hong C, Wang ET, Alexander C, Gregory KD, Pisarska MD. Pregnancy outcomes in very advanced maternal age pregnancies: the impact of assisted reproductive technology. Fertility and sterility. 2015 Jan 1;103(1):76-80. DOI: 10.1016/j.fertnstert.2014.09.037

[63] Hirshfeld-Cytron J, Van Loendersloot LL, Mol BW, Goddijn M, Grobman WA, Moolenaar LM, Milad MP. Cost-effective analysis of oocyte cryopreservation: stunning similarities but differences remain. Human reproduction. 2012 Dec 1;27(12):3639-. DOI: 10.1093/humrep/des343

[64] Inhorn MC, Birenbaum-Carmeli D, Birger J, Westphal LM, Doyle J, Gleicher N, Meirow D, Dirnfeld M, Seidman D, Kahane A, Patrizio P. Elective egg freezing and its underlying socio-demography: a binational analysis with global implications. Reproductive Biology and Endocrinology. 2018 Dec;16(1):1-1. DOI: 10.1186/s12958-018-0389-z

[65] Kılıç A, Göçmen İ. Fate, morals and rational calculations: freezing eggs for non-medical reasons in Turkey. Social Science & Medicine. 2018 Apr 1;203:19-27. DOI: 10.1016/j.socscimed.2018.03.014

[66] Carroll K, Kroløkke C. Freezing for love: enacting 'responsible'reproductive citizenship through egg freezing. Culture, health & sexuality. 2018 Sep 2;20(9):992-1005. DOI: 10.1080/13691058.2017.1404643

[67] Gürtin ZB, Morgan L, O'Rourke D, Wang J, Ahuja K. For whom the egg thaws: insights from an analysis of 10 years of frozen egg thaw data from two UK clinics, 2008-2017. Journal of assisted reproduction and genetics. 2019 Jun;36(6):1069-1080. DOI: 10.1007/s10815-019-01429-6

[68] Mohammadi L, Aranda D, Martínez-Martínez S. The narratives of fertility clinic's websites in Spain. Profesional de la Información. 2019 Mar 8;28(2). DOI: 10.3145/epi.2019.mar.19

[69] Wennberg AL, Rodriguez-Wallberg KA, Milsom I, Brännström M. Attitudes towards new assisted reproductive technologies in Sweden: a survey in women 30-39 years of age. Acta obstetricia et gynecologica Scandinavica. 2016 Jan;95(1):38-44. DOI: 10.1111/aogs.12781

[70] Stoop D, Nekkebroeck J, Devroey P. A survey on the intentions and attitudes towards oocyte cryopreservation for non-medical reasons among women of reproductive age. Human Reproduction. 2011 Mar 1;26(3):655-661. DOI: 10.1093/humrep/deq367

[71] de Groot M, Dancet E, Repping S, Goddijn M, Stoop D, van der Veen F, Gerrits T. Perceptions of oocyte banking from women intending to circumvent age-related fertility decline. Acta obstetricia et gynecologica Scandinavica. 2016 Dec;95(12):1396-1401. DOI: 10.1111/aogs.13019

[72] O'Brien Y, Martyn F, Glover LE, Wingfield MB. What women want? A scoping survey on women's knowledge, attitudes and behaviours towards ovarian reserve testing and egg freezing. European Journal of Obstetrics & Gynecology and Reproductive Biology. 2017 Oct 1;217:71-76. DOI: 10.1016/j.ejogrb.2017.08.024

[73] Tozzo P, Fassina A, Nespeca P, Spigarolo G, Caenazzo L.

Understanding social oocyte freezing in Italy: a scoping survey on university female students' awareness and attitudes. Life sciences, society and policy. 2019 Dec;15(1):1-4. DOI: 10.1186/s40504-019-0092-7

[74] Schick M, Sexty R, Ditzen B, Wischmann T. Attitudes towards social oocyte freezing from a socio-cultural perspective. Geburtshilfe und Frauenheilkunde. 2017 Jul;77(7):747. https://www.ncbi.nlm.nih.gov/pmc/articles/PMC5514017/

[75] FMedRÄG. BGBl. 2015.

[76] im Gesundheitswesen O. Bundesministerium für Arbeit, Soziales, Gesundheit und Konsumentenschutz.

[77] Martin LJ. Anticipating infertility: Egg freezing, genetic preservation, and risk. Gender & Society. 2010 Aug;24(4):526-545. DOI: 10.1177/0891243210377172

[78] Mertes H. Egg banking in anticipation of age-related fertility decline: using medical technology for better, not for worse (Doctoral dissertation, Ghent University). https://biblio.ugent.be/publication/8522913/file/8522914

Chapter 7

Efficiency of Autologous Egg Cryopreservation: Eight Years' Experiences and Clinical Outcomes

Cassie T. Wang, Xiangli Niu, Qiuyan Ruan and Wei-Hua Wang

Abstract

Oocyte cryopreservation is one of the state-of-art technologies in human reproductive medicine, which brings opportunities for women to preserve their fertility. In the present study, we analyzed the efficiency and outcomes of 8 years' autologous egg cryopreservation: Frozen oocytes were warmed from 120 cycles and oocyte survival, fertilization, blastocyst development, clinical pregnancy, embryo implantation, live birth rates and birth weights were collected based on the patients' ages of <35, 35–37 and > 37 years old. The details of oocyte cryopreservation and the efficiency were further analyzed based on different patient categories. During the study period, 849 oocytes from 120 cycles were warmed. Oocyte survival, fertilization, and blastocyst development were not affected by women's ages at the time of cryopreservation. However, number of patients without blastocyst formation was significantly ($P < 0.05$) higher in patients >37 years old (31.2%) than that in patients <35 years old (13.1%). Higher live birth rates were observed in patients <35 (51.1%) and 35–37 (46.7%) years old than in patients >37 years old (28.6%) after fresh embryo transfer. Some patients did not have blastocysts mainly due to low fertilization by poor sperm or small number of oocytes warmed. These results indicate that the efficiency of oocyte cryopreservation, evaluated by live birth and embryo implantation rates is affected by women's age, number of oocytes warmed and sperm quality.

Keywords: Oocyte cryopreservation, Fertility preservation, Fresh embryo transfer, Frozen embryo transfer, Implantation

1. Introduction

Oocyte cryopreservation is one of the state-of-art technologies in human assisted reproductive technologies (ART), which provides opportunities for women to preserve their fertility. Recently, the demand for oocyte cryopreservation has increased significantly, especially in women who want to delay childbearing for medical or no medial indications [1–9].

It has been reported that survival, fertilization, embryo development and pregnancy rates of cryopreserved/warmed human oocytes are similar to those of fresh oocytes, especially in young women and oocyte donors [10, 11]. The rates of chromosomal abnormalities (embryonic aneuploidies), birth defects, or developmental deficits in offspring born from cryopreserved oocyte in vitro fertilization (IVF) were similar with those from fresh oocyte IVF [12]. However, fewer blastocysts were observed when cryopreserved oocytes were used for IVF as compared with fresh oocytes in patients who used autologous oocytes [13]. Furthermore, large clinical data reported by the Society for Assisted Reproductive Technology (SART) in USA indicated that fresh donor oocytes produced significantly higher live birth rate than cryopreserved donor oocytes [14] and the equivalency between fresh and cryopreserved oocytes still need more data to support [15].

As a new technology in human IVF, oocyte cryopreservation is still a challenge for IVF laboratories as it adds more laboratory manipulations on oocytes including cryopreservation and warming. Furthermore, the optimal time for oocytes to be cryopreserved after retrieval and for oocytes to be inseminated after warming may be different between patients. Therefore, differences in laboratory protocols may make the efficiency different and a case-specific protocol may be necessary to obtain the best outcome. More information remains to be collected whether oocyte cryopreservation will be widely offered to healthy women at any age as an approach to preserve fertility and delay childbirth [16, 17].

More women would like to give birth in their late 30s [4, 18]. However, women's fertility dramatically declines when they reach their late 30s, and further declines in their early 40s [4]. This phenomenon increases the demand for women to preserve their fertility by oocyte cryopreservation before their fertility declines [4, 18]. Although fertility preservation could benefit women who have hematologic diseases, breast cancer, some pelvic cancers and systematic diseases requiring chemotherapy, radiotherapy or bone marrow transplantation [2, 3, 19, 20], most users of this technology are healthy women who want to postpone childbearing [2, 3, 7, 8, 17, 18, 21, 22].

On the other hand, oocyte cryopreservation is offered not only to women for fertility preservation [7, 8, 21–23], it has also been offered to donor banks [24, 25], IVF patients as a backup technology. For example, in cases where semen sample may not be available on oocyte retrieval day, no motile sperm found in a semen sample, or there are not enough motile sperm for insemination of all oocytes retrieved. Some patients may produce a high number of oocytes and do not want to inseminate all, and some patients may want a limited number of oocytes to be fertilized [23]. Therefore, oocyte cryopreservation is required under various situations. Accordingly, the analysis of efficiency of clinical outcomes with cryopreserved oocytes becomes difficult.

The efficiency of human oocyte cryopreservation has been widely studied in donor oocytes and most data were collected from fresh embryo transfer [10, 11, 14, 15]. However, as preimplantation genetic testing for aneuploidies (PGT-A) and other genetic testing are very common in human IVF, it is required that biopsied embryos for testing are cryopreserved for later frozen embryo transfer (FET). Although cryopreservation by vitrification of human embryos from fresh oocytes does not affect embryo implantation [26–28], there is still no published evidence to address whether cryopreservation of embryos from frozen/warmed oocytes disturb embryo implantation or these embryos have a similar implantation as fresh embryos. Therefore, in the present study, we compared fresh blastocyst transfer and frozen/warmed blastocyst transfer to examine whether double cryopreservation (both oocyte and blastocyst cryopreservation) has a similar efficiency as single cryopreservation (oocyte cryopreservation) based on women's ages at the time of oocyte cryopreservation.

2. Methods

2.1 Ethics approval and consent to participate

All patients undergoing oocyte cryopreservation, warming for IVF, embryo culture, and embryo transfer signed informed consents for all laboratory and clinical procedures. All procedures were approved by Houston Fertility Institute's research and clinical committee. The data were retrospectively collected from the medical records and patients' information were not included in the data presentation, so the IRB was waived for this study.

2.2 Patients and data collection

Autologous oocyte cryopreservation was assessed in women whose oocyte cryopreservation and warming were performed between 2009 and 2017. Women's age at the time of oocyte cryopreservation was divided into 3 groups, <35, 35–37 and > 37 years old. Based on these age groups, data were compared between fresh blastocyst transfer and frozen/warmed blastocyst transfer.

There were mainly three reasons for patients to cryopreserve their oocytes: 1) all oocytes were cryopreserved because there was no motile sperm or no semen sample being collected at the time of oocyte retrieval; 2) partial oocytes were cryopreserved because no enough motile sperm was found to inseminate all of the oocytes, or patients required to inseminate a portion of oocytes and purposely required to cryopreserve remaining oocytes; and 3) all oocytes were cryopreserved for single women for fertility preservation. Therefore, the data were further analyzed based on these three categories.

2.3 Oocyte cryopreservation, warming and insemination

Oocyte cryopreservation and warming were based on the procedures previously reported [11] by using commercial vitrification and warming kits (Fujifilm-Irvine Scientific, CA, USA). Briefly, for cryopreservation, matured oocytes were vitrified 4–5 hours after retrieval with initial equilibration of the oocytes in equilibration solution (ES) for 9 mins, and then in vitrification solution (VS) for 90 seconds until vitrification in Cryotop.

For warming, Cryotops were removed from liquid nitrogen and the tips with oocytes were quickly placed in 1 ml thawing solution (TS) at 37°C for 1 min. Oocytes were then transferred to 0.5 ml dilution solution (DS) for 3 min and then to a 0.5 ml washing solution (WS) for 10 min with a solution change after 5 min. After warming, oocytes were washed in Global medium (IVFonline, CT, USA) supplemented with 10% serum protein substitute (SPS, IVFonline) and then cultured in the same medium until insemination. Oocyte survival was evaluated based on morphology after completion of the warming.

2.4 Insemination, fertilization assessment, embryo culture and fresh blastocyst transfer

All oocytes were inseminated by intracytoplasmic sperm injection (ICSI) 2–3 hours after warming. We chose this time for ICSI as it has been reported that most functions, such as meiotic spindle recovery, mitochondria activity and ATP level recovery in frozen/warmed oocytes, take about 2–3 hours after warming [29–31] and it has been found that ICSI time (9 ± 2 h) after oocyte retrieval in the vitrified human oocytes does not affect clinical outcomes [32].

Fertilization was examined 16–18 h after ICSI and normally fertilized zygotes were cultured in Global medium supplemented with 10% SPS at 37°C in a humidified atmosphere of 5.5% CO_2, 6% O_2 and balanced nitrogen until Day 7 (some patients' embryo culture was extended to Day 7 if morula or early blastocysts were observed at Day 6). On Day 3, embryo cleavage status was examined, and all embryos that divided to two cells and above were considered as cleaved embryos and were transferred to freshly prepared culture medium. On Day 5, embryo development was evaluated and the best 1 or 2 embryos were transferred.

2.5 Blastocyst biopsy for PGT-A

Blastocysts were biopsied at Days 5, 6 and 7 for PGT-A in some patients based on patients' requests and FET were performed in these patients if there were euploid blastocysts. After biopsy, blastocysts were vitrified individually, and biopsied samples were analyzed with DNA microarray or next generation sequencing by commercial genetic testing companies.

2.6 Blastocyst vitrification, warming and transfer

Blastocysts were vitrified and warmed using commercial vitrification and warming kits (Fujifilm-Irvine Scientific). For vitrification, both ES and VS were warmed in original vials at 37°C for at least 30 min before use. Briefly, collapsed blastocysts by a laser pulse were equilibrated in 100 µl drop (without oil cover) of ES for 2 min, and then 45 seconds in 100 µl drop (without oil cover) of VS (both steps were performed on a 37°C warming stage) before loading to vitrification devices. The devices were then immersed to liquid nitrogen for vitrification and all samples were stored in liquid nitrogen until warming for FET.

For warming, blastocysts were exposed to a TS at 37°C for 1 min, transferred to a DS for 3 min and finally to a WS for 10 min with a solution change after 5 min at room temperature. After completion of the warming process, blastocysts were cultured in Global medium supplemented with 10% SPS for 2–4 h before transfer. For blastocyst transfer, we selected the best quality of blastocyst for transfer regardless of Day 5, 6 or 7. However, if the blastocysts had the same quality, Day 5 blastocyst is preferred than Days 6 and 7 blastocysts. If embryos after PGT-A were transferred, we used same embryo selection criteria but only euploid blastocysts were transferred.

2.7 Patient preparation for fresh and frozen/warmed blastocyst transfer

All patients for embryo transfer received estradiol orally and transvaginally. Intramuscular administration of progesterone oil was initiated at about Day 14 of estradiol treatment. Endometrium thickness was measured on the day of progesterone administration. Embryo transfer occurred on the sixth or seventh day of progesterone administration and progesterone was continued until the first serum β-hCG test two weeks after transfer. Pregnancy was assessed 14 days after embryo transfer by a serum β-hCG assay. When the β-hCG was >5 mIU/ml, the patients were regarded as having a biochemical pregnancy and pregnancies were supported by continued estradiol and progesterone. Four weeks after embryo transfer, when a gestational sac and a heartbeat appeared ultrasonographically, the patients were diagnosed as having a clinical pregnancy. Live birth rates were calculated based on healthy baby delivery per transfer.

2.8 Statistical analysis

Interval data was analyzed by one-way analysis of ANOVA. The differences between groups were compared with chi square test. If the P value was less 0.05, the difference was considered to be statistically significant.

3. Results

As shown in **Figure 1**, 849 oocytes from 120 patients were warmed, 61 cycles were from women <35 years old, 27 cycles were from women 35–37 years old, and 32 cycles were from women >37 years old. The resulting blastocysts were either fresh transfer (74 cycles) at Day 5 or cryopreserved at Day 5–7 (23 cycles) for later FET Twenty-two patients had frozen all blastocysts due to PGT-A, and one patient (45 years old) had plan for fresh blastocyst transfer but did not have blastocyst at Day 5, so blastocyst transfer was canceled. However, one embryo developed to blastocyst at Day 7, so it was frozen and then processed for frozen/warmed blastocyst transfer.

A total of 67 blastocysts from 22 patients were biopsied and 55.2% (37) blastocysts were euploid after PGT-A. Euploid blastocysts in 16 patients and a Day 7 blastocyst without PGT-A in 1 patient were transferred in FET cycles.

Twenty-three cycles did not have embryo transfer due to no blastocyst formation, including no fertilization, no cleavage or arrested embryo development before blastocyst stage.

Women's ages at the time of oocyte cryopreservation on post-warming outcomes were shown in **Table 1**. It was found that average numbers of oocytes warmed

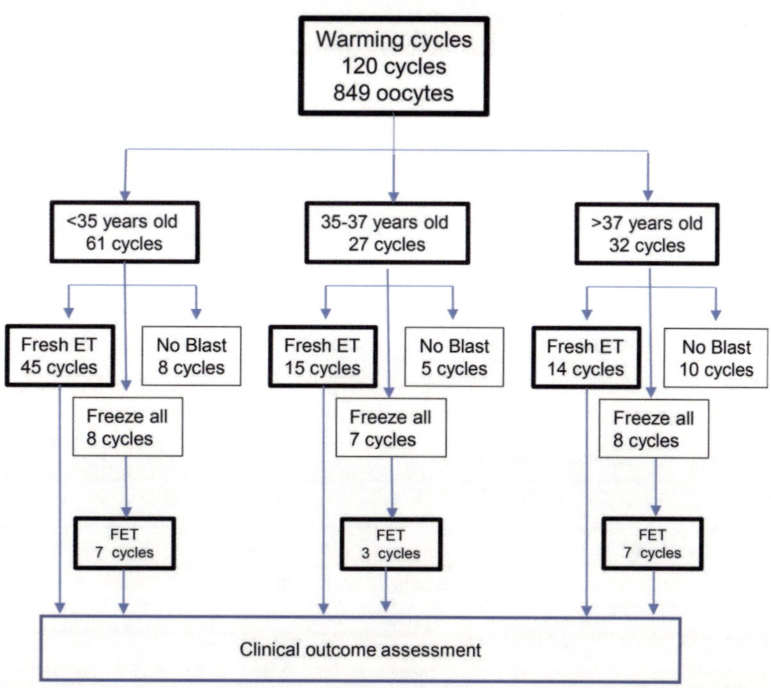

Figure 1.
Diagram of patient population and cycle information. Patients were grouped based on ages of <35, 35–37 or > 37 years old at the time of oocyte cryopreservation. Only the first embryo transfer (either fresh or FET) was included in the data analysis.

Age	<35	35–37	>37
Cases	61	27	32
No. of oocytes warmed	439	195	215
Mean No. of oocytes	7.2 ± 6.0	7.2 ± 5.5	6.7 ± 3.7
No. of oocytes survived (%)	410 (93.4)	177 (90.8)	204 (94.9)
No. of oocytes fertilized (%)	292 (71.2)	128 (72.3)	149 (73.0)
No. of oocytes cleaved (%)	278 (95.2)	118 (92.2)	140 (94.0)
No. of blastocysts (%)	158 (56.8)	64 (54.2)	69 (49.3)
No. of patients without blastocysts (%)*	8 (13.1)[a]	5 (18.5)	10 (31.2)[b]

No. of patients without blastocysts includes all cases in which oocytes were not fertilized after ICSI, fertilized oocytes did not cleave, and cleaved embryos did not develop to blastocyst stage.
[ab]*Values are significantly different with different superscripts in the same row, $P < 0.05$.*

Table 1.
Women's ages at the time of oocyte cryopreservation on post-warming laboratory outcomes.

(7.2 ± 6.0, 7.2 ± 5.5 and 6.7 ± 3.7, respectively), proportions of oocytes survived (93.4, 90.8 and 94.9%, respectively), fertilized (71.2, 72.3 and 73.0%, respectively), cleaved (95.2, 92.2 and 94.0%, respectively) and developed to blastocysts (56.8, 54.2 and 49.3%, respectively) were similar ($P > 0.05$) among patients <35, 35–37 and > 37 years old. However, cancelation rates, which were determined by no available blastocyst for transfer were significantly ($P < 0.05$) higher in patients >37 years old (31.2%) than in patients <35 years old (13.1%).

As significant differences in the cancelation rates were present in the three age groups, we further analyzed the detailed reasons of the cancelation. As shown in **Table 2**, it was found that oocyte survival after warming did not cause any cancelation, and all patients had survived oocytes after warming. However, cancelation was observed in 30.4% (7/23) patients without fertilization after ICSI, in 8.7%

Age	<35	35–37	>37	Total
No. of cases with no survived oocyte after warming (%)	0 (0)	0 (0)	0 (0)	0 (0)
No. of cases with no fertilization after ICSI (%)	5 (62.5)	1 (20)	1 (10)	7 (30.4)
No. of cases with no cleavage after fertilization (%)	0 (0)	1 (20)	1 (10)	2 (8.7)
No. of cases with no blastocyst (%)	3 (37.5)	3 (60)	8 (80)	14 (60.9)

No statistical differences were found between different age groups, $P > 0.05$.

Table 2.
Detailed reason analysis of patients without blastocysts.*

No. of oocytes warmed	Patients' age			Total
	<35	35–37	>37	
1–3	4 (50)	1 (20)	3 (30)	8 (34.8)
4–8	3 (37.5)	4 (80)	5 (50)	12 (52.1)
>8	1 (12.5)	0 (0)	2 (20)	3 (13.0)

No statistical differences were found between different age groups, $P > 0.05$.

Table 3.
Relationship between number of oocytes warmed and no blastocyst formation.*

(2/23) patients without embryo cleavage and in 60.9% (14/23) patients without blastocyst development that was the main reason of cancelation. However, no statistical differences were found among three age groups.

Age	<35	35–37	>37
No. of transfer	45	15	14
No. of clinical pregnancy (%)	24 (53.3)	7 (46.7)	6 (42.9)
Mean No. of embryos transferred	1.6 ± 0.6	1.8 ± 0.5	1.71 ± 0.47
Implantation rate (%)	39.2	29.6	25.0
No. of live birth (%)	23 (51.1)	7 (46.7)	4 (28.6)
Mean birth weight (g)	3037 ± 805	3462 ± 674	2856 ± 516

$^{*}P > 0.05$ in all comparison groups within the same age group between transfers (only fresh embryo transfers were compared).

Table 4.
Women's ages at the time of oocyte cryopreservation on post-warming clinical outcomes.*

Patient categories	All oocyte freezing (No motile sperm & no sperm)*	Partial oocyte freezing**	All oocyte freezing for fertility preservation***
No. of cases	37	67	16
Age	35.5 ± 5.7	33.4 ± 4.5	36.8 ± 3.7
No. of oocytes warmed	363	336	150
Mean No. of oocytes warmed	9.8 ± 5.8^{a}	5.0 ± 3.7^{b}	9.4 ± 4.4^{a}
No. of oocyte survived (%)	339 (93.4)	307 (91.3)	145 (96.7)
No. of oocyte fertilized (%)	$251\ (74.0)^{ab}$	$207\ (67.4)^{b}$	$111\ (76.6)^{a}$
No. of oocyte cleaved (%)	235 (93.6)	194 (93.7)	107 (96.4)
No. of blastocysts (%)	132 (56.2)	112 (57.7)	47 (43.9)
No. of cancelation (%)	5 (13.5)	14 (21.8)	4 (8.7)
No. of transfers	32	50	9
Mean No. embryos transferred	1.4 ± 0.8	1.6 ± 0.5	1.7 ± 0.5
No. of clinical pregnancy (%)	$17\ (53.1)^{ab}$	$18\ (36)^{b}$	$8\ (88.9)^{a}$
No. of live birth (%)	$15\ (46.9)^{ab}$	$18\ (36)^{b}$	$7\ (77.8)^{a}$
Implantation rate (%)	$21/53\ (39.6)^{ab}$	$21/79\ (26.6)^{a}$	$11/15\ (73.3)^{b}$

$^{ab}P < 0.05$ at least in the same row with different superscripts.
**Semen samples were not able to collect or samples did not have motile sperm, all oocytes were frozen.*
***Semen sample had motile sperm but sperm number was not enough to fertilize all of the oocytes or patients wanted to fertilize partial oocytes and to freeze the remaining oocytes.*
****All oocytes were frozen for fertility preservation.*

Table 5.
Patient categories for oocyte cryopreservation and clinical outcomes.

As shown in **Table 3**, when oocyte number (1–3, 4–8 and > 8 oocytes per warming cycle) and cancelation were analyzed, it was found that no blastocyst formation was found in all groups: 34.8% with 1–3 oocytes, 52.1% with 4–8 oocytes and 13.0% with >8 oocytes. There is increased tendency that less cancelation was observed if more than 8 oocytes were warmed. However, no statistical differences were found among three age groups or three oocyte number groups.

As shown in **Table 4**, when fresh blastocyst transfers were compared in terms of clinical pregnancy, mean no. of embryo transferred, embryo implantation, live birth and birth weight in three age groups, there were no statistical difference be observed although the rates were lower in the patients at age of >37. FET cases in each age group were small (7, 3 and 7 cases for age of <35, 35–37 and > 37, respectively), the clinical pregnancies (2, 2 and 2 cases, respectively) and live births (2, 2 and 2 cases, respectively) were not included in the comparisons.

When the data were analyzed based on three categories of patients for oocyte cryopreservation, as shown in **Table 5**, it was found that the number of oocytes warmed and reasons for oocyte cryopreservation had significant impact on clinical outcomes. The patients who had partial oocyte cryopreservation had significantly ($P < 0.05$) fewer oocytes to be warmed (5.0 ± 3.7) as comparing with patients who had all oocyte cryopreservation, including patients for backup oocyte cryopreservation (9.8 ± 5.8) and women for fertility preservation (9.4 ± 4.4). There was no statistical difference in the oocyte survival (91.3–96.7%) among three categories, however, significantly ($P < 0.05$) lower rates in fertilization (67.4 vs. 76.6%), clinical pregnancy (36.0 vs. 88.9%), live birth (36.0 vs. 77.8%) and embryo implantation (26.6 vs. 73.3%) were observed in patients with partial oocyte cryopreservation as compared with women for fertility preservation. Other comparisons, including women's age, cleavage, blastocyst formation, cancelation, and mean no. of embryos transferred in all groups did not show statistical differences.

4. Discussion

It has been demonstrated that oocyte cryopreservation does not compromise in vitro development and pregnancy rates as compared with fresh oocytes [1, 9–12]. Because of its reliability and efficiency, oocyte cryopreservation allows young cancer patients to have their oocytes collected prior to the initiation of chemo- or radiotherapy for the treatment of various malignant diseases, with the expectation of having their oocytes fertilized after recovery [2, 3, 19, 20]. It also would permit healthy women to have their oocytes collected and preserved for use in the future [4, 7, 8, 16–18] and for donor oocyte bank establishment [24, 25, 33].

It has been found that live birth rate was reduced significantly in women >37 years old after fresh oocyte IVF and the reduced live birth rate was mainly caused by embryonic aneuploidies [34–37]. Therefore, women's age at the time of oocyte cryopreservation is the most important factor affecting live birth rates. Present and previous data [3, 9, 16–18] suggest that women should preserve their oocytes before 37 years old if they plan to rely on oocyte cryopreservation to have a live birth. However, for the women who are more than 37 years old, it is still possible to have their oocytes to be cryopreserved for future use, but success mainly relies on oocyte quality and number [3, 9, 13].

In the present study, when we analyzed the efficiency of oocyte cryopreservation in women at different age groups, we found that live birth rates can reach to 51.1, 46.7 and 28.6% in women <35, 35–37, and > 37 years old, respectively, with their first embryo transfer (fresh), which is comparable to live birth rates with embryo transfer from fresh oocytes in our clinic or other published data [2, 3, 9, 23, 25]. A decreased tendency in live birth rate was observed in women >37 years as compared with women ≤37 years old. This is true because embryo quality (competence to develop to blastocysts and chromosome status) decreases when women reach >37 years old [37, 38]. Even when high quality blastocysts were transferred, embryo implantation rates also dropped, which eventually reduced live birth rates. Furthermore, morphological assessment of embryos does not always choose chromosomally normal embryos, thus high miscarriage rates were found in this population [35, 36]. In the present study, most patients had fresh blastocyst transfer without PGT-A. Actually frozen/warmed euploid blastocyst transfer after PGT-A did not further increase embryo implantation in all age groups in the present study. Similar outcomes have recently been found when embryos (with or without PGT-A) from fresh oocytes were transferred [39, 40], especially the benefits of PGT-A were not found in patients <37 years old. However, large data analysis of pregnancy outcomes in women aged 35–40 years demonstrated a significant improvement in clinical pregnancy rate and live birth rate with the use of PGT-A per embryo transfer [41]. Thus, it is difficult to explain the differences between reports.

Cancelation is very common in human ART, especially in poorly responding and/or older patients. In the present study, we cultured all embryos to Days 5–7 to allow embryos to develop to blastocyst stage and found that more patients >37 years old had to cancel embryo transfer due to lack of blastocyst development than patients <35 years old, and this indicates that oocyte quality in older patients are poorer than that in young patients. Although number of oocytes is also a reason for cancelation of a cycle, oocyte quality may be the main reason. Other factors should also be considered as the reasons for cancelation. For example, some canceled cycles had previous failed IVF cycles with the same cohort of fresh oocytes or had failed cycles due to severe male factor infertility. From laboratory results, it was found that no fertilization (mainly due to male factor infertility) and no embryo cleavage also caused cycle cancelation. Therefore, the reason(s) for cycle cancelation is complicated and multiple factors should be considered to explain the cause of failed blastocyst development.

Blastocyst transfer has been one of the most practical embryo selection strategies in human ART [42, 43], which could reduce number of embryos to be transferred and multiple pregnancy [43–45]. Our clinic has adopted blastocyst transfer for all patients, even in patients with a limited number of oocytes. However, we still do not know if pregnancy can be improved by early-stage embryo transfer for oocyte warming cycles. As some fertilized oocytes (as high as 10%) did not cleave during the culture, it is unknown whether embryo development arrest can be overcome by transferring early stage of embryos to uterus. It would also be possible that embryo arrest is caused by damages of some intra-oocyte structures during oocyte cryopreservation and warming, as embryo arrest is less than 1% in human IVF with fresh oocytes in our laboratory. Thus, current oocyte cryopreservation and warming technology needs further improving.

In the present study, we also found that average birth weight and proportions of babies with low birth weight after fresh embryo transfer were comparative to average weight of babies from fresh oocytes [42, 45, 46]. However, low birth weight was observed in babies from frozen/warmed blastocyst transfer in the present study although there are no statistical differences as compared with babies from fresh blastocyst transfer. This is certainly different from those with fresh oocyte IVF in which birth weights were higher in babies from FET than babies from fresh embryo transfer [47]. Because this is the first time that we noticed the difference in birth weight between fresh blastocyst transfer and frozen/warmed blastocyst transfer from frozen/warmed oocytes and the case number is also very limited, further data collection is necessary to reveal whether low birth weight after transfer of frozen/warmed blastocysts resulting from frozen/warmed oocytes is a common phenomenon.

Oocyte cryopreservation has been widely provided to women for various purposes. In the present study, we found that the efficiency was different among three different patient categories. Women used oocyte cryopreservation as fertility preservation had higher live birth rate as compared with patients who initially underwent infertility treatment. For infertility patients, live birth rates between partial oocyte cryopreservation/warming and all oocyte cryopreservation/warming were not significantly different although fewer oocytes had less opportunity to have a live birth, which was similar as that predicted by other researchers [3], especially when cumulated live birth rates were calculated [9].

However, for patient own oocytes, there are many factors, such as age and ovarian and hormone status. Some patients with oocyte cryopreservation may be due to lack of (enough) sperm for insemination, thus the time for oocyte cryopreservation may be delayed (after insemination of partial oocytes or after waiting for attempt of sperm collection). Occyte cryopreservation is usually performed 3–5 h after egg retrieval [2, 9, 11], thus it is still unknown whether delayed cryopreservation affects oocyte survival, fertilization, and embryo development. We did not examine these factors in the present study because the case numbers are very small in each category. For these patients, male factor infertility may also affect oocyte fertilization and embryo development and implantation.

We found that embryo development is slower with frozen oocytes as compared with fresh oocytes. Recently, Cobo et al. used time-lapse scope to track oocyte fertilization and embryo development, they found that pronuclear formation is about 1 h delayed in frozen oocytes as compared with fresh oocytes [48]. We also found that Day 5 blastocyst rates were lower but overall blastocyst rates (Days 5–7) were same between fresh and frozen donor oocytes in a previous study [11, 49].

A comprehensive analysis should be done whether an oocyte warming cycle can eventually result in a live birth. Many factors, such as oocyte quality, numbers of oocytes warmed, previous IVF outcomes, male factor infertility and others, should be carefully evaluated because women will rely on cryopreserved oocyte IVF to have a live birth in the future. It should be realized that if a fresh oocyte IVF cycle fails (no embryo available for transfer after IVF or no live birth after embryo transfer), the patients can attempt the second or more cycles to achieve a live birth. However, if an oocyte warming cycle fails to have a live birth, it may be too late for the patients to attempt the second or more oocyte retrieval cycles, especially when women use oocyte cryopreservation as their fertility preservation.

5. Conclusions

In conclusion, many factors affect the successful application of oocyte cryopreservation for women who want to preserve their fertility. Women's age at the time of oocyte cryopreservation is one of the most important factors to consider. Based on our current and previously published data, we can conclude that oocyte cryopreservation for fertility preservation can be done at any time during a woman's reproductive age. Similar as fresh oocyte IVF, the overall efficiency of oocyte cryopreservation is dependent up on women's age and reproductive health at the time of oocyte cryopreservation.

Conflict of interests

The authors declare that they have no conflict of interests.

Author details

Cassie T. Wang[1], Xiangli Niu[2], Qiuyan Ruan[2] and Wei-Hua Wang[1]*

1 Prelude-Houston Fertility Laboratory, Houston, TX, USA

2 Research Center for Reproductive Medicine, Reproductive Hospital of Guangxi Zhuang Autonomous Region, Nanning, Guangxi, China

*Address all correspondence to: wangweihua11@yahoo.com

References

[1] Crawford S, Boulet SL, Kawwass JF, Jamieson DJ, Kissin DM. Cryopreserved oocyte versus fresh oocyte assisted reproductive technology cycles, United States, 2013. Fertil Steril. 2017; 107:110-118.

[2] Garcia-Velasco JA, Domingo J, Cobo A, Martínez M, Carmona L, Pellicer A. Five years' experience using oocyte vitrification to preserve fertility for medical and nonmedical indications. Fertil Steril. 2013; 99:1994-9.

[3] Doyle JO, Richter KS, Lim J, Stillman RJ, Graham JR, Tucker MJ. Successful elective and medically indicated oocyte vitrification and warming for autologous in vitro fertilization, with predicted birth probabilities for fertility preservation according to number of cryopreserved oocytes and age at retrieval. Fertil Steril. 2016; 105:459-66.e2.

[4] Stoop D, Cobo A, Silber S. Fertility preservation for age-related fertility decline. The Lancet. 2014; 384:1311-1319.

[5] Rybak EA, Lieman HJ. Egg freezing, procreative liberty, and ICSI: the double standards confronting elective self-donation of oocytes. Fertil Steril. 2009; 92:1509-1512.

[6] Sunde A, Balaban B. The assisted reproductive technology laboratory: toward evidence-based practice? Fertil Steril. 2013; 100:310-318.

[7] Mertes H, Pennings, G. Social oocyte freezing: For better, not for worse. Reprod Biomed Online. 2011; 23:824-829.

[8] Cobo A, García-Velasco JA. Why all women should freeze their eggs. Curr Opin Obstet Gynecol. 2016; 28:206-210.

[9] Cobo A, García-Velasco JA, Coello A, Domingo J, Pellicer A, Remohí J. Oocyte vitrification as an efficient option for elective fertility preservation. Fertil Steril. 2016; 105:755-64.e8.

[10] Cobo A, Kuwayama M, Pérez S, Ruiz A, Pellicer A, Remohí J. Comparison of concomitant outcome achieved with fresh and cryopreserved donor oocytes vitrified by the Cryotop method. Fertil Steril. 2008; 89: 1657-1664.

[11] Wang CT, Liang L, Witz C, Williams D, Griffith J, Skorupski J, Haddad G, Gill J, Wang W. Optimized protocol for cryopreservation of human eggs improves developmental competence and implantation of resulting embryos. J Ovarian Res. 2013; 6:15.

[12] Mature oocyte cryopreservation: A guideline. Fertil Steril. 2013; 99:37-43.

[13] Goldman KN, Noyes NL, Knopman JM, McCaffrey C, Grifo JA. Oocyte efficiency: does live birth rate differ when analyzing cryopreserved and fresh oocytes on a per-oocyte basis? Fertil Steril. 2013; 100:712-717.

[14] Kushnir VA, Darmon SK, Barad DH, Gleicher N. New national outcome data on fresh versus cryopreserved donor oocytes. J Ovarian Res. 2018; 11:2.

[15] Kushnir VA, Gleicher N. Fresh versus cryopreserved oocyte donation. Curr Opin Endocrinol Diabetes Obes. 2016; 23:451-457.

[16] Eleanor L. Stevenson M, Hurt J, Trotter KJ. Oocyte cryopreservation for fertility preservation in healthy women. Nursing for Women's Health. 2017; 21:384-393.

[17] Dondorp WJ, De Wert GM. Fertility preservation for healthy women: ethical aspects. Hum Reprod. 2009; 24:1779-1785.

[18] Mesen TB, Mersereau JE, Kane JB, Steiner AZ. Optimal timing for elective egg freezing. Fertil Steril. 2015; 103:1551-1556.

[19] Ethics Committee of the American Society for Reproductive Medicine. Fertility preservation and reproduction in cancer patients. Fertil Steril. 2005; 83:1622-1628.

[20] Meirow, D. Reproduction post-chemotherapy in young cancer patients. Mol Cell Endocrinol. 2000; 169:123-131.

[21] Goold I, Savulescu J. In favor of freezing oocytes for non-medical reasons. Bioethics. 2009; 23:47-58.

[22] Goldman, K.N. and Grifo, J.A. Elective oocyte preservation for deferred childbearing. Curr Opin Endocrinol Diabetes Obes. 2016; 23:458-464.

[23] Cobo A, García-Velasco JA, Coello A, Domingo J, Pellicer A, Remohí J. Oocyte vitrification as an efficient option for elective fertility preservation. Fertil Steril. 2016; 105:755-764.

[24] Graham J, Lim J, Tucker M. Establishing an oocyte cryobank network. Methods Mol Biol. 2017; 1568:195-203.

[25] Domingues TS, Aquino AP, Barros B, Mazetto R, Nicolielo M, Kimati CM, Devecchi T, Bonetti TCS, Serafini PC, Motta ELA. Egg donation of vitrified oocytes bank produces similar pregnancy rates by blastocyst transfer when compared to fresh cycle. J Assist Reprod Genet. 2017; 34:1553-1557.

[26] Liebermann J. Vitrification of human blastocysts: an update. Reprod Biomed Online. 2009; 19 Suppl 4:4328.

[27] Roy TK, Bradley CK, Bowman MC, McArthur SJ. Single-embryo transfer of vitrified-warmed blastocysts yields equivalent live-birth rates and improved neonatal outcomes compared with fresh transfers. Fertil Steril. 2014; 1025:1294-1301.

[28] Wong KM, Mastenbroek S, Repping S.Cryopreservation of human embryos and its contribution to in vitro fertilization success rates. Fertil Steril. 2014;102:19-26.

[29] Ciotti PM, Porcu E, Notarangelo L, Magrini O, Bazzocchi A, Venturoli S. Meiotic spindle recovery is faster in vitrification of human oocytes compared to slow freezing Fertil Steril. 2009; 91:2399-2407.

[30] Manipalviratn S, Tong ZB, Stegmann B, Widra E, Carter J, DeCherney A. September Time course of human oocyte ATP recovery after vitrification and thawing. Fertil Steril. 2008; 90: Suppl S272.

[31] Chen C, Han S, Liu W, Wang Y, Huang G. Effect of vitrification on mitochondrial membrane potential in human metaphase II oocytes. J Assist Reprod Genet. 2012; 29:1045-1050.

[32] Bárcena P, Rodríguez M, Obradors A, Vernaeve V, Vassena R. Should we worry about the clock? Relationship between time to ICSI and reproductive outcomes in cycles with fresh and vitrified oocytes. Hum Reprod. 2016; 31:1182-1191.

[33] Quaas AM, Pennings G. The current status of oocyte banks: domestic and international perspectives. Fertil Steril. 2018; 110:1203-1208.

[34] Harton GL, Munné S, Surrey M, Grifo J, Kaplan B, McCulloh DH, Griffin DK, Wells D; PGD Practitioners Group. Diminished effect of maternal age on implantation after preimplantation genetic diagnosis with array comparative genomic hybridization. Fertil Steril. 2013; 100:1695-1703.

[35] Taranissi M, El-Toukhy T, Gorgy A. Verlinsky Y. Influence of maternal age on the outcome of PGD for aneuploidy screening in patients with recurrent implantation failure. Reprod Biomed Online. 2005; 10:628-632.

[36] Franasiak JM, Forman EJ, Hong KH, Werner MD, Upham KM, Treff NR, Scott RT Jr. The nature of aneuploidy with increasing age of the female partner: a review of 15,169 consecutive trophectoderm biopsies evaluated with comprehensive chromosomal screening. Fertil Steril. 2014; 101:656-663.

[37] Platteau P, Staessen C, Michiels A, Van Steirteghem A, Liebaers I, Devroey P. Preimplantation genetic diagnosis for aneuploidy screening in women older than 37 years. Fertil Steril. 2005; 84:319-324.

[38] Bettio D, Venci A, Levi Setti PE. Chromosomal abnormalities in miscarriages after different assisted reproduction procedures. Placenta. 2008; 29:126-128.

[39] Munné S, Kaplan B, Frattarelli JL, Child T, Nakhuda G, Shamma FN, Silverberg K, Kalista T, Handyside AH, Katz-Jaffe M, Wells D, Gordon T, Stock-Myer S, Willman S. STAR Study Group. Preimplantation genetic testing for aneuploidy versus morphology as selection criteria for single frozen-thawed embryo transfer in good-prognosis patients: a multicenter randomized clinical trial. Fertil Steril. 2019; 112:1071-1079.

[40] Kang HJ, Melnick AP, Joshua D. Stewart JD, Xu KP, Rosenwaks Z. Preimplantation genetic screening: who benefits? Fertil Steril. 2016;106: 597-602.

[41] Society for Assisted Reproductive Technology. SART national summary report: final CSR for 2016. https://www.sartcorsonline.com/rptCSR_Public MultYear. aspx?reportingYear=2016.

[42] Sunderam S, Kissin DM, Zhang Y, Folger SG, Boulet SL, Warner L, Callaghan WM, Barfield WD. Assisted Reproductive Technology Surveillance-United States, 2016. MMWR Surveill Summ. 2019; 68:1-23.

[43] Pandian Z, Templeton A, Serour G, Bhattacharya S. Number of embryos for transfer after IVF and ICSI: A Cochrane review. Hum Reprod. 2005; 20: 2681-2687.

[44] Maheshwari A, Hamilton M, Bhattacharya S. Should we be promoting embryo transfer at blastocyst stage? Reprod Biomed Online. 2016; 32:142-146.

[45] Litzky JF, Boulet SL, Esfandiari N, Zhang Y, Kissin DM, Theiler RN, Marsit CJ. Birthweight in infants conceived through in vitro fertilization following blastocyst or cleavage-stage embryo transfer: a national registry study. J Assist Reprod Genet. 2018; 35:1027-1037.

[46] Noyes N, Porcu E, Borini A. Over 900 oocyte cryopreservation babies born with no apparent increase in congenital anomalies. Reprod Biomed Online. 2009; 18:769-776.

[47] Spijkers S, Lens JW, Schats R, Lambalk CB. Fresh and frozen-thawed embryo transfer compared to natural conception: Differences in Perinatal Outcome Gynecol Obstet Invest. 2017; 82:538-546.

[48] Cobo A, Coello A, Remohí J, Serrano J, de Los Santos JM, Meseguer M. Effect of oocyte vitrification on embryo quality: time-lapse analysis and morphokinetic evaluation. Fertil Steril. 2017; 108:491-497.

[49] Niu X, Wang CT, Li R, Haddad G, Wang W. Is day 7 culture necessary for in vitro fertilization of cryopreserved/warmed human oocytes? Reprod Biol Endocrinol. 2020 Jan 18;18(1):4. doi: 10.1186/s12958-020-0565-9.

Chapter 8

Understanding Male Infertility for Promising ART

Mahrukh Hameed Zargar, Faisel Ahmad, Mohammad Lateef and Tahir Mohiuddin Malla

Abstract

Infertility is a serious problem of not being able to conceive despite regular intercourse for more than a year. Natural conception is seen to be achieved in 80%–85% of couples. About 15% of couples suffer infertility with male factor contributing to almost 50% of cases. Paradoxically, on traditional assessment, the underlying etiology of male contribution towards infertility remains unrecognized in 30% of the patients and thereby grouped as idiopathic. Diagnostics of male infertility cannot therefore be limited to usual semen analysis only. The spectrum of the recent research encourages the experts in the field to approach the Clinical, Molecular and cytogenetic shades associated with the problem besides secondary factors like life style and environment. Clinical assessment sums the medical history and physical examination of the affected individual. Molecular and cytogenetic analysis help gain new insights in understanding the problem and thereby an advantage for a successful assisted reproductive treatment (ART). Given the cost and burden ART puts in and prior to application of any invasive techniques, understanding precisely the etiology associated with male infertility is essential for the fertility specialist to circumvent inefficient or any unproductive steps in the fertilization process besides helping in counseling patients on their chance of success with the use of reproductive technology.

Keywords: Male infertility, Assisted reproduction, xenobiotics, oxidative stress

1. Introduction

Male infertility is a multifactor problem, the sensitivity of the infertility plus the relative paucity of information around male infertility gravitate scientific senses to think and extensively explore the aetiologies associated with it [1]. To bring the underlying causes to surface one can approach the problem viz-a-viz many different contours- Clinical examination, Molecular analysis and cytogenetic assays, life style and environmental factors. While standard Clinical assessment sums the medical history and physical examination of the affected individual, Molecular analysis help gain new insights in understanding the problem and thereby a boon in diagnosis [2]. Cytogenetic version that aims to provide the karyotype spectrum of idiopathic infertile men precisely provides lead in efficient counseling of couples and further gaining the mileage in reproductive assistance [3]. Important to mention here that apart from the aforementioned three factors, available data in literature provide evidences of environmental factors playing an instrumental role in male infertility, the natural and synthetic chemicals after interacting with endocrine system disturb fertility of men [3]. With the advance of industrial revolution, Fifty years down the li ne has seen a mushroom growth of chemical industries in developed and developing countries both. All this has finally resulted in the excessive release of xenobiotics into the environment [4]. Male reproductive system is very sensitive to these factors (environmental) that impair the fertility. Factors related to life style such as smoking, temperature and alcohol also prove detrimental to male fertility [4]. Oxidative Stress (OS) has an important role to play in human reproduction. It arises mainly due to excessive ROS production or impaired antioxidants defense mechanism [5].

To squeeze the width of obscurity associated with male infertility and to further infiltrate deep in possibility of finding compatibility of causes in resolving the issue at assisted reproductive level, the experts of the field have to imperatively rely on finding the spots that are even remotely linked to the infertility [6]. All this necessitates the investigation that spans between the congenital, acquired and idiopathic factors contributing to the infertility. The research thereby cannot be limited to routine investigations that include the semen analysis, hormonal profile and usual physical examination.

Looking at this escalating problem from the standard semen analysis, males are being considered as unproductive while failing to meet the standard WHO parameters, Apart from the possible aetiologies in the likes of oligospermia (low sperm concentration), asthenospermia (low sperm motility) and teratospermia, (distorted morphology), semen analysis also rules out the possibility of underprivileged semen as the cause of failure of sperm capacitation that ultimately leads to infertility [7]. One study at the reproduction Biology laboratory from the university Hospital of the Marseille (France) carried between 1988 and 2007, incorporated the semen analysis of 10932 male partners of infertile couples figured the declining trends in sperm concentration (1.5% /year). Data further mentions the decline in sperm count (1.6%/year), total motility (0.4%/year), rapid motility (5.5%/year) [7]. In gaining the understanding of infertility, routine examination subscribes to the findings that traverses between the cryptorchidism (uni or bilateral), testicular trauma, genitourinary infections, gonad toxic medication that includes the anabolic drugs, exposure to radiations involving both occupational as well as therapeutics, testicular torsions, anorchia, gynaecomastia, abnormal testicular volume and varicocele. In evaluation of hormonal profile, men with testicular deficiencies show hypergonadotrophic hypogonadism, increased levels of follicle stimulating (FSH) and luteinising hormone (LH) with low levels of testosterone. All these play havoc on the normal development of spermatogonia thereby prove very detrimental to the reproductive health of men [8].

2. Clinical factors and male infertility

Anatomical disorders distract the ability of man to produce viable sperms. Fertility centres regularly work with the specialists to diagnose the anatomical causes responsible for Male infertility [8]. Some of the common forms of anatomical factors include.

2.1 Varicocele

The anatomical issues can surface as varicocele, a condition in which the enlargement of testicular veins adversely affects the sperm quality and production. In certain cases varicocele can even impair the development of testicles. Varicocele can lead to the increased state of the temperature of testes and thereby causes the reflux of metabolites (toxic) of adrenal vein to the left kidney [9]. It is reported that 40 percent of infertile men have varicocele being diagnosed as the primary reason of the ailment.

2.2 Obstruction

Tube blockage is one more reason for the infertility in men. Obstruction in the tubes that pave way to the passage of sperm from the testicle to penis can have underlying causes like previous infections, pelvic surgeries, and cystic fibrosis associated with it. In case a severe duct obstruction is found, patients are advised to undergo the invasive procedure like transurethral resection to pave way for the normal course of ejaculate besides proving very important for the maintenance of sperm parameters [10].

2.3 Erectile dysfunction

Most prevalent reason for erectile dysfunction includes neurovascular problems, or psychological factors [11]. The main symptom involves the inability to keep an erection firm enough for intercourse. Though, most men experience difficulty in keeping the erection but erectile dysfunction is only considered a concern if it impairs the satisfactory sexual performance [11]. Erectile dysfunction is usually caused by anxiety, fatigue, or consumption of alcohol [12]. Drugs like sildenafil are used to raise the blood flow to the penis to aid the cause of the erection [13]. Possible causes include the tapering of penis blood vessels, increased blood pressure, raised cholesterol, hormonal issues or even the side effects of the other prescribed medicines.

2.4 Hypospadiasis

Another problem associated with the infertile men is hypospadiasis. More common in infants with a family history for hypospadiasis [14]. It is a condition of opening of penis on the underside rather than the tip. Hypospadasis is a birth defect with urethral opening on the underside of the penis instead of being terminal [15]. Early symptoms of hypospadiasis can be the downward curve of the penis (chordee), baby may spray while urinating. The appearance of hooded penis with only the top half of the penis being covered with foreskin [16]. Hypospadiasis affects one of every 250 male at birth. Hypospadiasis can be glandular, cornal, distal penile,proximal,scrotal or even perineal [17] (**Figure 1**).

2.5 Orchitis

Orchitis is a condition of the inflammation of the testicles. It can affect one or both the testicles. Common cause of orchitis can be a bacteria or a virus, most often the underlying cause is the bacterial infection (Sexually Transmitted Infection) [18]. Mumps virus can also be the reason of orchitis. Bacterial infection is more commonly seen in patients struggling with epididymitis on the hind end of testicle intended for the storage and passage of the sperms (epididymo- architis) [19].

2.6 Cryptorchidism

Crptorchidism is a serious developmental disorder while in either one or both the testes fail to descend into the scrotum from abdomen [19]. It is the most common defect of the male reproductive tract pooled in the scientific literature. Almost

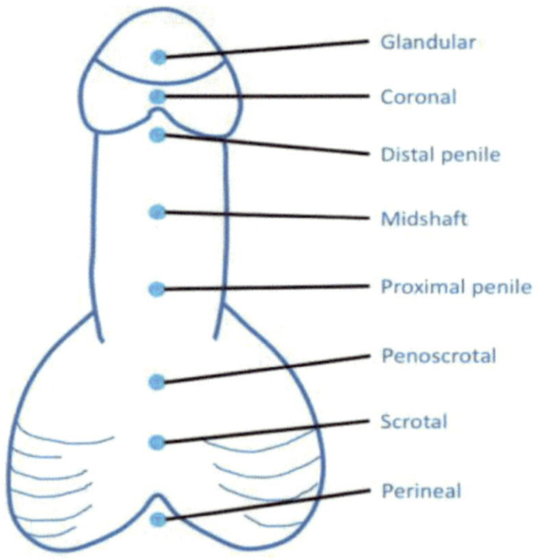

Figure 1.
Hypospadiasis. Image source, Charles G Macias, 2015 (International journal of pediartics endocrinology).

3% of full term and 30% of premature infant boys have been reported to born with at least one undescended testis. Absent testis from usual scrotal position can be present anywhere along the path of the descent, in the inguinal canal, ectopic, hypo plastic or dysgenetic.

2.7 Bilateral congenital anorchia

Congenital anorchia often called as prepubertal castrate or vanishing testis syndrome. It is a condition with one or both testes absent in the otherwise normal male (phenotypically and genotypically) [20]. The prevalence of bilateral congenital anorchia is reported to be 1 in 20,000 and that of unilateral congenital anorchia being 1in 5000 males. Anorchia is a case of absence of testicular tissue, monorchia a condition in which only one testis is absent and polyorchia although exceedingly rare refers to the presence of one or more supernumerary testis.

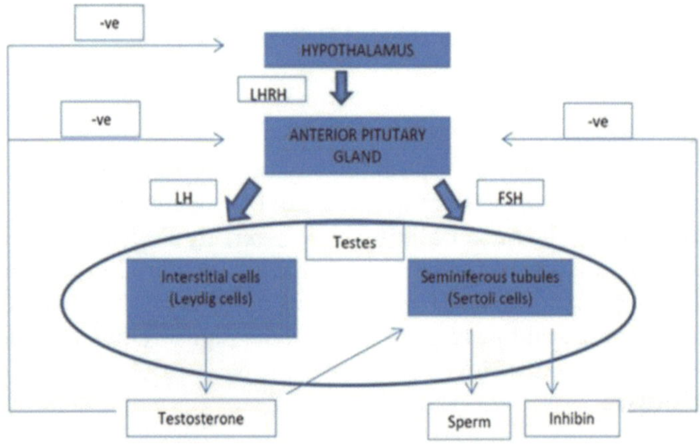

Figure 2.
The hormonal role in reproductive development. https://www.urologynews.uk.com/features/features/post/male-infertility.

2.8 Hormonal defects

The reproductive hormone axis of males often called as hypothalamic–pituitary axis keeps three important domains. Hypothalamic, pituitary and testicular glands (gonad axis) [21]. The axis regularly works to provide the optimum concentration of hormones much required for smooth reproductive development of males. **Figure 2** sums up the role of hormones in the reproductive development of human males. Malfunction of this system pave way to infertility. Absence of the normal levels of hormones like GnRH leads to the lack of testosterone and is potent enough to cause a group of disorders like hypogonadotrophic hypogonadism [22]. One of the common examples in this case is Kallman syndrome, linked with impaired sense of smell and immaturity. Another common defect that occurs in the gonadal axis includes the inability of pituitary to produce the required levels of luteinizing hormones and Follicular stimulating Hormone that impairs the stimulation of the testes and has direct bearings on the production of the sperms and testosterone [23].

3. Life style and male infertility

There has been an association established between the life style factors and male infertility. Factors like the dietary measures, smoking, regular exposure to hot surfaces, common insomnia, liquor boozing, advanced ages, illicit drugs, obesity and prolonged exposure to the mobile phone led electromagnetic radiation play vital roles in causing male infertility [4].

3.1 Smoking

Smoking pays heavily with the fertile health of the man. Cigarette has addictive ingredients like nicotine, tar, carbon monoxide, polycyclic aromatic hydrocarbons or benzene like volatile organic compound besides heavy metals like cadmium and lead [24]. Smoking is associated with the deterioration of semen quality. Smokers have raised levels of reactive oxygen species (ROS) at levels that can overpower the cell anti oxidant defenses [25]. With increase in ROS the spermatozoa is exposed to oxidative stress that causes the impairment in the sperm physiology that ultimately ends up in infertility. **Figure 3** shows the role of ROS in impairing the male infertility. Without the activation of (ChK1), the overall decline in sperm repairing is affected by large [26].

It ultimately leads to increase in the sperm apoptosis, thereby compromising semen quality. The paternal smoking prior to conception proves an increased risk for various developmental disorders in the offspring. During the pregnancy time maternal smoking potentially causes severe effects on male offspring fertility by lessen the germ cell population.

3.2 Alcohol

Alcohol action on male reproductive system is through hypothalamus- pituitary-gonadal axis (HPG). Alcohol impairs the production of hormones like GnRH, FSH, LH and testosterone besides impairing the function of leydig and Sertoli cells [27]. All this leads to the impaired development of spermatozoa. Acute ethanol intake affects the testicular Steriodogenic activities; it further has a negative impact on the anti oxidant enzyme activities resulting in response to the raised oxidative stress. Studies also reveal the link between the alcohol administration by male partners in couples facing the primary infertility and sperm Terotogeny. **Figure 4** summarizes the role of Alcohol in impairing the production of hormones.

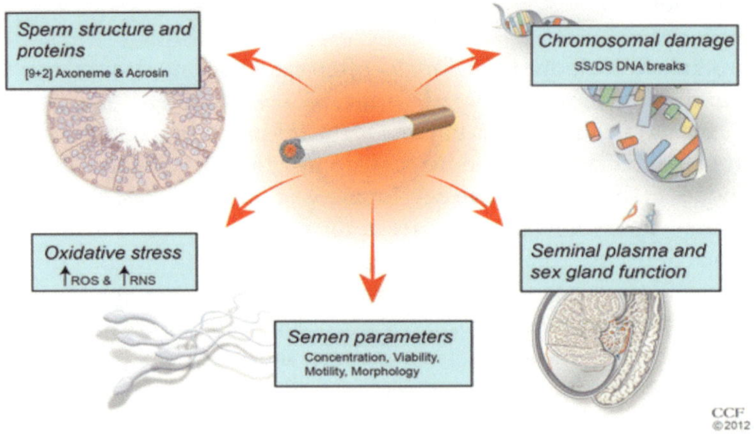

Figure 3.
The effects of smoking on male infertility. Adapted from, Omar Haque Joseph A. Vitale Ashok Agarwal Stefan S. du Plessis.

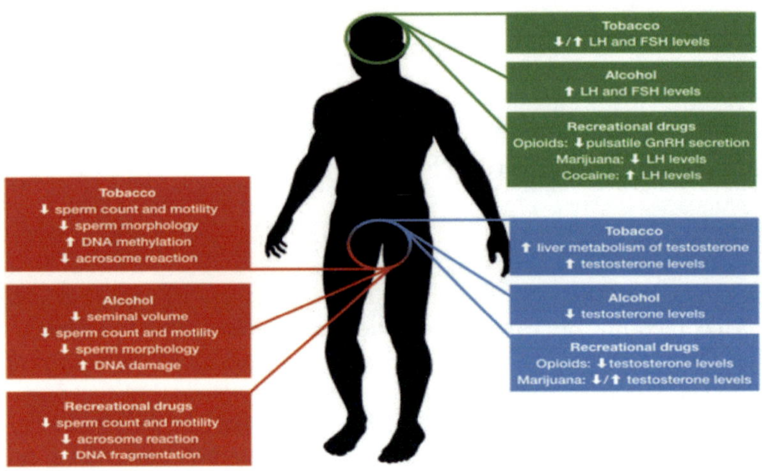

Figure 4.
The role of alcohol in impairing the production of hormones. Image source, Andrea Sansone reproductive biology and endocrinology volume 16, Article Number 3(2018).

3.3 Drugs

Drugs like Marijuana, narcotics and anabolic –androgenic steroids (AAS) have a negative correlation with male infertility [27]. These recreational drugs as we count them have adverse impact history on HPG axis, testicular anatomy and sperm functioning. Marijuana Phytocannabinoids obstructs the cannabinoids in binding with the cannabinoid and vaniloid receptors that negatively influences the ECS (Endogenous cannabinoid system) and thereby consequently impair male infertility [28].

3.4 Anaboilic androgenic steroids

Anabolic Androgenic steroids (AAS) are used by males to boost the sport activity or athletic performance. The AAS induced hypogonadism has seen a surge among young men over years [28]. Increased levels of Testosterone due to administration of AAS imply a negative feedback on hypothalamic –pituitary gonad axis leading to the containment of spermatogenesis, testicular atrophy and finally infertility [29].

It further results in the transitory Azoospermia with a recovery period of no less than two years. Besides inducing the Azospermia, Anabolic Androgenic Steroid abuse also promote the failure of libido besides erectile dysfunction.

3.5 Obesity

Despite the advances in understanding the male infertility, studies show the 30% of male infertility corresponds to idiopathic sperm abnormalities [30]. Important to mention here that a variety of conditions affect semen parameters- Medical condition like liver failure,renal diseases, cystic fibrosis, chronic obstructive pulmonary disease are few names to be mentioned here. The Medical etiologies impact fertility and therby causes the effects on hormonal levels, sexual function or testicular function and spermatogenesis. In maintaining the quality semen parameters, sexual function and fertility potential man's state of health needs to be optimized by large. Obesity is linked with male infertility primarly and mainly due to hormonal changes. Bierick et al. has come up with an inverse relationship between body mass index (BMI) and testosterone, testosterone to estradiol, ejaculate volume, sperm concentration and morphology. In this regard many authors reported higher rates of Azospermia and oligospermia among obese men compared with men of normal weight. It is also pooled in the literature that couples with a female partner of normal BMI and obese male partner are more susceptible to have prolonged time to conceive compared with couples with male partners of normal weight. Studies also bring on forth that couples with an obese male partner seeking Assisted reproductive technology (ART) have decreased pregnancy rates and increased pregnancy lost mainly because of prevalent DNA fragmentation [31].

Mass Adipose tissue in obese individuals leads to conversion of testosterone to estrogen which potentially affects the HPG axis therby causing the reduction in the release of gonadotrophin [32]. Apart from this, the raised leptin production by white adipose tissue causes the fall in testosterone production. Further studies reveal the increased scrotal adiposity as one of the major reasons of testicular heat stress and causes oxidative stress. It can potentially impair the spermatogenesis, integrity of DNA and sperm-oocyte interaction.

3.6 Diet

Diet plays an instrumental part in maintenance of semen quality. There is amble evidence in literature supporting the fact that balanced diet improves the rates of semen quality and fecundity in males. Diet can have either the Mediterranean, western or prudent composure. While former is enriched with omega-3 fatty acids, antioxidants, vitamins and low in saturated and trans-fatty acids [33]. All these are collectively and inversely related to the low semen quality. A more prudent diet that largely comprises of white meat, fruits and vegetables is positively associated with the overall wellbeing of sperms.

4. Environment and male Infertility

Relating environment to the infertility is not a new measure, it is a known fact that our environment is contaminated [34]. The natural and synthetic chemicals obviously interact with the endocrine system. Studies reveal the potential of some substances in inhabiting the specific enzymes in Steriodogenesis like ketoconazole and cyanoketone. In the synthesis of epoxy resins and poly carbonate, Bisphenol A (BPA) is widely used so is potent enough in causing harm to the fertility in men.

BPA is involved in designing of the plastic bottles often used in containers meant for beverage and water storage. Acting as a metabolic and endocrine disruptor, BPA can imitate the action of endrogen estrogen. Studies mention the presence of partial doses leading to the precocious puberty. In some cases even the prostatic hyperplasia and low sperm count has been recorded as a result of exposure to bisphenol. The other severe factor that is established to be hazardous to the reproductive health of men is the exposure to heavy metals. The pooled data available in literature reveals that even the trace concentration due to contaminated water or food can accumulate in the body. Surveys reveal the hostility of heavy metals like lead (Pb), Mercury (Hg) and cadmium (Cd) with the male reproductive system [35]. It impairs the hypothalamic–pituitary axis therby spermatogenesis that leads to impaired semen quality.

Another risk factor that has surfaced in the scientific literature is agricultural related pesticides. Prolonged exposure to the pesticides and other chlorinated hydrocarbons affects the reproductive system. The very parameters of sperm density and motility, mitochondrial DNA, sperm morphology are affected by exposure to these chemicals [36]. There have been evidences reported about the enormous risk of fetal death from congenital anomalies, particularly where father is having the longer exposure to the common agricultural use pesticides. Pesticide exposure affects the fertilizing ability of sperm even in men seeking IVF treatment.

5. Genetic factors and male infertility (Y chromosome infertility)

15 percent of male infertility cases have genetic factors associated either with the chromosomal abnormality or single –gene mutations. Men with Azospermia have reported chromosomal abnormalities in 14% of cases [37]. The most common being the Klinefelter syndrome, 47, XXY leads to the impaired spermatogenesis. Patients with severe oligozoospermia show translocation, the most common being the Robertson and Bilateral translocation. Autosomal inversions are almost eight times seen in the men with infertility issues. Y chromosome deletions in the long arm region termed AZF mostly occur in Azospermic men. **Figure 5** showing the AZF region with three zones AZFa, AZFb, AZFc, micro deletion occur in palindrome sequences. Y chromosome micro deletion affects the 10% of infertile men [1]. Deletion of AZFa results in the sertoli cell phenotype. Intra AZFb deletion is prevalent in Azospermic men. Deletions corresponding to AZFc region are most severe and can lead to the issues like sertoli cell syndrome and Oligospermia. Some gene mutations with pathological syndrome are also involved in the male infertility. In cases of severe testiculopathies in infertile men deletions pertaining to the long arm on Y chromosome are commonly reported in the available literature.

5.1 Primary ciliary dyskinesia (PCD)

PCD is a blanket term most commonly used to describe a condition of many closely related disorders caused due to the impaired motility of Ciliary Structures [39]. Although not obligatory but it has been reported in the literature that affected males suffer infertility mainly due immotile spermatozoa. Important to mention here that Ultra structural defects are mainly due to the absence of dynin arms and malformed radial spokes.

5.2 Kartagener syndrome

Men suffering from KS syndrome have joint disorders like bronchiectasis, Chronic Sinusitis and Sperm immotility. Kartagener syndrome is often recognized

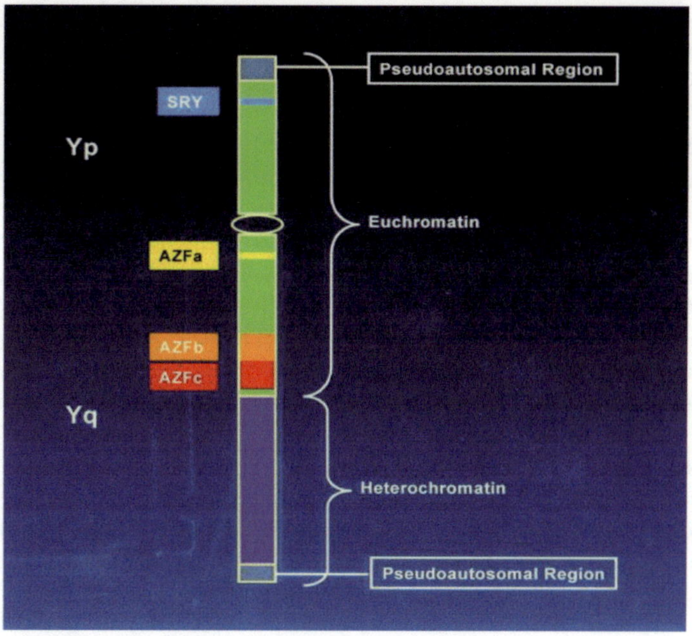

Figure 5.
Structure of Y chromosome [38].

as a subset of a larger Ciliary disorder. In this syndrome the genetic defects leads to impaired Ciliary motility mainly responsible for causing recurrent chest and ear infection besides infertility has also been reported in the scientific literature [40].

5.3 Persistent mullerian duct syndrome

It is seen during the early embryonic development that regression of Mullerian duct is mediated mainly due to the anti-mullerian hormone (AMH) often called as Mullerian inhabiting substance (MIS) [39]. Gene for this hormone has been mapped to 19p13 and mutations in it can cause the persistent Mullerian syndrome. Normally virilised Men with persistent Mullerian duct syndrome show the presence of both fallopian tubes and a uterus.

5.4 Aarskog-Scott syndrome

Aarkskog-Scott syndrome is an X-linked recessive disorder with genital, facial and skeletal abnormalities. Affected men also possess facial features including hypertelorism, eyelid ptosis, irregular auricular shape with prominently broad nasal bridge. Other features associated with Aarskog –scott syndrome are cryptorchidism, subfertility, mild cutaneous syndactyly [41].

5.5 Kallmann syndrome

Kallman syndrome affected ones show characteristic combination of anosmia and hypogonadotrophic hypogonadism [42]. Affected men show impaired secretion of GnRH (Gonadotrophic releasing hormone) with low concentration of follicle stimulating hormone (FSH) and testosterone. Some other complications of men suffering with Kallman syndrome are unilateral renal aplasia, mirror movements of extremities and pescavas. Unilateral renal aplasia is a commonly seen in affected men, kidney tends to be hypertrophied, ectopic and likely to contract infection. The inheritance pattern of Kallmann syndrome is X-linked recessive in mo st families. Gene corresponding to KS (X –linked) is mapped to Xp22.3 with 200000 bp genomic DNA.

5.6 Leydig cell hypoplasia

Development of male genitals begins at the 9th week of gestation. Fetal leydig's cells are stimulated by human chorionic gonadotrophin (hCG) to secrete the male sex hormone testosterone [43]. With the progress in the pregnancy towards the later stage, the very function of hCG is taken over by luteinizing hormone. Leydig cell hypoplasia is a rare disorder in which the fetal leydig's cells turn insensitive to the hCG. It results in the feminization of the external genitials. LHCGR gene with eleven exons is found to be involved in it.

5.7 XY gonadal dysgenesis

XY gonadal dysgenesis also called as swyer syndrome. It is a type of hypogonadism with 46,XY karyotype. People with this syndrome have non-functional gonads. Affected ones are born with the appearance of a normal female on anatomical aspects with an exception of having non functional gonads [42] With their body producing no noticeable changes before puberty, defects in reproductive system remains unsuspected until no puberty is evident. Usually they are being considered as the girl child until they fail to have menstrual periods (primary amenorrhea). Major consequences of XY gonadal dysgenesis if left without treament are severe. Deprivation of estrogen in affected ones leads to the underdevelopment of breasts and uterus. Gonads miserably fail to produce progesterone and thereby lead to the unpredictable menstrual periods. Ovulation too is not seen, so conceiving children too is not possible unless and until there is an intervention [44].

6. Recent reports

The recent reports suggest the possibilities of undiagnosed but potentially treatable defects of male infertility. With adequate investment in the DNA, RNA and protein research, the percentage of the patients being classified as cases of idiopathic can be brought down.

6.1 Advanced sperm tests

Sperm owe various internal components that are very important for normal embryo development and pregnancy in general. Out of these internal features DNA is one of the primary to be discussed here, DNA is conventenally used to resolve the cause for the infertility when other examination or tests fail to deliver. At present, DNA is being evaluated in clinics in two different ways. Determining Y chromosome deletions (Y-micro deletion) and screening the appearance or chromosome numbers by karyotyping [45]. Only some abnormalities in sperm DNA can be diagnosed using these tests. So, additional DNA tests are eqally important for proper diagnostics. Other advanced tests analyze DNA: DNA fragmentation and oxidative stress. DNA fragmentation assessment can benefit couples that have not had success with previous IVF/ICSI cycles or have had repeated miscarriages.

6.2 Magnetic assisted cell sorting (MACS)

Magnetic assited cell sorting help in selecting sperm with high-quality DNA, and retrieval of testicular sperm (known as testicular sperm extraction, TESE, or testicular sperm aspiration, TESA) to be later used with ICSI (intra cytoplasmic sperm injection) [46].

6.3 Male oxidative stress disorder (MOSI)

In case an Oxidative stress is suspected, most often oral antioxidant therapy is employed. Both DNA fragmentation and oxidative stress tests are being validated by the contemporary studies [47]. This advanced format of sperm testing of DNA provides the detailed information towards the understanding of overall health and function of the sperms.

6.4 Experimental sperm tests

Diagnostic experimental tests focusing on recently discovered essential sperm components are being designed and investigated by scientists [48].

6.5 RNA: sperm transcripts

Sperm head, nucleus, and residual cytoplasm of the sperm are known regions that possess RNAs (RNA elements and messenger RNA). Sperm RNA is concerned in regulating the epigenetic code of the embryo. Currently no treatment is available for defects in the RNAs that can corner the disease, but it does provide an important clue in understanding the concern of infertility [49].

6.6 Proteins: sperm proteome

Sperm being transcriptionally and translationally inert cells are always dependent on already existing proteins. Using mass spectroscopy one can identify the sperm proteome which can play an important role in determining status of male fertility [50]. A Deviant or aberrant expression of sperm proteins influence molecular dynamics associated with the overall motility, sperm capacitation, acrosomal reaction, and sperm-oocyte interaction in unexplained male infertility cases. Identifying deficiencies in the expression or function of any protein may be resolved by introducing the protein itself, its DNA, or RNA during ICSI.

6.7 Activation factors

Phospholipase C zeta (PLCζ) an oocyte activation factor in human reproductive biology, are a type of sperm protein play an crucial role in initiating embryo development. Deficiencies in PLCζ can be treated with $Ca2+$, which increases ICSI treatment outcome.

6.8 Clinical prespective

Experts of reproducive health have an important goal while identifying male infertility with the use of standard clinical or experimental diagnostics. It includes the identification of aberrant anatomical features or treatable causes like oxidative stress and DNA fragmentation or any irreversible conditions that could still be treated with ART, defects in the RNA and centrioles. The indepth understanding the underlying cause of male infertility may change the course of action for couples that have had several rounds of failed ART treatment. Fertility preservation is yet another option available where eggs can be freezed to give clinicians the wrist to correct the male infertility. As such these future diagnostic tests may be relevant even if there are no obvious treatment strategies because it may help the experts predict the productivity of ART.

6.9 Y-chromosome microdeletion (YCM)

Genes located in the Y chromosome are involved in important male fertility related functions like spermatogenesis, endocrine and physiological factors. The microdeletions sites are located on q arm of Y chromosome, specifically Azoospermia Factor (AZF) region, hence called Yq microdeletions. These deletions are mostly in the form of complete/incomplete, recombination; mutations and Copy Number Variations (CNV) and vary in frequency depending on region, ethnicity, lifestyles and other epigenetic factors. Available data on thousands of Y chromosome analysis reveal that the frequency of microdeletions are affected by sample size, selection criteria of subjects, different geographical regions, ethnicity, Oxidative Stress (OS), Deoxyribonucleic Acid (DNA) fragmentation and food styles in addition to genetic defects. It has been hence noticed that screening of Yq microdeletion is an important criterion and its correlation with spermeograms is very necessary to infer degree of infertility in men [51]. Such cases strongly suggested to undergo genetic counseling before adoption of ARTS as deletions increase risk of genetic anomalies, low birth weight and congenital malformations in New Births (NB) of Intracytoplasmic Sperm Injection and Testicular Sperm Ejaculates (ICSI/TESE) adopted cases. Thus, Y deletion evaluation reckons the diagnosis of type of male infertility and its prevention in the next generation propagation through ARTs.

7. Conclusion

Patients who aspire to seek the reproductive assistance to achieve parenthood need to go through a mandatory, systematic clinical screening. The evaluation of patients for infertility demands a comprehensive medical history that includes the basic physical examination to rule out the possibilities of anatomical constraints if any. A review of the past medical record, congenital abnormalities, previous conception, environmental exposure besides molecular and cytogenetic assay must be taken a serious note of before opting for ART. This chapter is only a small step rather a precise attempt towards the understanding of problem of male infertility for promising ART.

Author details

Mahrukh Hameed Zargar[1]*, Faisel Ahmad[2], Mohammad Lateef[2]
and Tahir Mohiuddin Malla[3]

1 Department of Advanced Human Genetics, Sheri –Kashmir Institute of Medical Sciences, (SKIMS), Srinagar, J&K, India

2 Department of Zoology Central University of Kashmir, J&K, India

3 Cancer Diagnostics and Research Centre, Sheri –Kashmir Institute of Medical Sciences,(SKIMS), Srinagar, J&K, India

*Address all correspondence to: mhameedz@gmail.com

References

[1] Colaco, S. & Modi, D. Genetics of the human Y chromosome and its association with male infertility. Reprod. Biol. Endocrinol. **16**, 1-24 (**2018**).

[2] Tahmasbpour, E., Balasubramanian, D. & Agarwal, A. A multi-faceted approach to understanding male infertility: gene mutations, molecular defects and assisted reproductive techniques (ART). J. Assist. Reprod. Genet. **31**, 1115-1137 (**2014**).

[3] Shaffer, R. M. *et al.* Improving and expanding estimates of the global burden of disease due to environmental health risk factors. Environ. Health Perspect. **127**, 105001 (**2019**).

[4] Leisegang, K. & Dutta, S. Do lifestyle practices impede male fertility? Andrologia **53**, e13595 (**2021**).

[5] Nowicka-Bauer, K. & Nixon, B. Molecular changes induced by oxidative stress that impair human sperm motility. Antioxidants **9**, 134 (**2020**).

[6] Gürtin, Z. B. The ART of Making Babies. (**2013**).

[7] Sharma, A. Male infertility; evidences, risk factors, causes, diagnosis and management in human. Ann. Clin. Lab. Res. **5**, 188 (**2017**).

[8] Pourmoghadam, Z., Aghebati-Maleki, L., Motalebnezhad, M., Yousefi, B. & Yousefi, M. Current approaches for the treatment of male infertility with stem cell therapy. J. Cell. Physiol. **233**, 6455-6469 (**2018**).

[9] Majzoub, A., Cho, C.-L., Agarwal, A. & Esteves, S. C. Scrotal Hyperthermia, Hormonal Disturbances, Testicular Hypoperfusion, and Backflow of Toxic Metabolites in Varicocele. in *Varicocele and Male Infertility* 27-35 (Springer, **2019**).

[10] Comparetto, C. & Borruto, F. Human papillomavirus infection: Overview. Handb. Hum. Papillomavirus Preval. Detect. Manag. Smith–New York Nova Sci. Publ. Inc **1**, 1-137 (**2013**).

[11] Modh, R. A., Mulhall, J. P. & Gilbert, S. M. Sexual dysfunction after cystectomy and urinary diversion. Nat. Rev. Urol. **11**, 445 (**2014**).

[12] Yaacov, D., Nelinger, G. & Kalichman, L. The Effect of Pelvic Floor Rehabilitation on Males with Sexual Dysfunction: A Narrative Review. *Sex. Med. Rev.* (**2021**).

[13] Goel, B. & Maurya, N. K. Aphrodisiac Herbal therapy for Erectile Dysfunction. Arch. Pharm. Pract. **11**, (**2020**).

[14] Haraux, E. *et al.* Maternal exposure to domestic hair cosmetics and occupational endocrine disruptors is associated with a higher risk of hypospadias in the offspring. Int. J. Environ. Res. Public. Health **14**, 27 (**2017**).

[15] Elumalai, G. & Ezzeddin, E. A. "HYPOSPADIAS" ITS EMBRYOLOGICAL BASIS AND CLINICAL IMPORTANCE. *Elixir Int. J.* **102**, 44481-44487 (**2017**).

[16] Heyerick, L. HYPOSPADIAS REPAIR IN ADULTS. (Ghent University, **2018**).

[17] Donaire, A. E. & Mendez, M. D. Hypospadias. StatPearls Internet (**2020**).

[18] Liu, W., Han, R., Wu, H. & Han, D. Viral threat to male fertility. Andrologia **50**, e13140 (**2018**).

[19] Onyiriuka, A. N., Kuhnle-Krahl, U., Sadoh, W. E. & Elusiyan, J. B. External genital anomalies in newborns in two

Nigerian hospitals: A pilot study of the birth prevalence. Int. J. Child Adolesc. Health **9**, 187-193 (**2016**).

[20] SAENGER, L. ° f HY* Testis-— Plocentuf HCG. *Diagn. Androl.* **4**, 31 (**2012**).

[21] Syriou, V., Papanikolaou, D., Kozyraki, A. & Goulis, D. G. Cytokines and male infertility. Eur. Cytokine Netw. **29**, 73-82 (**2018**).

[22] Dwyer, A. A. & Quinton, R. The metabolic syndrome in central hypogonadotrophic hypogonadism. Metab. Syndr. Consequent Endocr. Disord. **49**, 156-169 (**2018**).

[23] Bharadwaj, S. & Vasan, S. S. Male Endocrine Disorders. *Donald Sch. Textb. Hum. Reprod. Gynecol. Endocrinol.* 273 (**2018**).

[24] Shi, X. Effect of Lifestyle, Environmental and Genetic Factors on Semen Quality of Subjects in Hong Kong. (The Chinese University of Hong Kong (Hong Kong), **2019**).

[25] Dutta, S., Majzoub, A. & Agarwal, A. Oxidative stress and sperm function: A systematic review on evaluation and management. Arab J. Urol. **17**, 87-97 (**2019**).

[26] Martin, J. H., Aitken, R. J., Bromfield, E. G. & Nixon, B. DNA damage and repair in the female germline: contributions to ART. Hum. Reprod. Update **25**, 180-201 (**2019**).

[27] Durairajanayagam, D. Lifestyle causes of male infertility. Arab J. Urol. **16**, 10-20 (**2018**).

[28] Tatem, A. J., Beilan, J., Kovac, J. R. & Lipshultz, L. I. Management of Anabolic Steroid-Induced Infertility: Novel Strategies for Fertility Maintenance and Recovery. World J. Mens Health **38**, 141-150 (**2019**).

[29] Athey, N. C. *Anabolic androgenic steroids: measuring level of knowledge and perceived explanations for its use*. (California State University, Long Beach, **2010**).

[30] Jonathan, F. Recent advances in understanding and managing male infertility. *F1000Research* **8**, (**2019**).

[31] Pathak, U. I., Gabrielsen, J. S. & Lipshultz, L. I. Cutting-edge evaluation of male infertility. Urol. Clin. **47**, 129-138 (**2020**).

[32] Davidson, L. M., Millar, K., Jones, C., Fatum, M. & Coward, K. Deleterious effects of obesity upon the hormonal and molecular mechanisms controlling spermatogenesis and male fertility. Hum. Fertil. **18**, 184-193 (**2015**).

[33] Safarinejad, M. R. & Safarinejad, S. The roles of omega-3 and omega-6 fatty acids in idiopathic male infertility. Asian J Androl **14**, 514-515 (**2012**).

[34] Ma, Y. *et al.* Effects of environmental contaminants on fertility and reproductive health. J. Environ. Sci. **77**, 210-217 (**2019**).

[35] Gur, S. & Sikka, S. C. Environmental Risk Factors Related to Male Reproductive Health in Turkish Society. *Bioenvironmental Issues Affect. Mens Reprod. Sex. Health* 41-52 (**2018**).

[36] De Falco, M., Forte, M. & Laforgia, V. Estrogenic and anti-androgenic endocrine disrupting chemicals and their impact on the male reproductive system. Front. Environ. Sci. **3**, 3 (**2015**).

[37] Gunes, S. & Esteves, S. C. Role of genetics and epigenetics in male infertility. Andrologia **53**, e13586 (**2021**).

[38] Janet M Choi, MD, Male Factor I volume 81, Issue 2,P337- 3 41,February 01,(2004)

[39] Fgeer, S. A. S. Serum Level of Anti-mullerian Hormone among Sudanese Females with Sickle Cell Anemia in Khartoum and Western Kordofan States. (Sudan University of Science & Technology, (**2016**).

[40] D'Argenio, V., Dittfeld, L., Lazzeri, P., Tomaiuolo, R. & Tasciotti, E. Unraveling the Balance between Genes, Microbes, Lifestyle and the Environment to Improve Healthy Reproduction. Genes **12**, 605 (**2021**).

[41] Teebi, A. S., Rucquoi, J. K. & Meyn, M. S. Aarskog syndrome: report of a family with review and discussion of nosology. Am. J. Med. Genet. **46**, 501-509 (**1993**).

[42] Scherer, G. *et al.* Three novel SRY mutations in XY gonadal dysgenesis and the enigma of XY gonadal dysgenesis cases without SRY mutations. Cytogenet. Genome Res. **80**, 188-192 **(1998)**.

[43] Rey, R. A. & Grinspon, R. P. Normal male sexual differentiation and aetiology of disorders of sex development. Best Pract. Res. Clin. Endocrinol. Metab. **25**, 221-238 **(2011)**.

[44] Creatsas, G., Deligeoroglou, E., Tsimaris, P., Pantos, K. & Kreatsa, M. Successful pregnancy in a Swyer syndrome patient with preexisting hypertension. Fertil. Steril. **96**, e83–e85 **(2011)**.

[45] 45.Swanson, G.M.; Estill, M.; Diamond, M.P.; Legro, R.S.; Coutifaris, C.; Barnhart, K.T.; Huang, H.; Hansen, K.R.; Trussell, J.C.; Coward, R.M.; et al. Human chromatin remodeler cofactor, RNA interactor, eraser and writer sperm RNAs responding to obesity. Epigenetics 2019, 15, 32-46

[46] 46.Estill, M.S.; Hauser, R.; Krawetz, S.A. RNA element discovery from germ cell to blastocyst. Nucleic Acids Res. **2019**, 47, 2263-2275

[47] 47.Estill, M.; Hauser, R.; Nassan, F.L.; Moss, A.; Krawetz, S.A. The effects of di-butyl phthalate exposure from medications on human sperm RNA among men. Sci. Rep. **2019**, 9, 12397.

[48] Panner Selvam, M.K.; Agarwal, A. Update on the proteomics of male infertility: A systematic review. Arab. J. Urol. **2018**, 16, 103-112.

[49] 49.Panner Selvam, M.K.; Agarwal, A.; Pushparaj, P.N.; Baskaran, S.; Bendou, H. Sperm Proteome Analysis and Identification of Fertility-Associated Biomarkers in Unexplained Male Infertility. Genes **2019**, 10, 522.

[50] 50.Agarwal, A.; Parekh, N.; Panner Selvam, M.K.; Henkel, R.; Shah, R.; Homa, S.T.; Ramasamy, R.; Ko, E.; Tremellen, K.; Esteves, S.; et al. Male Oxidative Stress Infertility (MOSI): Proposed Terminology and Clinical Practice Guidelines for Management of Idiopathic Male Infertility. World J. Men's Health **2019**, 37, 296-312.

[51] Colaco S, Modi D. Genetics of the human Y chromosome and its association with male infertility. Reprod Biol Endocrinol. **2018**;16(1):14..

Chapter 9

Effect of Heavy Metals on Tyrosine Kinases Signaling during Sperm Capacitation

Bhawna Kushwaha, Rohit Beniwal, Aradhana Mohanty, Ajay Kumar Singh, Raj Kumar Yadav and Satish Kumar Garg

Abstract

Sperm capacitation is the key event prior to fertilization. Success rate of currently used assisted reproductive technology like *in-vitro* fertilization is 50% dependent on sperm maturation or capacitation. *In-vivo* capacitation occur almost in female reproductive tract in response to various signaling or enzymatic molecules. Interestingly, both early and late events of capacitation are centrally regulated by protein kinase A (PKA). Influx of Ca^{2+} and HCO3-transmembrane drive leads to change in pH and intracellular cAMP which ultimately activate PKA regulated capacitation. PKA phosphorylates several target proteins that are presumed to initiate different signaling pathways. Some divalent heavy metals like lead, mercury, arsenic and cadmium mimic Ca^{++} entry and its functions and ultimately affect capacitation by inhibiting or inducing tyrosine phosphorylation. In this chapter we review the mechanism of heavy metals by which they affect the tyrosine phosphorylation during sperm capacitation.

Keywords: Tyrosine Phosphorylation, Spermatozoa, Capacitation, Heavy Metals

1. Introduction

Heavy metals are known to be harmful to humans, animals as well as plants in large amounts. Heavy metals are distributed throughout the environment from both natural sources (inorganic form) and human activities (organic form) and thus accumulating in biosphere including humans and animals' body [1, 2]. Most of these non-degradable toxic elements, such as Arsenic (As), Cadmium (Cd), Chromium (Cr), Copper (Cu), Mercury (Hg), Nickel (Ni), Lead (Pb), and Zinc (Zn), are listed as hazardous contaminants by the EPA [3, 4]. Potential health hazards as toxic manifestations and subtle effects of heavy metals are matter of concern because of daily and wide-spread exposure of humans and animals' consequent to their daily life. The molecular mechanisms for metal carcinogens are still poorly understood. Mercury containing compounds have been used for thousands of years in preservation of various vaccines, treatment of syphilis, skin creams, dental amalgams, and extraction of gold [5]. Direct application of cadmium, lead and arsenic in soil fertilizers and fungicides, leather tanning, waste-water treatment facilities, paper mills and disposal of solid wastes as well as batteries and thermometers in landfills are the chief sources within the environment which may influence animal and human health [6]. The cause of male infertility in 50% cases is still not clear; thus, it is very important to flash a light on role of heavy metals in infertility [7]. Some malformations of male reproductive system, such as cryptorchidism, hypospadias, and prostate and testicular cancers may originate from exposure to endocrine disruptors [8, 9]. In addition, metals can cause hormonal imbalance by affecting the neuroendocrine system, disrupting the secretion of androgens from Leydig cells or inhibin-B from Sertoli cells [10]. Evidence also exists linking mercury with erectile dysfunction [11, 12]. Loss of libido have been reported in men acutely exposed to metallic mercury vapor [13]. Choy et al. [14] did a study in Hong Kong on 150 infertile couples undergoing *In-vitro* fertilization versus 20 fertile couples. The infertile couples had significantly higher blood mercury levels than the fertile group. About 1/3 of the infertile men and 1/4 of the infertile females had high mercury levels and they attributed it to seafood consumption. Considering the fact that they looked only at blood, fish may have been the culprit. However, fish is not usually a major direct source of exposure. Nevertheless, this study reinforces the fact that mercury levels need to be investigated when dealing with infertility, both in males and females. Evidently, metal dependent and/or species-dependent differences in signaling mechanisms seem to exist in mediating toxic effects of metals; however, further studies on these aspects are required.

Arsenic is reported in human tissues ranging 100–6000 ppb [15]. Arsenic toxicity has been reported in case of respiratory, dermatological, cardiovascular disorders including diabetes and obesity [16–19]. Cd is also reported to have toxic effects including endocrine nephrotoxicity, carcinogenity, and neurotoxicity [20–22]. These heavy metals affect the these heavy metals effect the molecular mechanism of tyrosine kinase that plays a central role in the response of cells to various kinds of stresses or growth factors and acts as switch in many cellular functions. For example, in regulation of cell proliferation regulation of cell proliferation, differentiation, cell-cycle regulation, and cell signal transduction [23] specifically in cAMP-dependent pathway, which is a hallmark event of capacitation, that leads to sperm hyperactivation which is necessary for fertilization [24]. Dysfunctional tyrosine phosphorylation mechanisms linked to abnormal cell signaling, frenzied cell growth leading to development of leukemia, lymphoma, multiple endocrine neoplasia type 2, small lung cancer, breast cancer, and colon cancer [25, 26]. Proteins are building blocks of the living systems and alterations in protein function indicate the response to abnormal or stress condition [27].

Tyrosine kinase-dependent pathways are mediated by the activities of receptor (RTKs) and non-receptor tyrosine kinases (NTKs) [28, 29]. The RTK are transmembrane-spanning receptor and an intrinsic protein and further classified as EGF receptor (EGFR), PDGF receptor (PDGFR), FGFR, VEGF receptor (VEGFR), while NRTKs act as substrates of RTKs, include Src family members [30] and, are classified as SRC, ABL, FAK and Janus kinase [31]. Upon stimulation, RTKs undergo autophosphorylation on the tyrosine residues located in their own carboxy terminus and induce conformational changes. This enhances kinase activities and creates binding sites for cellular substrates through SH2 domain interactions [30]. Some proteins which get phosphorylated at tyrosine residue during capacitation are A Kinase Anchoring Protein-4, dihydrolipoamide dehydrogenase, pyruvate dehydrogenase-A2, glycerol-3-phosphate dehydrogenase-2, pyruvate dehydrogenase, and phospholipid hydroperoxide glutathione peroxidase [32–38]. The molecular events of the acrosome reaction overlap substantially with those of capacitation, including phosphorylation of similar tyrosine proteins, influx of Ca^{2+}, and increased cAMP and PKA levels. The role of ROS in the in-vivo acrosome reaction involves the spermatozoa's actions on ZP via phosphorylation of plasma membrane proteins. *In-vitro* activation of the acrosome reactions (AR) is also reported against stressors like heavy metals, O^{2-}, H_2O_2, and NO. Cyclic-AMP regulation and Ca^{2+} influx are the key events of capacitation. In-vitro exposure of goat's spermatozoa to mercuric chloride is reported to increase the intracellular Ca^{2+} release and alter the cAMP levels that leads to spontaneous acrosome reaction and inhibition of tyrosine phosphorylation [39, 40]. The primary downstream target of cAMP is protein kinase-A (PKA), whose activity increases during sperm capacitation [41]. Sperm motility stimulant, pentoxifylline (PF) significantly increased sperm hyperactivation and induced an early onset of sperm capacitation via various cell-signaling molecules such as cAMP, Ca^{2+} and protein kinases in hamsters [42]. Targeted disruption of the sperm-specific catalytic subunit, i.e., Ca^{2+} of protein kinase- A (PKA), led to hypo-tyrosine phosphorylation of sperm proteins accompanied by a lack of hyperactivation in mice spermatozoa [43].

In mammals, fertilization requires the release of spermatozoa into female reproductive tract. After ejaculation, to become fully fertilization competent, mammalian sperm must undergo a combination of sequential maturation process in female reproductive tract. Austin [44], demonstrated independently that sperm acquire fertilization capacity only after residing in the female reproductive tract for a finite period of time in a process known as sperm capacitation. Capacitation include variations in sperm intracellular ions concentrations, plasma membrane fluidity as a result of changes in localization of membrane antigens and removal of cholesterol [45]. In particular, capacitation has been associated with a cAMP/PKA-dependent increase in protein tyrosine phosphorylation [46]. Capacitation involves modifications occurring both in the head (i.e., preparation for the acrosome reaction) and the tail (i.e., motility changes such as hyperactivation) which renders sperm to penetrate the egg following acrosome reaction (exocytosis of acrosomal contents). The physiological event of mammalian sperm capacitation had been recognized for a long time, but the molecular players regulating capacitation are still poorly understood. Interestingly, the process of capacitation can occur in-vitro in most species and the conditions required for sperm capacitation in-vitro include a balanced salt solution containing appropriate electrolytes concentrations (e.g., Na^+, K^+, Cl^-, $HCO3^-$, Mg^{2+}, Ca^{2+}, and $PO_4{}^{3-}$), metabolic energy sources (e.g., glucose, pyruvate and lactate) which support the high ATP consumption needed for motility and serum albumin as a a cholesterol acceptor. The important mediators of signal transduction pathways leading to capacitation include cAMP, Ca^{2+}, HCO^{3-}, inositol triphosphate (IP3), protein kinase A (PKA), protein tyrosine kinase (PTK), phospholipase-C (PLC).

Ca^{2+} is shown to play a very important role in sperm capacitation and acrosome reaction by influencing the activity of sperm adenylate cyclase and PLC [47]. Pentoxifylline (cAMP phosphodiesterase inhibitor) causes hyperactivated motility of hamster spermatozoa via increasing sperm cAMP level [48]. Inhibition of Protein kinase – A (PKA) activity led to an inhibition of cAMP dependent protein tyrosine phosphorylation in mice [46] and in hamster [49]. Mice that lack the sperm-specific PKA catalytic subunit Cα2, was infertile despite normal mating behavior, and their sperm shows defects in motility and capacitation-associated events such as the increased tyrosine phosphorylation [43]. This indicates that sperm capacitation and protein tyrosine phosphorylation are regulated through a PKA pathway, invoking an important role for tyrosine phosphorylation in sperm capacitation. Time dependent increase in protein tyrosine phosphorylation during capacitation has also been observed in cauda epididymis sperm [46]. As mature spermatozoa lack de novo gene expression, acquisition of fertilization competence is invariably dependent on post-translational modifications especially phosphorylation of pre-existing structural and intracellular proteins of spermatozoa during capacitation. AKAP4 was the first tyrosine phosphorylated protein identified in the humans [50], mouse [46] and hamster species [51]. The lack of AKAP4 gene expression results in loss of progressive sperm motility, leading to male infertility [52]. Similarly, tyrosine phosphorylated form of AKAP-3 recruits PKA to the sperm flagellum changing protein phosphorylation status and increasing sperm motility [53]. Phosphorylated AKAPs appears to interact with PKA and facilitate flagellar protein phosphorylation in a localization-specific manner. Chaperone protein VCP also undergoes tyrosine phosphorylation. VCP is important for membrane fusion, possibly involved in acrosome reaction [32, 33]. Dihydrolipoamide dehydrogenase (DHLD) [37], phospholipid hydroperoxide glutathione peroxidase (PHGPx) [38] and pyruvate dehydrogenase A2 (PDHA2) are among the metabolic-mitochondrial enzymes that are tyrosine phosphorylated and are localized to sperm flagellum; the inhibition of DHLD leads to decrease in sperm hyperactivation [54]. Calcium-binding tyrosine phosphorylation-regulated protein (CABYARa) and the Calcium/calmodulin-dependent protein kinase IV (CaMKIV) are other tyrosine phosphorylated proteins in humans and involved in calcium regulated protein tyrosine phosphorylation of sperm proteins [55, 56]. Thorough understanding of capacitation and molecular characterization of functionally important phosphorylated sperm proteins is required to benefit reproductive strategies, agriculture.

Sperm signaling pathways also required an optimal level of sperm-generated reactive oxygen species (ROS) for protein tyrosine phosphorylation [42]. The signaling pathway involving protein tyrosine phosphorylation is distinctly associated with hyperactivated motility during sperm capacitation in mice [46], humans [57], and hamsters [34, 35]. The number of Sertoli cells determine the number of sperms produced in adulthood, because each Sertoli cell can support only a finite number of germ cells that develop into sperm [58]. Cadmium (Cd) is reported to cross the blood-testis barrier and induce excessive oxidative stress in Sertoli cells leading to necrosis in mice spermatozoa [59]. Cd exposure led to halt the process of spermatogenesis and normal testicular development by inhibiting the synthesis of testosterone in adult mice [60]. Consequently, Cd caused remarkable drop in weight of testes and epididymis, sperm concentration, motility, and synchronously an elevation in dead and abnormal sperm [61]. Disruption of spermatogenesis in men at any stage of cell differentiation can decrease the total sperm count, increase the abnormal sperm count, impair the stability of sperm chromatin or damage sperm DNA [62], lowered epididymis sperm count, and testicular weight, aberrant chromosome numbers rather than the normal [63], chromosomes break, and lowered testosterone levels in male [64, 65]. Metal's accumulation in epididymis, prostate, and seminal fluid may impair progressive sperm motility [66, 67] and thus reproductive efficiency. Therefore, in this chapter we have discussed the effect of different heavy metals that effect male reproduction with special focus on sperm capacitation via a modification in tyrosine signaling mechanisms [68–71].

2. Effect of mercuric chloride on tyrosine phosphorylation

Reproductive toxicity of mercury has been described in several animal studies in which sperm motility, epididymal sperm count and normal sperm morphology decreased among rats, mice, fish, monkeys and humans after mercury exposure [72–75]. Evidence is usually limited to animal data or to in-vitro studies [76, 77]. The clinical and epidemiological findings are scarce and controversial, and often difficult to interpret because of multiple exposures to different agents and latency of effects. Human studies are few and contradictory too [78]. Seminal fluid mercury concentrations are correlated with abnormal sperm morphology and abnormal sperm motility [79]. Furthermore, infertile, and sub-fertile men have higher mercury levels than the fertile men [80] and tubular atrophy and Sertoli-cell-only syndrome has been observed among infertile patients that have been exposed to mercury [81]. Kushawaha et al. [39, 40] reported that in-vitro exposure of mercuric chloride (0.031 µg/mL) leads to significant increase in spontaneous acrosome reaction, intracellular Ca^{2+} and cAMP levels, and capacitation failure may be due to inhibition of 55, 70, and 80 kDa tyrosine phosphorylation of protein. Proteins of 80 and 105 kDa are the main substrates for enzymes and are important in acrosome reactions [82–84]. Sperm capacitation is a sequential process which involves several signaling pathways and ultrastructural changes such as modifications in membrane lipid composition, increased permeability to ions [85, 86] and phosphorylation of proteins on tyrosine (Tyr), serine (Ser) and threonine (Thr) residues [82, 87–89]. The cAMP/PKA-dependent increase in tyrosine phosphorylation of two fibrous sheath proteins, p80 and p105 related to A-kinase anchoring proteins (AKAPs), is one of the prominent events associated with capacitation [89, 90]. Martinez et al. [91] investigated the effects and underlying mechanisms of chronic mercury exposure at low levels on male reproductive system of rats. Three-month-old male Wistar rats were exposed to 4.6 µg/kg to 0.07 µg/kg/day subsequent dose of $HgCl_2$ for 60 days and they found that mercury treatment decreased daily sperm production, count, motility, and increased head and tail morphologic abnormalities. Moreover, mercury treatment decreased luteinizing hormone levels, increased lipid peroxidation in testis and decreased antioxidant enzymes activities (superoxide dismutase and catalase) in reproductive organs. According to the findings of in-vitro study by Arabi [92], $HgCl_2$ at 50 to 550 µM concentration affected the sperm membrane and DNA integrity, viability, and acrosomal status of normal bull spermatozoa. They recorded a sharp increase in lipid peroxidation/LPO rate; highest was at 550 µM mercury concentration, indicating the deleterious effect of mercury on sperm membrane intactness. There was also a strong negative correlation between LPO rate and % viable spermatozoa. Comet assay study revealed that mercury is capable of inducing DNA breaks in sperm nuclei. The correlation between LPO rate and % DNA breaks was 0.984 [92, 93]. Oxidative stress seemed to be the potential mechanism involved in mercury - induced male reproductive toxicity. Kinematic patterns of goldfish *Carassiusauratus* spermatozoa after mercury exposure (100 to 368 µM) studied by Van Look et al. [94]. They reported that sperm flagellar length was significantly shortened after instant exposure mercuric chloride, while curvilinear velocity (VCL) and the percentage of motile sperm were significantly decreased at mercuric chloride concentration of 1 and 10 mg/l (3.68 and 36.8 µM), respectively. After 24 h exposure to 0.001 mg/l (0.0037 µM) $HgCl_2$, flagellar length was significantly reduced in 38% of the spermatozoa. Following exposure to 0·1 mg/l (0·37 µM) mercuric chloride for 24 h, however, majority of the spermatozoa (98%) had significantly shortened flagella and increased sperm head length, width and area. Sperm motility was also significantly decreased at 0.1 mg/1(0.37 µM) mercuric chloride, probably due to significantly reduced flagellar length at this concentration. Several animal studies indicate that mercury is a male reproductive toxicant, but human studies are few and contradictory. Vergilio et al. [95] investigated the toxic effects of mercury chloride (1 µM - 30 µM) on testes and sperms of tropical fish (Gymnotuscarapo) and showed decrease in the sperm count (36.8%) after 20 µM/24 h treatment and subsequent decrease (48.7%) was observed after 20 µM/96 h. Hg (20 µM) also altered the sperm morphology in 24 h and 96 h where sperm head abnormalities were present.

Mocevic et al. [96] examined semen characteristics and serum levels of reproductive hormones in relation to environmental exposure to mercury. Blood and semen samples were collected from 529 male partners of pregnant women living in

Greenland, Poland and Ukraine between May 2002 and February 2004 [97]. Total content of mercury in whole blood was 9.2 ng/ml in Greenland (0.2–385.8 ng/ml), 1.0 ng/ml in Poland (0.2–6.4 ng/ml21) and 1.0 ng/ml in Ukraine (0.2–4.9 ng/ml). They found a significantly positive association between blood levels of mercury and serum concentration of inhibin B in men from Greenland (β = 50.074, 95% confidence interval (CI) = 50.021 to 0.126) and in an analysis including men from all three regions (β = 50.067, 95% CI = 50.024 to 0.110). The association may be due to beneficial effects of polyunsaturated fatty acids (PUFAs), which are contained in seafood and fish. No significant association (P < .0.05) was found between blood concentrations of mercury and any of the other measured semen characteristics (semen volume, total sperm count, sperm concentration, morphology and motility) and reproductive hormones (free androgen index (FAI), follicle-stimulating hormone (FSH), luteinizing hormone (LH), testosterone and LH_3 testosterone) in any region. These findings did not provide evidence that environmental mercury exposure in Greenlandic and European men with median whole blood concentration up to 10 ng/ml had adverse effects on biomarkers of male reproductive health. Overall, studies have found that mercury accumulates in testes, inhibits enzymes necessary for sperm production, affects DNA in sperm, causes aberrant number of chromosomes in cells, and induces chromosomes breaks; all of which can cause infertility, spontaneous abortion, or birth defects. From the foregoing scientific data it is apparent that mercury is a metal of great global concern and has the potential to alter reproductive functions in males thus, still further investigation on protein phosphorylation during capacitation are warranted.

3. Effect of cadmium (Cd) on tyrosine phosphorylation

Cd possesses oxidation state +2 just like mercury and calcium with half-life of 15–30 years with low execration rate. It can accumulate into the non-smoking population via fumes, dust, contaminated food and water and it is widely use in cancer drugs [98, 99]. Tobacco plant absorbs Cd specially into leaves which is then used in smoking [100]. Apart from this 0.5 mg of Cd is radially reported into per kg fertilizer which is then accumulate into the fruits, vegetables and grains [101, 102]. Cd is reported to accumulate in various tissues via bloodstream [103]. Ca shows a high affinity toward sulfhydryl (–SH and GHS) and disulphide groups (-S-S) of the proteins and result in increased production of ROS [104]. Epigenetic changes like DNA methylation are reported to associated with the in-vivo Cd exposure in three-month-old rats. Short time exposure of Cd for 24 h–1 week induces hypomethylation, while longer times (8–10 weeks) induce hypermethylation [105]. In-vivo orally administered Cd (1, 2 or 4 mg kg^{-1}) to 3–7-days postpartum rats for 30 min did not showed any effect on sperm motility, but significantly decrease the rate of fertilization and embryo development indicating that Cd affects the epigenetic factors [106, 107]. Cd is also reported to induced germ cell apoptosis, loss of daily sperm production, and decreased sperm motility might be responsible for the decline of male fertility [108, 109] specifically spontaneous acrosome reaction in mouse [109–111], rats [112], ram [113], rabbit [114] and sheep [115, 116] sperms. Research indicates that oxidative stress and apoptosis are the major players which affects the in the post-translation modifications like phosphorylation and methylation [117, 118]. Ca^{2+}/calmodulin-dependent kinase II (CaMK-II) which is sensitive to concentration of intracellular calcium and calmodulin, are involve in apoptotic pathway [119–121] and responsible for phosphorylation of serine/thrionine residue of tyrosine kinase [119]. Wang et al. [122] reported that 10 μM Cd inhibited the sperm motility, GAPDH activity, AMPK activity and ATP production, and induced tyrosine phosphorylation of 55–57KDa proteins. These results suggest that Cd-induced tyrosine phosphorylation of 55–57KDa proteins particularly localized in the middle piece of sperm that may inhibit or interfere with mitochondria and ultimately affect the motility of sperm. Exposure of adult rats to 2 mg/kg Cd for 24 hr. induced the ROS and catalase activity and also inhibit the TGF- β3 response and p38 MAPK phosphorylation [123, 124]. Role of tyrosine-phosphorylated dihydrolipoamide dehydrogenase (DLD) was reported in capacitation, hyperactivation and acrosome reaction in hamster [37, 125] after Cd exposure of 1.2 mg/kg BW that induce tyrosine phosphorylation of DLD leads to lower the dehydrogenase activity, and thus affect the mitochondria and sperm motility. Only few studies are reported the effect of Cd during sperm capacitation. As capacitation process involve the influx of Ca^{2+} ions, thereby in presence of Cd which is also having similar charge as Ca, may mimic or replace the Ca entry by competitive binding and, thus affecting the capacitation process. More research is warranted to find out the molecular mechanism of Cd toxicity on capacitation in different species with different doses.

4. Effect of arsenic on tyrosine phosphorylation

Arsenic is mainly present in four forms namely arsenate (As(V)), arsenite (As (III)), MMA (monomethylarsonic acid), and DMA (dimethylarsenic acid) [126]. Trace quantities of arsenic were found in drinking water of rats, hamsters, goats, chickens and humans [127]. Arsenic-induced male infertility is reported to cause abnormal sperms, decreased sperm count, and decreased sperm motility in both humans and animals [128–130]. Exposure of the cells to arsenic increased total cellular tyrosine phosphorylation of 110–120, 90, 70, 56, and 40 kDa proteins [131]. Arsenic-induced tyrosine-phosphorylation in EGFR [132]. It is not known how arsenic induces the activation of EGFR either by the conformational changes or by dimerization of EGFR, which results in the activation of EGFR [133]. It was proposed that arsenic might activate EGFR through generation of ROS that, in turn, triggered the conformational changes in the receptor [134, 135]. The arsenic-induced activation of EGFR recruits Sh-c and phosphorylates its tyrosine residues, which results in enhancement of the interactions between Sh-c and Grb2. Signals are then relayed to the downstream signaling proteins [132]. Inhibition of EGFR kinase blocked arsenic-induced activation of MAPKs [136]. Arsenic may activate with the vicinal sulfhydryl groups of the Src molecule, (2) direct interactions with extracellular matrix proteins to induce integrin rearrangements, or (3) the generation of ROS [137, 138]. Biscardi and colleagues found that Src was able to phosphorylate EGFR at two unique tyrosine residues, distinct from the autophosphorylation sites, to activate EGFR in association with the activation of other cell signaling proteins [139, 140]. Arsenic induces Src and that activates downstream proteins e.g., MAPKs via EGFR-dependent and EGFR-independent pathways [138, 141]. Shim et al. [142] reported that arsenic inhibits Ca^{2+} influx into antigen-activated mast cells and inhibit tyrosine phosphorylation. These results indicate that the target of arsenic is upstream of the Ca^{2+} influx which is a major pathway of sperm capacitation as well. Thus, further detailed studies are warranted to find out the effects of arsenic on sperm capacitation mechanism.

Six months exposure to sodium arsenite (1, 5, or 25 mg/L) reduced Voltage-dependent anion channel protein 3 (VDAC3), which leads to impaired capacitation and fertilization process in male rats [143, 144]. cAMP activates the serine/threonine Kinase and cAMP-dependent protein kinase catalytic subunit alpha (PRKACA), which in turn activates tyrosine through phosphorylation. Blocking of

PRKACA altered the tyrosine phosphorylation at the protein level which results in impairment of capacitation of sperm [143, 144]. Arsenic exposure on the proteome and metabolome in rat testis leads to 36 up-regulated and 34 down-regulated proteins and 13 metabolites (8 high and 5 low). Theses altered proteins were related to spermatogenesis, fertilization, fertility, and mating behavior which may be mediated by the ERK/AKT/NF-κB-dependent signaling pathway [143, 144]. However, these studies indicate the toxic effect of arsenic, but arsenic-induced male reproductive toxicity, particularly effect on capacitation and tyrosine phosphorylation mechanisms are still far from being completely understood.

5. Effect of lead (Pb) on tyrosine phosphorylation

It is well known that there has been a worldwide decrease in human male fertility in recent years. One of the main factors affecting this is environmental pollution. Lead is one of the major heavy metal contaminants that threatens the health of animals and human beings at global level. It is a naturally occurring element and widely used in acid batteries, paints, smelters, and paper printing. It accumulates into human and animal blood, bone and soft tissues with a half-life of 35 days in blood and 20–30 years in bone via contaminated food, and drinking water [145]. Pb has also been reported to accumulate in the epididymus and some glands [146, 147] and is considered a male reproductive toxicant [148]. The mechanism of toxicity of Pb is still not very clear. Pb mainly targets events of spermatogenesis and spermatozoa function via free radical generation, apoptosis, motility, and DNA fragmentation, and ultimately declines the rate of fertilization [149]. Recently Hassan et al. [150] reported that exposure of 20 mg PbAc/kg bwt, orally in rats for 45 days resulted in significant decrease in testis weight, spermatozoa count, testosterone levels, and antioxidant enzymes levels. Histological study indicated that Pb -exposed group was devoid of germ cells and maturation arrest with the formation of giant primary spermatocytes. Some studies reported that Pb has the ability to displace zinc and results in alteration in Ca^{2+} mediated process [151].

Capacitation is highly Ca^{2+} dependent process which means lead exposure could inhibit or induce the capacitation. Only few studies are reported about the effect of Pb on tyrosine phosphorylation during capacitation. Yuanqiao et al. [152] reported that 10–100 μM lead acetate dose-dependently inhibited total and progressive motility measures, capacitation and progesterone-induced acrosome reaction in humans. It also decreased the intracellular concentrations of cyclic adenosine monophosphate (cAMP) and intracellular calcium (Ca^{2+})i, and reduced the tyrosine phosphorylation of sperm proteins, all of which are thought to be key factors in regulation of capacitation. These findings suggest that lead inhibits human sperm functions by reducing the levels of sperm intracellular cAMP, (Ca^{2+})i and tyrosine phosphorylation of sperm proteins *in-vitro*. Voltage-dependent Ca^{2+} channels, known as Catsper, are mainly involved in regulation of capacitation by mediating Ca^{2+} influx [153]. Therefore, it can be postulated that Pb exposure decreases intracellular Ca^{2+} by inhibiting progesterone -induced acrosome reaction via voltage-dependent channels. Further concentration and time dependent studies are warranted to explicate the effects of Pb on sperm capacitation and tyrosine signaling mechanism.

6. Conclusions

Heavy metals affect tyrosine phosphorylation during capacitation of spermatozoa and lead to male infertility. Alteration in tyrosine signaling might be a result of various stress conditions which are produced by heavy metals in cells like oxidative stress, apoptosis, mitochondrial damage, calcium influx and change in osmolarity of cells. Particularly Hg, Pb, As and Cd inhibit or induce tyrosine phosphorylation of sperm proteins. There are several factors including animal species and strains, gender, age, stress, genetic disorders, nutritional status, smoking, alcohol consumption, use of medicines, and concomitant exposure to other chemicals or even physical factors which will influence both the metabolism and the dose–response relationships including reproduction that affects biological processes specifically signaling mechanism. Therefore, extensive research is warranted focusing on tyrosine phosphorylation signaling during sperm capacitation using large sample size or population with minimum dose which are reported in human blood after exposure of lead, mercury, arsenic and cadmium. It is now generally accepted that the mammalian testes are very sensitive to heavy metals, and these induce changes in the testicular biochemical functions via ROS and DNA damage that ultimately affect the fertilizing ability particularly capacitation in spermatozoa.

Acknowledgements

We are thankful to IntechOpen for inviting corresponding author to write this chapter.

Funding information

No financial assistance was provided from any source to write this chapter.

Conflict of interest

The authors declare that they have no conflict of interest.

Author details

Bhawna Kushwaha[1*], Rohit Beniwal[1,2], Aradhana Mohanty[1,2], Ajay Kumar Singh[1], Raj Kumar Yadav[3] and Satish Kumar Garg[3]

1 National Institute of Animal Biotechnology, Hyderabad, Telangana, India

2 Graduate studies, Regional Centre for Biotechnology, Faridabad, India

3 Pandit Deen Dayal Upadhyaya Pashu Chikitsa Vigyan Vishwavidyalaya Evam Go-Anusandhan Sansthan, Mathura, India

*Address all correspondence to: bhawnarajput31jan@gmail.com

References

[1] Qiu, Yao-Wen. "Bioaccumulation of heavy metals both in wild and mariculture food chains in Daya Bay, South China." *Estuarine, Coastal and Shelf Science* 163 (2015): 7-14.

[2] Zhang, Tao, Jujun Ruan, Bo Zhang, Shaoyou Lu, Chuanzi Gao, Lifei Huang, Xueyuan Bai, Lei Xie, Mingwei Gui, and Rong-liang Qiu. "Heavy metals in human urine, foods and drinking water from an e-waste dismantling area: Identification of exposure sources and metal-induced health risk." *Ecotoxicology and environmental safety* 169 (2019): 707-713.

[3] Cobbina, Samuel J., Yao Chen, Zhaoxiang Zhou, Xueshan Wu, Ting Zhao, Zhen Zhang, Weiwei Feng et al. "Toxicity assessment due to sub-chronic exposure to individual and mixtures of four toxic heavy metals." Journal of Hazardous Materials 294 (2015): 109-120.

[4] Toth, G., T. Hermann, M. R. Da Silva, and L. Montanarella. "Heavy metals in agricultural soils of the European Union with implications for food safety." Environment international 88 (2016): 299-309.

[5] Clarkson, Thomas W., and Laszlo Magos. "The toxicology of mercury and its chemical compounds." Critical reviews in toxicology 36, no. 8 (2006): 609-662.

[6] World Health Organization. *Health guidelines for the use of wastewater in agriculture and aquaculture: report of a WHO scientific group [meeting held in Geneva from 18 to 23 November 1987]*. World Health Organization, 1989.

[7] Wirth, Julia J., and Renee S. Mijal. "Adverse effects of low level heavy metal exposure on male reproductive function." Systems biology in reproductive medicine 56, no. 2 (2010): 147-167.

[8] Henkel, Ralf. "Environmental contamination and testicular function." In *Bioenvironmental Issues Affecting Men's Reproductive and Sexual Health*, pp. 191-208. Academic Press, 2018.

[9] Iavicoli, Ivo, Luca Fontana, and Antonio Bergamaschi. "The effects of metals as endocrine disruptors." Journal of Toxicology and Environmental Health, Part B 12, no. 3 (2009): 206-223.

[10] Jensen, Tina Kold, Jens Peter Bonde, and Michael Joffe. "The influence of occupational exposure on male reproductive function." *Occupational Medicine* 56, no. 8 (2006): 544-553.

[11] Schrag, S. Don, and Robert L. Dixon. "Occupational exposures associated with male reproductive dysfunction." *Annual review of pharmacology and toxicology* 25, no. 1 (1985): 567-592.

[12] Wijesekara, G. U. S., D. M. S. Fernando, S. Wijerathna, and N. Bandara. "Environmental and occupational exposures as a cause of male infertility." (2016).

[13] Lauwerys, Robert, Harry Roels, Pierre Genet, Guy Toussaint, André Bouckaert, and Serge De Cooman. "Fertility of male workers exposed to mercury vapor or to manganese dust: a questionnaire study." *American Journal of Industrial Medicine* 7, no. 2 (1978): 171-176.

[14] Choy, C.M., Yeung, Q.S., Briton-Jones, C.M., Cheung, C.K., Lam, C.W. and Haines, C.J. Relationship between semen parameters and mercury concentrations in blood and in seminal fluid from subfertile males in Hong Kong. Fertil.Steril, no. 78(2002b):426-428.

[15] Hutchinson, Lee M., Benett M. Trinh, Rachel K. Palmer, Christopher A. Preziosi, Jonathan H. Pelletier, Hannah M. Nelson, and Julie A. Gosse. "Inorganic arsenite inhibits IgE receptor-mediated degranulation of

mast cells." Journal of Applied Toxicology 31, no. 3 (2011): 231-241.

[16] Abernathy, Charles O., Yung-Pin Liu, David Longfellow, H. Vasken Aposhian, Barbara Beck, Bruce Fowler, Robert Goyer et al. "Arsenic: health effects, mechanisms of actions, and research issues." Environmental health perspectives 107, no. 7 (1999): 593-597.

[17] Paul, Somnath, Nandana Das, Pritha Bhattacharjee, Mayukh Banerjee, Jayanta K. Das, Nilendu Sarma, Ajoy Sarkar et al. "Arsenic-induced toxicity and carcinogenicity: a two-wave cross-sectional study in arsenicosis individuals in West Bengal, India." *Journal of exposure science & environmental epidemiology* 23, no. 2 (2013): 156-162.

[18] Smith, Allan H., Elena O. Lingas, and Mahfuzar Rahman. "Contamination of drinking-water by arsenic in Bangladesh: a public health emergency." Bulletin of the World Health Organization 78 (2000): 1093-1103.

[19] Xia, Yajuan, Timothy J. Wade, Kegong Wu, Yanhong Li, Zhixiong Ning, X. Chris Le, Binfei Chen, Yong Feng, Judy L. Mumford, and Xingzhou He. "Well water arsenic exposure, arsenic induced skin-lesions and self-reported morbidity in Inner Mongolia." *International journal of environmental research and public health* 6, no. 3 (2009): 1010-1025.

[20] Bernhoft, Robin A. "Cadmium toxicity and treatment." *The Scientific World Journal* 2013 (2013).

[21] Waalkes, Michael P., Larry K. Keefer, and Bhalchandra A. Diwan. "Induction of proliferative lesions of the uterus, testes, and liver in Swiss mice given repeated injections of sodium arsenate: possible estrogenic mode of action." Toxicology and applied pharmacology 166, no. 1 (2000): 24-35.

[22] Yang, Hong, and Yan Shu. "Cadmium transporters in the kidney and cadmium-induced nephrotoxicity." International journal of molecular sciences 16, no. 1 (2015): 1484-1494

[23] Gozin, Alexia, Elisabeth Franzini, Valérie Andrieu, Lydie Da Costa, Emmanuelle Rollet-Labelle, and Catherine Pasquier. "Reactive oxygen species activate focal adhesion kinase, paxillin and p130cas tyrosine phosphorylation in endothelial cells." Free Radical Biology and Medicine 25, no. 9 (1998): 1021-1032.

[24] Visconti, Pablo E. "Understanding the molecular basis of sperm capacitation through kinase design." *Proceedings of the National Academy of Sciences* 106, no. 3 (2009): 667-668.

[25] Chen, Ming Hui, Risto Kerkelä, and Thomas Force. "Mechanisms of cardiac dysfunction associated with tyrosine kinase inhibitor cancer therapeutics." *Circulation* 118, no. 1 (2008): 84-95.

[26] Kolibaba, Kathryn S., and Brian J. Druker. "Protein tyrosine kinases and cancer." *Biochimica et Biophysica Acta (BBA)-Reviews on Cancer* 1333, no. 3 (1997): F217-F248.

[27] Zhong, Zhenyu, Elsa Sanchez-Lopez, and Michael Karin. "Autophagy, inflammation, and immunity: a troika governing cancer and its treatment." Cell 166, no. 2 (2016): 288-298.

[28] Kemble, David J. A biochemical study on the regulation of the Src and FGFR family of protein tyrosine kinases. University of Rhode Island, 2009.

[29] Siveen, K.S., Prabhu, K.S., Achkar, I.W., Kuttikrishnan, S., Shyam, S., Khan, A.Q., Merhi, M., Dermime, S. and Uddin, S., 2018. Role of non-receptor tyrosine kinases in hematological malignances and its targeting by natural products. Molecular cancer, 17(1), pp.1-21.

[30] Blume-Jensen, Peter, and Tony Hunter. "Oncogenic kinase signalling." Nature 411, no. 6835 (2001): 355-365.

[31] Dubois, Marie-Françoise, and Olivier Bensaude. "MAP kinase activation during heat shock in quiescent and exponentially growing mammalian cells." FEBS letters 324, no. 2 (1993): 191-195.

[32] Ficarro, Scott, Olga Chertihin, V. Anne Westbrook, Forest White, Friederike Jayes, Petr Kalab, Jarrod A. Marto et al. "Phosphoproteome analysis of capacitated human sperm: evidence of tyrosine phosphorylation of a kinase-anchoring protein 3 and valosin-containing protein/p97 during capacitation." *Journal of Biological Chemistry* 278, no. 13 (2003a): 11579-11589.

[33] Ficarro, Scott, Olga Chertihin, V. Anne Westbrook, Forest White, Friederike Jayes, Petr Kalab, Jarrod A. Marto et al. "Phosphoproteome analysis of capacitated human sperm: evidence of tyrosine phosphorylation of a kinase-anchoring protein 3 and valosin-containing protein/p97 during capacitation." *Journal of Biological Chemistry* 278, no. 13 (2003b): 11579-11589.

[34] Jha, Kula Nand, and S. Shivaji. "Identification of the major tyrosine phosphorylated protein of capacitated hamster spermatozoa as a homologue of mammalian sperm a kinase anchoring protein." *Molecular Reproduction and Development* 61, no. 2 (2002a): 258-270.

[35] Jha, Kula Nand, and S. Shivaji. "Identification of the major tyrosine phosphorylated protein of capacitated hamster spermatozoa as a homologue of mammalian sperm a kinase anchoring protein." *Molecular Reproduction and Development* 61, no. 2 (2002b): 258-270.

[36] Kota, Janaiah, Chalonda R. Handy, Amanda M. Haidet, Chrystal L. Montgomery, Amy Eagle, Louise R. Rodino-Klapac, Danielle Tucker et al. "Follistatin gene delivery enhances muscle growth and strength in nonhuman primates." *Science translational medicine* 1, no. 6 (2009): 6ra15-6ra15.

[37] Mitra, Kasturi, and S. Shivaji. "Novel tyrosine-phosphorylated post-pyruvate metabolic enzyme, dihydrolipoamide dehydrogenase, involved in capacitation of hamster spermatozoa." *Biology of reproduction* 70, no. 4 (2004): 887-899.

[38] NagDas, Subir K., Virginia P. Winfrey, and Gary E. Olson. "Tyrosine phosphorylation generates multiple isoforms of the mitochondrial capsule protein, phospholipid hydroperoxide glutathione peroxidase (PHGPx), during hamster sperm capacitation." Biology of reproduction 72, no. 1 (2005): 164-171.

[39] Kushawaha, Bhawna, Rajkumar Singh Yadav, Dilip Kumar Swain, Pradeep K. Rai, and Satish Kumar Garg. "Mercury-induced inhibition of tyrosine phosphorylation of sperm proteins and altered functional dynamics of buck spermatozoa: An in vitro study." *Biological trace element research* (2020): 1-15.

[40] Kushawaha, Bhawna, Rajkumar Singh Yadav, Dilip Kumar Swain, Priyambada Kumari, Akhilesh Kumar, Brijesh Yadav, Mukul Anand, Sarvajeet Yadav, Dipty Singh, and Satish Kumar Garg. "Collapsed mitochondrial cristae in goat spermatozoa due to mercury result in lethality and compromised motility along with altered kinematic patterns." *Scientific reports* 11 (2021).

[41] Visconti, Pablo E., Linda R. Johnson, Maria Oyaski, Miguel Fornés, Stuart B. Moss, George L. Gerton, and Gregory S. Kopf. "Regulation, localization, and anchoring of protein kinase A subunits during mouse sperm capacitation." Developmental biology 192, no. 2 (1997): 351-363.

[42] Seshagiri, P. B., H. S. Lalitha, A. Mishra, and G. V. Sireesha. "Embryo-endometrial proteases during early mammalian development." (2003).

[43] Nolan, Michael A., Donner F. Babcock, Gunther Wennemuth, William Brown, Kimberly A. Burton, and G. Stanley McKnight. "Sperm-specific protein kinase A catalytic subunit Cα2 orchestrates cAMP signaling for male fertility." *Proceedings of the National Academy of Sciences* 101, no. 37 (2004): 13483-13488.

[44] Austin, C. R. "Observations on the penetration of the sperm into the mammalian egg." Australian journal of biological sciences 4, no. 4 (1951): 581-596.

[45] Yanagimachi, R. "Fertility of mammalian spermatozoa: its development and relativity." Zygote 2, no. 4 (1994): 371-372.

[46] Visconti, Pablo E., Janice L. Bailey, Grace D. Moore, Dieyun Pan, Patricia Olds-Clarke, and Gregory S. Kopf. "Capacitation of mouse spermatozoa. I. Correlation between the capacitation state and protein tyrosine phosphorylation." Development 121, no. 4 (1995): 1129-1137.

[47] Wertheimer, Eva V., Ana M. Salicioni, Weimin Liu, Claudia L. Trevino, Julio Chavez, Enrique O. Hernández-González, Alberto Darszon, and Pablo E. Visconti. "Chloride is essential for capacitation and for the capacitation-associated increase in tyrosine phosphorylation." Journal of Biological Chemistry 283, no. 51 (2008): 35539-35550.

[48] Jayaprakash, D., K. Santhosh Kumar, S. Shivaji, and P. B. Seshagiri. "Pentoxifylline induces hyperactivation and acrosome reaction in spermatozoa of golden hamsters: changes in motility kinematics." *Human reproduction (Oxford, England)* 12, no. 10 (1997): 2192-2199.

[49] Ain, Rupasri, K. Uma Devi, S. Shivaji, and P. B. Seshagiri. "Pentoxifylline-stimulated capacitation and acrosome reaction in hamster spermatozoa: involvement of intracellular signalling molecules." *Molecular human reproduction* 5, no. 7 (1999): 618-626.

[50] Carrera, Alfonso, Jiri Moos, Xiao Ping Ning, George L. Gerton, Jan Tesarik, Gregory S. Kopf, and Stuart B. Moss. "Regulation of protein tyrosine phosphorylation in human sperm by a calcium/calmodulin-dependent mechanism: identification of A kinase anchor proteins as major substrates for tyrosine phosphorylation." Developmental biology 180, no. 1 (1996): 284-296.

[51] Lefievre, Linda, Kula N. Jha, E. V. E. de LAMIRANDE, Pablo E. Visconti, and Claude Gagnon. "Activation of protein kinase A during human sperm capacitation and acrosome reaction." *Journal of andrology* 23, no. 5 (2002): 709-716.

[52] Miki, Kiyoshi, William D. Willis, Paula R. Brown, Eugenia H. Goulding, Kerry D. Fulcher, and Edward M. Eddy. "Targeted disruption of the Akap4 gene causes defects in sperm flagellum and motility." Developmental biology 248, no. 2 (2002): 331-342.

[53] Luconi, M., I. Porazzi, P. Ferruzzi, S. Marchiani, G. Forti, and E. Baldi. "Tyrosine phosphorylation of the a kinase anchoring protein 3 (AKAP3) and soluble adenylate cyclase are involved in the increase of human sperm motility by bicarbonate." Biology of reproduction 72, no. 1 (2005): 22-32.

[54] Kumar, Vivek, Nandini Rangaraj, and Sisinthy Shivaji. "Activity of pyruvate dehydrogenase A (PDHA) in hamster spermatozoa correlates positively with hyperactivation and is associated with sperm capacitation." Biology of reproduction 75, no. 5 (2006): 767-777.

[55] Hansen Naaby, Soren, Arabinda Mandal, Michael J. Wolkowicz, Buer Sen, V. Anne Westbrook, Jagathpala Shetty, Scott A. Coonrod et al. "CABYR, a novel calcium-binding tyrosine

phosphorylation-regulated fibrous sheath protein involved in capacitation." *Developmental biology* 242, no. 2 (2002): 236-254.

[56] Marín-Briggiler, Clara I., Kula N. Jha, Olga Chertihin, Mariano G. Buffone, John C. Herr, Mónica H. Vazquez-Levin, and Pablo E. Visconti. "Evidence of the presence of calcium/calmodulin-dependent protein kinase IV in human sperm and its involvement in motility regulation." Journal of Cell Science 118, no. 9 (2005): 2013-2022.

[57] Leclerc, Pierre, Eve de Lamirande, and Claude Gagnon. "Cyclic adenosine 3′, 5′ monophosphate-dependent regulation of protein tyrosine phosphorylation in relation to human sperm capacitation and motility." Biology of reproduction 55, no. 3 (1996): 684-692.

[58] Sharpe, Richard M., Chris McKinnell, Catrina Kivlin, and Jane S. Fisher. "Proliferation and functional maturation of Sertoli cells, and their relevance to disorders of testis function in adulthood." REPRODUCTION CAMBRIDGE- 125, no. 6 (2003): 769-784.

[59] Thompson, Jennifer, and John Bannigan. "Cadmium: toxic effects on the reproductive system and the embryo." Reproductive toxicology 25, no. 3 (2008): 304-315.

[60] Ji, Yan-Li, Hua Wang, Ping Liu, Qun Wang, Xian-Feng Zhao, Xiu-Hong Meng, Tao Yu et al. "Pubertal cadmium exposure impairs testicular development and spermatogenesis via disrupting testicular testosterone synthesis in adult mice." Reproductive Toxicology 29, no. 2 (2010): 176-183.

[61] El-Demerdash, Fatma M., Mokhtar I. Yousef, Fatma S. Kedwany, and Hoda H. Baghdadi. "Cadmium-induced changes in lipid peroxidation, blood hematology, biochemical parameters and semen quality of male rats: protective role of vitamin E and β-carotene." Food and chemical toxicology 42, no. 10 (2004): 1563-1571.

[62] Boujbiha, Mohamed Ali, Khaled Hamden, Fadhel Guermazi, Ali Bouslama, Asma Omezzine, Abdelaziz Kammoun, and Abdelfattah El Feki. "Testicular toxicity in mercuric chloride treated rats: association with oxidative stress." *Reproductive toxicology* 28, no. 1 (2009): 81-89.

[63] Huang, Kai, Han Li, Bin Zhang, Tongzhang Zheng, Yuanyuan Li, Aifen Zhou, Xiaofu Du et al. "Prenatal cadmium exposure and preterm low birth weight in China." Journal of exposure science & environmental epidemiology 27, no. 5 (2017): 491-496.

[64] Lee, I. P., and R. L. Dixon. "Factors influencing reproduction and genetic toxic effects on male gonads." Environmental health perspectives 24 (1978): 117-127.

[65] Toft, Gunnar, and Louis J. Guillette Jr. "Decreased sperm count and sexual behavior in mosquitofish exposed to water from a pesticide-contaminated lake." Ecotoxicology and environmental safety 60, no. 1 (2005): 15-20.

[66] Marchlewicz, M., M. Protasowicki, L. Rozewicka, M. Piasecka, and M. Laszczyńska. "Effect of long-term exposure to lead on testis and epididymis in rats." Folia histochemica et cytobiologica 31, no. 2 (1993): 55-62.

[67] Wang, Yi-Xin, Peng Wang, Wei Feng, Chong Liu, Pan Yang, Ying-Jun Chen, Li Sun et al. "Relationships between seminal plasma metals/metalloids and semen quality, sperm apoptosis and DNA integrity." Environmental pollution 224 (2017): 224-234.

[68] Si, Yuming, and Makoto Okuno. "Role of tyrosine phosphorylation of flagellar proteins in hamster sperm hyperactivation." Biology of reproduction 61, no. 1 (1999): 240-246.

[69] Smith, Allan H., and Craig M. Steinmaus. "Health effects of arsenic and chromium in drinking water: recent human findings." Annual review of public health 30 (2009): 107-122.

[70] Tóth, G., T. Hermann, M. R. Da Silva, and L. Montanarella. "Heavy metals in agricultural soils of the European Union with implications for food safety." Environment international 88 (2016): 299-309.

[71] Zhang, Jingcheng, Pengxiang Qu, Chuan Zhou, Xin Liu, Xiaonan Ma, Mengyun Wang, Yongsheng Wang, Jianmin Su, Jun Liu, and Yong Zhang. "MicroRNA-125b is a key epigenetic regulatory factor that promotes nuclear transfer reprogramming." Journal of Biological Chemistry 292, no. 38 (2017): 15916-15926.

[72] Ghaffari, Mohammad Ali, and Behrooz Motlagh. "In vitro effect of lead, silver, tin, mercury, indium and bismuth on human sperm creatine kinase activity: a presumable mechanism for men infertility." *Iranian biomedical journal* 15, no. 1-2 (2011): 38.

[73] Hayati, Alfiah, Erika Wulansari, Dhea Sanggita Armando, Ari Sofiyanti, Muhammad Hilman Fu'adil Amin, and Manikya Pramudya. "Effects of in vitro exposure of mercury on sperm quality and fertility of tropical fish Cyprinus carpio L." *The Egyptian Journal of Aquatic* Research 45, no. 2 (2019): 189-195.

[74] Mohamed, Mostafa K., Thomas M. Burbacher, and N. Karle Mottet. "Effects of methyl mercury on testicular functions in Macaca fascicularis monkeys." *Pharmacology & toxicology* 60, no. 1 (1987): 29-36.

[75] Orisakwe, Orish E., Onyenmechi J. Afonne, Eddy Nwobodo, Lasbrey Asomugha, and Chudi E. Dioka. "Low-dose mercury induces testicular damage protected by zinc in mice." European Journal of Obstetrics & Gynecology and Reproductive Biology 95, no. 1 (2001): 92-96.

[76] Massanyi, Peter, Martin Massanyi, Roberto Madeddu, Robert Stawarz, and Norbert Lukac. "Effects of Cadmium, Lead, and Mercury on the Structure and Function of Reproductive Organs." Toxics 8, no. 4 (2020): 94.

[77] Siu, Erica R., Dolores D. Mruk, Catarina S. Porto, and C. Yan Cheng. "Cadmium-induced testicular injury." Toxicology and applied pharmacology 238, no. 3 (2009): 240-249.

[78] Henriques, Magda Carvalho, Susana Loureiro, Margarida Fardilha, and Maria Teresa Herdeiro. "Exposure to mercury and human reproductive health: A systematic review." Reproductive toxicology 85 (2019): 93-103.

[79] Choy, Christine MY, Christopher WK Lam, Lorena TF Cheung, Christine M. Briton-Jones, L. P. Cheung, and Christopher J. Haines. "Infertility, blood mercury concentrations and dietary seafood consumption: a case–control study." *BJOG: An International Journal of Obstetrics & Gynaecology* 109, no. 10 (2002): 1121-1125.

[80] Dickman, M. D., and K. M. C. Leung. "Mercury and organochlorine exposure from fish consumption in Hong Kong." Chemosphere 37, no. 5 (1998): 991-1015.

[81] Keck, Christoph, Martin Bergmann, Erik Ernst, Cornelia Müller, Sabine Kliesch, and Eberhard Nieschlag. "Autometallographic detection of mercury in testicular tissue of an infertile man exposed to mercury vapor." Reproductive Toxicology 7, no. 5 (1993): 469-475.

[82] Baldi, Elisabetta, Michaela Luconi, Lorella Bonaccorsi, Monica Muratori, and Gianni Forti. "Intracellular events and signaling pathways involved in sperm acquisition of fertilizing capacity and acrosome reaction." Front Biosci 5, no. 1 (2000): 110-123.

[83] De Lamirande, E., and C. Gagnon. "The extracellular signal-regulated kinase (ERK) pathway is involved in human sperm function and modulated by the superoxide anion." Molecular human reproduction 8, no. 2 (2002): 124-135.

[84] Fu, Jieli, Yuhua Li, Lirui Wang, Linqing Zhen, Qiangzhen Yang, Peifei Li, and Xinhong Li. "Bovine serum albumin and skim-milk improve boar sperm motility by enhancing energy metabolism and protein modifications during liquid storage at 17 C." Theriogenology 102 (2017): 87-97.

[85] Demarco, Ignacio A., Felipe Espinosa, Jennifer Edwards, Julian Sosnik, Jose Luis De la Vega-Beltran, Joel W. Hockensmith, Gregory S. Kopf, Alberto Darszon, and Pablo E. Visconti. "Involvement of a Na+/HCO 3– cotransporter in mouse sperm capacitation." *Journal of Biological Chemistry* 278, no. 9 (2003): 7001-7009.

[86] Krasznai, Zoltán, Masaaki Morisawa, Zoárd Tibor Krasznai, Sachiko Morisawa, Kazuo Inaba, Zsuzsa Kassai Bazsáné, Bálint Rubovszky, Béla Bodnár, Antal Borsos, and Teréz Márián. "Gadolinium, a mechano-sensitive channel blocker, inhibits osmosis-initiated motility of sea-and freshwater fish sperm, but does not affect human or ascidian sperm motility." *Cell motility and the cytoskeleton* 55, no. 4 (2003): 232-243.

[87] Grasa, Patricia, Carmen Colas, Margarita Gallego, Luís Monteagudo, Teresa Muino-Blanco, and José Alvaro Cebrián-Pérez. "Changes in content and localization of proteins phosphorylated at tyrosine, serine and threonine residues during ram sperm capacitation and acrosome reaction." *Reproduction* 137, no. 4 (2009): 655.

[88] Liguori, L., E. De Lamirande, A. Minelli, and C. Gagnon. "Various protein kinases regulate human sperm acrosome reaction and the associated phosphorylation of Tyr residues and of the Thr-Glu-Tyr motif." Molecular human reproduction 11, no. 3 (2004): 211-221.

[89] Urner, Françoise, and Denny Sakkas. "Protein phosphorylation in mammalian spermatozoa." Reproduction 125, no. 1 (2003): 17-26.

[90] Visconti, P. E., V. A. Westbrook, O. Chertihin, I. Demarco, S. Sleight, and A. B. Diekman. "Novel signaling pathways involved in sperm acquisition of fertilizing capacity." Journal of reproductive immunology 53, no. 1-2 (2002): 133-150.

[91] Martinez, Caroline S., Alyne G. Escobar, João Guilherme D. Torres, Daniela S. Brum, Francielli W. Santos, María J. Alonso, Mercedes Salaices et al. "Chronic exposure to low doses of mercury impairs sperm quality and induces oxidative stress in rats." *Journal of Toxicology and Environmental Health, Part A* 77, no. 1-3 (2014): 143-154.

[92] Arabi, M. "The role of mercury in the etiology of sperm dysfunction in holstein bulls." Asian-australasian journal of animal sciences 19, no. 3 (2006): 335-340.

[93] Arabi, M., and M. S. Heydarnejad. "In vitro mercury exposure on spermatozoa from normospermic individuals." Pakistan Journal of Biological Sciences 10, no. 15 (2007): 2448-2453.

[94] Van Look, K. J. W., and D. E. Kime. "Automated sperm morphology analysis in fishes: the effect of mercury on goldfish sperm." Journal of Fish Biology 63, no. 4 (2003): 1020-1033.

[95] Vergílio, C. S., R. V. Moreira, C. E. V. Carvalho, and E. J. T. Melo. "Effects of in vitro exposure to mercury on male gonads and sperm structure of the tropical fish tuvira G ymnotus carapo (L.)." *Journal of fish diseases* 37, no. 6 (2014): 543-551.

[96] Mocevic, Emina, Ina O. Specht, Jacob L. Marott, Aleksander

Giwercman, Bo AG Jönsson, Gunnar Toft, Thomas Lundh, and Jens Peter Bonde. "Environmental mercury exposure, semen quality and reproductive hormones in Greenlandic Inuit and European men: a cross-sectional study." Asian journal of andrology 15, no. 1 (2013): 97.

[97] Chan, Celia HY, Ernest HY Ng, Cecilia LW Chan, and Timothy HY Chan. "Effectiveness of psychosocial group intervention for reducing anxiety in women undergoing in vitro fertilization: a randomized controlled study." Fertility and sterility 85, no. 2 (2006): 339-346

[98] Batlle-Bayer, Laura, Alba Bala, Elodie Lemaire, Jaume Albertí, Isabel García-Herrero, Rubén Aldaco, and Pere Fullana-i-Palmer. "An energy-and nutrient-corrected functional unit to compare LCAs of diets." Science of The Total Environment 671 (2019): 175-179.

[99] Jarup, Lars. "Cadmium overload and toxicity." Nephrology Dialysis Transplantation 17, no. suppl_2 (2002): 35-39

[100] Dias, Maria Celeste, Cristina Monteiro, José Moutinho-Pereira, Carlos Correia, Berta Gonçalves, and Conceição Santos. "Cadmium toxicity affects photosynthesis and plant growth at different levels." *Acta physiologiae plantarum* 35, no. 4 (2013): 1281-1289.

[101] Chaney, Rufus L. "Food safety issues for mineral and organic fertilizers." Advances in Agronomy 117 (2012): 51-116.

[102] Singh, Priyanka, Husna Siddiqui, Fareen Sami, Yamshi Arif, Andrzej Bajguz, and Shamsul Hayat. "Cadmium: A Threatening Agent for Plants." In Plant Responses to Soil Pollution, pp. 59-88. Springer, Singapore, 2020.

[103] Satarug, Soisungwan. "Cadmium sources and toxicity." (2019): 25.

[104] Matovic, Vesna, Aleksandra Buha, Danijela Đukić-Ćosić, and Zorica Bulat. "Insight into the oxidative stress induced by lead and/or cadmium in blood, liver and kidneys." Food and Chemical Toxicology 78 (2015): 130-140.

[105] Takiguchi, Masufumi, William E. Achanzar, Wei Qu, Guying Li, and Michael P. Waalkes. "Effects of cadmium on DNA-(Cytosine-5) methyltransferase activity and DNA methylation status during cadmium-induced cellular transformation." Experimental cell research 286, no. 2 (2003): 355-365.

[106] Geng, Hui-Xia, and Lai Wang. "Cadmium: Toxic effects on placental and embryonic development." Environmental toxicology and pharmacology 67 (2019): 102-107.

[107] Zhu, Qiqi, Xiaoheng Li, and Ren-Shan Ge. "Toxicological effects of cadmium on mammalian testis." Frontiers in Genetics 11 (2020): 527.

[108] Meeker, John D., Mary G. Rossano, Bridget Protas, Michael P. Diamond, Elizabeth Puscheck, Douglas Daly, Nigel Paneth, and Julia J. Wirth. "Cadmium, lead, and other metals in relation to semen quality: human evidence for molybdenum as a male reproductive toxicant." Environmental health perspectives 116, no. 11 (2008): 1473-1479.

[109] Oliveira, Helena, Marcello Spanò, Conceição Santos, and Maria de Lourdes Pereira. "Adverse effects of cadmium exposure on mouse sperm." Reproductive Toxicology 28, no. 4 (2009): 550-555.

[110] Rana, S. V. S. "Perspectives in endocrine toxicity of heavy metals—a review." Biological trace element research 160, no. 1 (2014): 1-14.

[111] Shojaeepour, Saeedeh, Fariba Sharififar, Tahereh Haghpanah, Maryam Iranpour, Masoud Imani, and Shahriar Dabiri. "Panax ginseng ameliorate toxic effects of cadmium on germ cell apoptosis, sperm quality, and oxidative stress in male Wistar rats." Toxin Reviews (2021): 1-13.

[112] Obembe, Olawale O., and Yunus Raji. "Effects of aqueous extract of Moringa oleifera seed on cadmium-induced reproductive toxicity in male Wistar rats." African health sciences 18, no. 3 (2018): 653-663.

[113] Leoni, Giovanni, Luisa Bogliolo, Gianni Deiana, Fiammetta Berlinguer, Irma Rosati, Pier Paolo Pintus, Sergio Ledda, and Salvatore Naitana. "Influence of cadmium exposure on in vitro ovine gamete dysfunction." Reproductive toxicology 16, no. 4 (2002): 371-377.

[114] Roychowdhury, A., and A. K. Gautam. "Alteration of human sperm and other seminal constituents after lead exposure." Indian journal of physiology and allied sciences, no. 49 (1995): 68-73.

[115] Heidari, Amir Hassan, Mohammad Javad Zamiri, Mohammad Naser Nazem, Mohammad Reza Jafarzadeh Shirazi, Amir Akhlaghi, and Zarbakht Ansari Pirsaraei. "Detrimental effects of long-term exposure to heavy metals on histology, size and trace elements of testes and sperm parameters in Kermani Sheep." *Ecotoxicology and Environmental Safety* 207 (2021): 111563.

[116] Saleh, Ramadan A., and ASHOK AGARWAL HCLD. "Oxidative stress and male infertility: from research bench to clinical practice." Journal of andrology 23, no. 6 (2002): 737-752.

[117] Kiziler, Ali Riza, Birsen Aydemir, Ilhan Onaran, Bulent Alici, Hamdi Ozkara, Tevfik Gulyasar, and Mehmet Can Akyolcu. "High levels of cadmium and lead in seminal fluid and blood of smoking men are associated with high oxidative stress and damage in infertile subjects." *Biological trace element research* 120, no. 1 (2007): 82-91.

[118] Li, Jin-Long, Rui Gao, Shu Li, Jin-Tao Wang, Zhao-Xin Tang, and Shi-Wen Xu. "Testicular toxicity induced by dietary cadmium in cocks and ameliorative effect by selenium." Biometals 23, no. 4 (2010): 695-705.

[119] Choong, Grace, Ying Liu, and Douglas M. Templeton. "Interplay of calcium and cadmium in mediating cadmium toxicity." Chemico-biological interactions 211 (2014): 54-65.

[120] Templeton, Douglas M., and Ying Liu. "Multiple roles of cadmium in cell death and survival." Chemico-biological interactions 188, no. 2 (2010): 267-275.

[121] Zhao, Li-lin, Yan-fei Ru, Miao Liu, Jia-nan Tang, Ju-fen Zheng, Bin Wu, Yi-hua Gu, and Hui-juan Shi. "Reproductive effects of cadmium on sperm function and early embryonic development in vitro." PloS one 12, no. 11 (2017): e0186727.

[122] Wang, Xinghao, Ruijuan Qu, Jiaoqin Liu, Zhongbo Wei, Liansheng Wang, Shaogui Yang, Qingguo Huang, and Zunyao Wang. "Effect of different carbon nanotubes on cadmium toxicity to Daphnia magna: The role of catalyst impurities and adsorption capacity." Environmental Pollution 208 (2016): 732-738.

[123] Nair, Ambily Ravindran, Olivier DeGheselle, Karen Smeets, Emmy Van Kerkhove, and Ann Cuypers. "Cadmium-induced pathologies: where is the oxidative balance lost (or not)?." *International journal of molecular sciences* 14, no. 3 (2013): 6116-6143.

[124] Rinaldi, Mariagrazia, Antonio Micali, Herbert Marini, Elena B. Adamo, Domenico Puzzolo, Antonina Pisani, Vincenzo Trichilo, Domenica Altavilla, Francesco Squadrito, and Letteria Minutoli. "Cadmium, organ toxicity and therapeutic approaches: a review on brain, kidney and testis damage." *Current medicinal chemistry* 24, no. 35 (2017): 3879-3893

[125] Li, Xinhong, Lirui Wang, Yuhua Li, Na Zhao, Linqing Zhen, Jieli Fu, and Qiangzhen Yang. "Calcium regulates motility and protein phosphorylation by changing cAMP and ATP concentrations

in boar sperm in vitro." Animal reproduction science 172 (2016): 39-51.

[126] Kitchin KT, Wallace K. 2008. Evidence against the nuclear in situ binding of arsenicals—oxidative stress theory of arsenic carcinogenesis. Toxicol Appl Pharmacol232(2):252-25718671993.

[127] Mazumder, D.N.G. (2008) Chronic arsenic toxicity and human health. Indian J Med Res 128:436-447.

[128] Centeno, J.A., Mullick, F.G., Martinez, L., Page, N.P., Gibb, H., Longfellow, D. (2002) Pathology related to chronic arsenic exposure. Environ Health Perspect 110:883-886.

[129] Pant, N., Murthy, R.C. and Srivastava, S.P. (2004) Male reproductive toxicity of sodium arsenite in mice. Hum Exp Toxicol 23:399-403.

[130] Sarkar, M., Biswas, N.M. and Ghosh, D. Effect of sodium arsenite on testicular 5-3,17-HSD activities in albino rats: Dose and duration dependent responses. Medical Science and Research, no 19(1991):789-790.

[131] Hossain, Khaled, Anwarul A. Akhand, Masashi Kato, Jun Du, Kozue Takeda, Jianghong Wu, Kei Takeuchi, Wei Liu, Haruhiko Suzuki, and Izumi Nakashima. "Arsenite induces apoptosis of murine T lymphocytes through membrane raft-linked signaling for activation of c-Jun amino-terminal kinase." The Journal of Immunology 165, no. 8 (2000): 4290-4297.

[132] Chen, Wei, Jennifer L. Martindale, Nikki J. Holbrook, and Yusen Liu. "Tumor promoter arsenite activates extracellular signal-regulated kinase through a signaling pathway mediated by epidermal growth factor receptor and Shc." Molecular and Cellular Biology 18, no. 9 (1998): 5178.

[133] Wu, Weidong, Lee M. Graves, Ilona Jaspers, Robert B. Devlin, William Reed, and James M. Samet. "Activation of the EGF receptor signaling pathway in human airway epithelial cells exposed to metals." American Journal of Physiology-Lung Cellular and Molecular Physiology 277, no. 5 (1999): L924-L931.

[134] Hu, Yuxin, Jin Li, Bin Lou, Ruirui Wu, Gang Wang, Chunwei Lu, Huihui Wang, Jingbo Pi, and Yuanyuan Xu. "The role of reactive oxygen species in arsenic toxicity." Biomolecules 10, no. 2 (2020): 240.

[135] Suc, Isabelle, Olivier Meilhac, Isabelle Lajoie-mazenc, Jean Vandaele, Günther Jurgens, Robert Salvayre, and Anne Nègre-salvayre. "Activation of EGF receptor by oxidized LDL." The FASEB Journal 12, no. 9 (1998): 665-671.

[136] Wu, Weidong, Ilona Jaspers, Wenli Zhang, Lee M. Graves, and James M. Samet. "Role of Ras in metal-induced EGF receptor signaling and NF-κB activation in human airway epithelial cells." American Journal of Physiology-Lung Cellular and Molecular Physiology 282, no. 5 (2002): L1040-L1048.

[137] Kodigepalli, Karthik M., Punashi S. Dutta, Kyle A. Bauckman, and Meera Nanjundan. "SnoN/SkiL expression is modulated via arsenic trioxide-induced activation of the PI3K/AKT pathway in ovarian cancer cells." FEBS letters 587, no. 1 (2013): 5-16.

[138] Simeonova, Petia P., Shiyi Wang, Tracy Hulderman, and Michael I. Luster. "c-Src-dependent activation of the epidermal growth factor receptor and mitogen-activated protein kinase pathway by arsenic: Role in carcinogenesis." Journal of Biological Chemistry 277, no. 4 (2002): 2945-2950.

[139] Biscardi, Jacqueline S., Ming-Chei Maa, David A. Tice, Michael E. Cox, Tzeng-Horne Leu, and Sarah J. Parsons. "c-Src-mediated phosphorylation of the epidermal growth factor receptor on Tyr845 and Tyr1101 is associated with

modulation of receptor function." Journal of Biological Chemistry 274, no. 12 (1999): 8335-8343.

[140] Tice, D.A., Biscardi, J.S., Nickles, A.L. and Parsons, S.J., 1999. Mechanism of biological synergy between cellular Src and epidermal growth factor receptor. Proceedings of the National Academy of Sciences, *96*(4), pp.1415-1420.

[141] Renu, Kaviyarasi, Harishkumar Madhyastha, Radha Madhyastha, Masugi Maruyama, Sathishkumar Vinayagam, and Abilash Valsala Gopalakrishnan. "Review on molecular and biochemical insights of arsenic-mediated male reproductive toxicity." Life sciences 212 (2018): 37-58.

[142] Shim, Juyoung, Rachel H. Kennedy, Lisa M. Weatherly, Lee M. Hutchinson, Jonathan H. Pelletier, Hina N. Hashmi, Kayla Blais, Alejandro Velez, and Julie A. Gosse. "Arsenic inhibits mast cell degranulation via suppression of early tyrosine phosphorylation events." Journal of Applied Toxicology 36, no. 11 (2016): 1446-1459.

[143] Huang, Qingyu, Lianzhong Luo, Ambreen Alamdar, Jie Zhang, Liangpo Liu, Meiping Tian, Syed Ali Musstjab Akber Shah Eqani, and Heqing Shen. "Integrated proteomics and metabolomics analysis of rat testis: mechanism of arsenic-induced male reproductive toxicity." Scientific reports 6, no. 1 (2016a): 1-12.

[144] Q. Huang, L. Luo, A. Alamdar, J. Zhang, L. Liu, M. Tian, S.A.M.A.S. Eqani, H. Shen, Integrated proteomics and metabolomics analysis of rat testis: mechanism of arsenic-induced male reproductive toxicity, Sci. Rep. 6 (2016b) 32518, https://doi. org/10.1038/srep32518.

[145] Gavaghan, H., 2002. Lead, unsafe at any level. Bulletin of the World Health Organization, *80*, pp.82-82.

[146] Li, Na, Yu-hua Hou, Dan-dan Ma, Wei-xin Jing, Hans-Uwe Dahms, and Lan Wang. "Lead accumulation, oxidative damage and histopathological alteration in testes and accessory glands of freshwater crab, Sinopotamon henanense, induced by acute lead exposure." Ecotoxicology and environmental safety 117 (2015): 20-27.

[147] Oldereid, N. B., Y. Thomassen, A. Attramadal, B. Olaisen, and K. Purvis. "Concentrations of lead, cadmium and zinc in the tissues of reproductive organs of men." Reproduction 99, no. 2 (1993): 421-425.

[148] Rahman, Zeeshanur, and Ved Pal Singh. "The relative impact of toxic heavy metals (THMs)(arsenic (As), cadmium (Cd), chromium (Cr)(VI), mercury (Hg), and lead (Pb)) on the total environment: an overview." *Environmental monitoring and assessment* 191, no. 7 (2019): 1-21.

[149] Gandhi, Jason, Rafael J. Hernandez, Andrew Chen, Noel L. Smith, Yefim R. Sheynkin, Gargi Joshi, and Sardar Ali Khan. "Impaired hypothalamic-pituitary-testicular axis activity, spermatogenesis, and sperm function promote infertility in males with lead poisoning." *Zygote* 25, no. 2 (2017): 103-110.

[150] Hassan, Eman, Khaled Kahilo, Tarek Kamal, Marwa Hassan, and Mohamed Saleh Elgawish. "The protective effect of epigallocatechin-3-gallate on testicular oxidative stress in lead-induced toxicity mediated by Cyp19 gene/estradiol level." Toxicology 422 (2019): 76-83.

[151] Bridges, Christy C., and Rudolfs K. Zalups. "Molecular and ionic mimicry and the transport of toxic metals." Toxicology and applied pharmacology 204, no. 3 (2005): 274-308.

[152] He, Yuanqiao, Qianxing Zou, Houyang Chen, Shiqi Weng, Tao Luo, and Xuhui Zeng. "Lead inhibits human sperm functions by reducing the levels of intracellular calcium, cAMP, and

tyrosine phosphorylation." The Tohoku journal of experimental medicine 238, no. 4 (2016): 295-303.

[153] Tamburrino, L., S. Marchiani, E. Vicini, B. Muciaccia, M. Cambi, S. Pellegrini, G. Forti, M. Muratori, and E. Baldi. "Quantification of CatSper1 expression in human spermatozoa and relation to functional parameters." Human Reproduction 30, no. 7 (2015): 1532-1544.

Chapter 10

Rare Sperm Freezing

Desislava Dyulgerova-Nikolova and Tanya Milachich

Abstract

Gamete cryobanking has been widely incorporated in present assisted reproductive technology (ART). Preserving male gametes for future fertility is considered to be an easy and accessible way to insure one's reproduction. Despite the fact that the method could not secure success, sperm freezing could be the only chance to father biological offspring. In cases when severe male factor (SMF) infertility is diagnosed (retrograde ejaculation, virtual azoospermia, obstructive azoospermia, cryptozoospermia) and providing fresh semen samples for assisted reproduction may alter chances to achieve pregnancy, rare sperm cryopreservation could contribute for conceiving. Isolation, selection and cryopreservation of single sperm cells from semen samples is a challenging procedure. Different approaches and devices could be used in order to extract utmost spermatozoa. Aiming to highest cryosurvival rates sperm freezing protocols should be carefully considered. For some men, rare sperm cryopreservation might be the only alternative for parenting biological offspring. Thus, the latter technique should be widely discussed, developed and practiced in assisted reproduction.

Keywords: cryopreservation, fertility preservation, single sperm selection, sperm sorting devices, cryptozoospermia, sperm genetics

1. Introduction

Gamete cryobanking has been considerably incorporated in present assisted reproductive technology (ART). Preserving fertility through banking is an accessible and relatively reliable procedure that gives opportunity for men to parent their own biological child. Most of the clinics providing fertility treatment have their individual cryobanks and offer fertility preservation counseling. Network structures for gamete and tissue storage have also been developed. Some of the affirmed ones would be the Danish network (www.rigshospitalet.dk), *Ferti*PROTECT ® (www.fertiprotect.com), German-Austrian-Swiss centralized and decentralized network between the countries, Oncofertility® Concortium (www.oncofertility.northwestern.edu) for knowledge exchange in the field of fertility preservation [1]. The complexity of fertility preservation generates necessity for close interaction between the patients, reproductive specialist, reproductive biologist, urologist, oncologist, etc. In order to provide accurate and prompt counseling and treatment, each clinical case should be considered in full and timely.

Retrieving, freezing, storage and use of human oocytes, spermatozoa, embryos and ovarian and testicular tissue has been executively studied and explored in assisted reproduction (AR). Cryopreservation presents remarkable advance to men and women who have decided to postpone fertility. It turns out to be a safety plan for patient with subfertility and certain physiological or psychological conditions.

For patients with forthcoming cancer treatment it could be the only chance to have their own biological child.

Nowadays cryopreservation and cryobanking is inseparable branch to assisted reproduction and fertility preservation treatment.

2. Historical preview of sperm cryopreservation

First attempts to preserve human spermatozoa dates back to 1776 when Lazaro Spallanzani studied sperm cryopreservation by cooling it in snow. It was 1949 when Polge, Smith and Parkes discovered glycerol to be effective in protecting spermatozoa exposed to low temperatures [2]. This discovery, alongside with the first reports for achieving pregnancy by frozen and thawed spermatozoa in 1953 by Dr. Jerome K. Sherman [3], led to constant development and improvement of sperm freezing protocols and devices. In 1972 a slow freezing protocol, developed by D. Whittingham, S. Leibo, and P. Mazur, was introduced. Slow cooling with temperature drops in the range of 0.3 to 2 degrees Celsius per minute and consequent slow warming (4 to 25 degrees C° per minute) was performed. This protocol, applied to mouse embryos, resulted in 65% pregnancy rate and 40% full term pregnancy [4]. Recent challenge in cryobiology was freezing spermatozoa from strains of genetically engineered mice. A novel method using a cryoprotectant composed of 18% raffinose pentahydrate and 3% skim milk was presented [5, 6].

Not only protecting sperm cells at low temperatures, but preserving their structural (morphological), kinetic and functional characteristics is at aim when freezing semen samples. It is well known that cryopreservation has deleterious effect on sperm cells.

Although spermatozoa are relatively small in size and have large surface, cold shock and ice formation could damage different cell structures and organelles, as most affected structures are the plasmalema, acrosome and the tail [7]. Changes in membrane organization and permeability, formation of reactive oxygen species (ROS) and consequent DNA damage as a result to freezing hinders normal sperm activity and functions [8].

Semen cryopreservation strives high quality of the preserved samples. Thus, retaining sperm motility and viability, membrane integrity and intact DNA in thawed samples, has been formed as priority when developing freezing protocols. Cryoprotective medium, containing various additives – fatty acids, proteins, antioxidants, serum, essential oils derived from plants, nanoparticles and others, are also used in sperm freezing procedures.

3. Conditions requiring sperm preservation

Diversity of health conditions and personal or lifestyle circumstances could necessitate semen cryopreservation.

3.1 Sperm freezing for cancer patients

Five most common cancers diagnosed in men are prostate cancer, lung cancer, colorectal cancer, bladder cancer and melanoma. Testicular tumors, relatively rare condition on a per-population basis, are the most common malignancy in men aged 20 to 35 years [9, 10]. According to The National Cancer Institute one in two men will be diagnosed with cancer during their lifetime. Encouraging data for approximately

1.8% decrease in cancer death for male patients was recently published [11]. Modern medicine and constant scientific research in the field are the key to increasing the chances for long term survival (5 and above years). Quality of life after cancer treatment and when in remission is of great importance. Unfortunately, cancer by itself and chemo- and/or radiotherapy treatment, have adverse effect over the process of spermatogenesis. For most cured patients, after healing, sperm production recovers to a certain level in time. When bilateral orchiectomy was performed or high dosage of radiotherapy (24–25 Gy) was administrated permanent loss of fertility is inevitable [12]. Introducing cancer patients to fertility preservation before the treatment is required, especially for adolescents and young adults (aged 15–39 years) [13].

3.2 Sperm freezing for patients with retrograde ejaculation and hypospermia

Ejaculatory disorders could lead not only to psychological distress but may be the reason for 0.2–3% of infertility incidence in the couple. Co-ordination between epididymis, vas deferens, prostate, seminal vesicles, bladder neck and bulbourethral glands is required for the proper course of ejaculation. Various pharmacological, neurogenic or anatomic factors, disrupting the contraction of the bladder neck, may lead to retrograde ejaculation. In such cases semen is refluxed in the bladder and blends with the urine [14, 15]. As the urine normally has slightly acidic pH levels (average value - 6.0) compared to pH 7.1–8.0 of semen, the fusion of these fluids and pH fluctuations has adverse effect on spermatozoa [16]. Sperm cells retrieved from postejaculatory urine could be proceeded for assisted reproduction. Strict protocols for urine alkalization prior the procedure are mandatory. In some patients retrograde ejaculation results in hypospermia (abnormally low volume of less than 1.5 ml of the semen sample). Congenital absence of seminal vesicles and vas deferens, blockage of the ejaculatory duct, sympathetic nerves damage, and bladder neck surgery, insufficient levels of testosterone and short abstinence periods could also be the reason for hypospermia.

Retrograde ejaculation and hypospermia are linked to poor sperm parameters even cryptozoospermia. Freezing spermatozoa for fertility preservation in order to secure ART procedure would benefit any patient diagnosed with the described conditions.

3.3 Sperm freezing for patients with diabetes

Diabetes, a chronic autoimmune disease, is known to have detrimental effect to male fertility and sperm quality. Erectile dysfunction, retarded ejaculation and retrograde ejaculation could be persistent in patients with diabetes type 1 or 2. Reduced sperm quality and sperm DNA integrity impairment are also consequences to this health condition [17]. As all of the aforementioned are to affect fertility, cryopreservation of spermatozoa should be considered.

3.4 Sperm freezing for patients with Y-microdeletion and genetic aberrations

Alterations in autosomal genes, specific mutations/deletions of several X- or Y-chromosome genes, microdeletions in the azoospermic factor (AZF) regions of the Y chromosome and chromosomal anomalies can cause spermatogenic failure and affect male fertility.

Aberration in numerous autosomal genes result in fertility disturbance:

SYCP3 (synaptonemal complex protein 3) - meiotic arrest and consequent azoospermia.

PLK4 (Polo-like kinase 4) – Sertoli cell only (SCO) syndrome.

NANOS1 (**Nanos C2HC-Type Zinc Finger 1**) – SCO syndrome and oligoasthenoteratozoospermia.

HSF2 (heat-shock factor protein 2) - idiopathic azoospermia.

TAF4B (**TATA-Box Binding Protein Associated Factor 4b) - azoospermia.**

ZMYND15 **(Zinc Finger MYND-Type Containing 15) - azoospermia.**

SPATA16 (**Spermatogenesis-associated protein 16**) – globozoospermia.

KHLH10 (**Kelch Like Family Member 10**) – oligozoospermia.

SEPT12 (septin 12) - oligoasthenozoospermia or asthenoteratozoospermia.

GALNTL5 (**Polypeptide N-Acetylgalactosaminyltransferase Like 5**) – asthenozoospermia.

AURKC (**Aurora Kinase C**) - large-headed polyploid spermatozoa or macrozoospermia.

Alterations in X-chromosome located genes and fertility disturbance:

TEX11 (**Testis Expressed 11**) - meiotic arrest and consequent azoospermia.

RHOXF1 and RHOXF2/2B (human reproductive homeobox (RHOX) genes) - severe oligozoospermia.

ANOS1 (**Anosmin 1**) - anosmin-1 is involved in the migration of neurons producing gonadotropin-releasing hormone (GnRH). The latter controls the production of several hormones triggered to sexual development before birth and at puberty.

USP26 **(deubiquitinating enzyme gene)** - nucleotide variations in fertile and infertile men.

TAF7L (TATA-box binding protein associated factor 7) – reduced sperm count and motility, abnormal sperm morphology [18–20].

Y-microdeletion and fertility:

Y-chromosome microdeletions (YCMs) are the most common known structural chromosomal abnormalities for spermatogenic impairment. As high as 25–55% of the patients with hypospermia, sperm maturation arrest and SCO syndrome and 5–25% of the patients with severe oligozoospermia or azoospermia are established to have YCMs [21].

Deletions occur in three specific subregion - AZFa, AZFb and AZFc of the AZF in the long arm of the Y chromosome. Deletions in these regions are associated with:

AZFa region partial removal - hypo-spermatogenesis.

AZFa region complete deletion - inhibits the production and maturation of germ cells; SCO syndrome.

AZFb region deletions - pre-meiotic spermatogenic arrest or SCO syndrome; azoospermia, oligozoospermia.

AZFc region partial deletions - hypospermatogenesis.

AZFc region complete deletion - SCO syndrome and alterations in spermatocyte maturation [22].

Different studies indicate highest incidence of Y-microdeletion in the AZFc region, followed by AZFa+b + c; AZFb+c; AZFb; AZFa; and partial AZFa region deletion [23–25].

Passing genetic impairment to the offspring should be of high caution when sperm freezing and consequent ART is discussed.

3.5 Sperm freezing for patients with severe oligoasthenoteratozoospermia (OAT) or cryptozoospermia

Cryptozoospermia or virtual azoospermia and severe OAT may be the consequence to states of distinct origin. Extremly low sperm count in the ejaculate can occur for hormonal reasons, injuries, infections, varicocele, genetic abnormalities and improper descent of the testicle into the scrotum in newborn and infants. Lifestyle, occupational and environment factors have been proven to show adverse influence over male fertility. Obesity, alcohol consumption in regular and high potions, sedentary lifestyle are among the factors with high impact over semen parameters. As a prominent part of today's mode of life, stress should not be underestimated as it negatively affects male fertility. Occupational exposure to pesticides, chemicals, hormones, regular intake of enhancing drugs or therapeutic drug treatment may have an influence on the highly sensitive process of spermatogenesis. Environment radiation, tocsins, air and water pollution, phthalates, etc. are also linked to decrease in sperm count and motility as they may alter spermatogenesis [26–29].

In all groups under risk of infertility due to any of the preceding factors, freezing several sperm samples should be considered as a safety pool [30].

4. Sperm freezing protocols and efficiency

There are two main protocols for sperm freezing:

4.1 Slow freezing

The protocol for slow freezing of spermatozoa was suggested by Behram and Salewa in 1966 [31]. It is based on slow dehydration of the cells. Slow freezing could be performed either manually or by using programmed freezer. The sperm samples are cooled in a stepwise manner by lowering the temperature and adding cryoprotectants. Initially the temperature is lowered by 0.5°C/min and it should go down from room temperature to +5°C. The second step is to freeze the samples from +5°C to −80°C by lowering the temperature by 1–10°C/min. Finally the semen samples are transferred into liquid nitrogen (LN2) at −196°C.

Automatic freezers have been reported as reliable when freezing sperm is performed. One of the advantages of these devices is the perfect control over temperature changes as the process is performed through software. The three step protocol of slow freezing takes about 40 min [32].

In slow freezing, changes in lipid phase transition and increase in lipid peroxidation, consequent to saturation with cryoprotectants, could cause intracellular and extracellular physical and/or chemical damage to sperm membranes. Susceptible to cryopreservation induced damage are the viability, motility and the morphology of the post-thawed spermatozoa. Mitochondrial function, as well as DNA integrity, could be affected [33–36].

4.2 Rapid freezing: vitrification

Vitrification, as a method for cryopreservation, has been primarily used for cryobanking of oocytes and embryos. This method is based on direct exposure of the gametes to liquid nitrogen at −196°C. In comparison to slow freezing, where formation of intracytoplasmic ice crystals could damage different cell structures, during vitrification the liquid components of the cells set into a glass like amorphous solid and ice crystal structures are avoided (**Figure 1**) [37].

Regardless the protocol used for cryopreservation of spermatozoa, cryoprotective medium must be inset in order to reduce the stress induced while freezing or thawing cells.

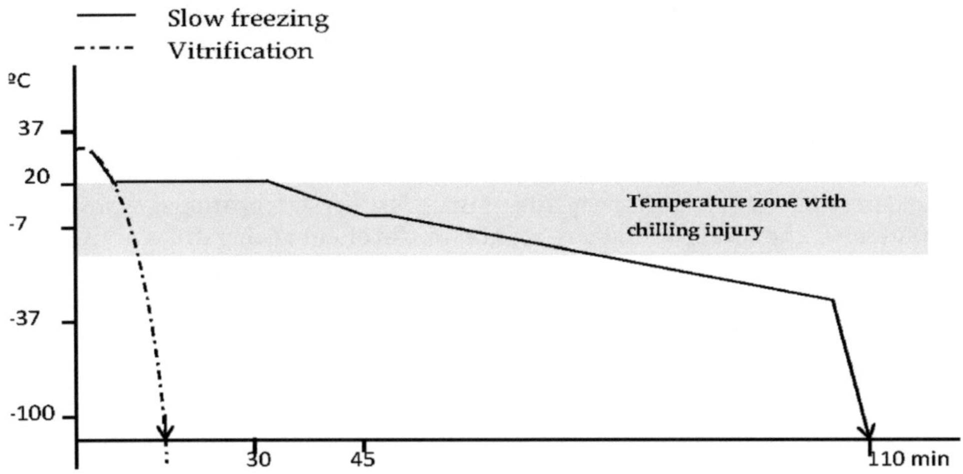

Figure 1.
Temperature changes in slow freezing and vitrification.

Permeable cryoprotectants can penetrate through cell membranes. They have intra- and extracellular activity. By forming osmotic gradient, water is ejected outside the cell, preventing it to form crystals. The cryoprotecting agents forms non-frozen channels in the medium in which sperm cells can be positioned while frozen. Glycerol, ethylene glycol, dimethyl sulfoxide (DMSO) and 1, 2 propanediol (PROH) are commonly used permeable cryoprotectants.

Non-permeable cryoprotectants cannot penetrate through the cell membrane. They can induce dehydration of the cells by increasing the concentration of extracellular solutes. Osmotic gradient is formed and the intracellular water is derived. Various sugars (raffinose, mannose, and trehalose) and proteins (lipoprotein, egg yolk) can be inset as *Non-permeable* cryoprotectants [38, 39].

5. Rare sperm freezing

Rare sperm freezing could be defined as a separate branch in sperm cryobiology. It has formed an important direction in the development of freezing protocols, methods and devices. The need for efficient freezing protocol for single sperm cells was evident at the very beginning, when pregnancies from epididymal and testicular sperm were reported [40–42]. In cases, where percutaneous epididymal aspiration (PESA) or testicular sperm extraction (TESE) is performed, freezing sperm cells would be of great benefit to the patient, as these procedures are traumatic and stressful to the organism. Most of the conditions described at *3. Conditions requiring sperm preservation* and poor semen quality are to request freezing of sporadic sperm cells.

Rare sperm freezing has some major advantages to standard protocols. In one hand this method gives chances for reliable fertility preservation in patient with severe male factor and sperm alterations. On the other hand, the successful freezing of single sperm cells and revolutionary methods such as intracytoplasmic sperm injection (ICSI), represent the opportunity for storage of larger quantity of samples for every men, as this premise increases the chances for fertilization of more oocytes retrieved in a cycle or secures larger number of ART cycles.

6. Rare sperm freezing protocols, carriers and devices

6.1 Biological carriers for rare sperm cryopreservation

6.1.1 Evacuated zona pellucida

Cryopreservation of single sperm cells in empty zona pellucida (ZP) was initially described in 1997 [43]. The biological carrier could be obtained by mouse or hamster pre-fertilization oocytes, human immature oocytes (e.g. germinal vesicle stage) prior fertilization, or embryos with abnormal fertilization and development after ICSI. The cumulus oophorus was removed via hyaluronidase and corona radiate was stripped by micropipettes. The oocyte was fixed with the holding pipette of the ICSI micromanipulator. By applying mechanical breach, chemical reagents (acidified Tyrode's solution) or highly focused laser beam, two small holes in the ZP were perforated. The cytoplasm of the oocyte must be aspirated and fully removed leaving the ZP empty of contents.

Sperm cells were obtained by centrifugation and placed in a droplet of 10% polyvinylpyrrolidone (PVP) solution. Using the ICSI needle each empty zona was injected with one to fifteen sperm cells. Slow freezing protocol and cryoprotective media of 8% glycerol solution in phosphate-buffered saline (PBS) and human serum albumin (3%) were preferred. The empty zonas were transfered in an individual sterile plastic straws of 0.25 ml. For easy location of their position they were situated between two small air bubbles.

Thawing of the biological carrier was implemented through exposure of the plastic straws to 30°C for 30 seconds in water bath. The content between the two air bubbles was extruded into droplets medium.

There are number of studies indicating that empty zona pellucida is an ideal carrier when it comes to freezing extremely small number of spermatozoa [44, 45]. Sperm recovery rate, compared to traditional freezing protocols, was higher, but motility recovery, DNA integrity and fertilization ability of sperm were similar in both methods [46]. From ethical point, it is important also to have an access to donated immature human oocytes and proper informed consent should be obtained (**Figure 2**).

Although this method shows high efficiency it is quite time and cost consuming and requires great precision with micromanipulation techniques and experience of the embryologist.

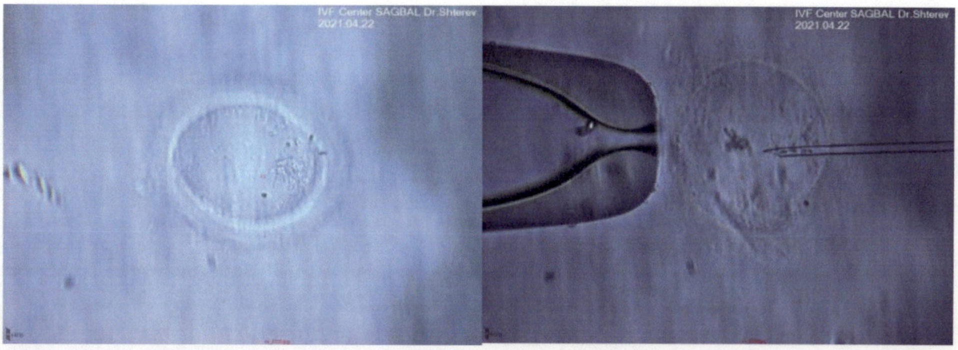

Figure 2.
Spermatozoa freezing in empty zona pellucida.

6.1.2 Volvox globator algae

Volvox gobator, a species of green algae of the genus *Volvox*, was described as a biological carrier for single sperm freezing and storage in 2004 [47]. The technique for loading rare sperm cells into the spherical algae is similar to the one used when freezing in ZP. Spermatozoa were injected in *Volvox globator* algae on a set of petri dish with media microdroplets and ICSI micromanipulator. In the pilot study, each Volvox sphere was loaded with eight male gametes. Cryoprotecting media containing 0.4% human serum albumin was supplemented. Each algae containing sperm was placed in a 0.2 mL plastic straw between two small air bubbles for easier location. Standard slow freezing protocol: 10 minutes at 4°C followed by 10 minutes of LN2 vapor and consequent submerging in LN2, was preferred.

Thawing of the biological carrier was performed through heating the plastic straws in a water bath at 25°C for 20 seconds. The content between the two air bubbles was extruded into droplets of medium. Sperm cells were subtracted through soft suction with the injection pipette at the micromanipulator set. The reported recovery rate (100%) and motility rate (at least 60%) were quite promising, but this method rises certain concerns. According to The United States *Food and Drug Administration (*FDA) and the European Tissue Directive regulations, there is no clear evidence that genetic material from the algae is not transferred and introduced into the oocyte with the injected sperm.

For the time being the use of non-human biological carrier in a clinical setting seems unacceptable. Still, there are countries with strict regulations prohibiting the destructive use of oocytes, and *Volvox globator* algae could be considered as an option for biological carrier when single sperm cryopreservation is nessesary [48].

Recently, non-biological carriers for rare sperm freezing, analogical to ZP and *Volvox globator* algae, were developed. Microcapsules composed of alginic acid, agarose or hollow hyaluronan -phenolic hydroxyl (HA-Ph) were tested with loading, freezing and thawing techniques adopted from the abovementioned biological carriers. First attempts were conducted in 2006, when sperm cells were frozen in polymerized alginic acid drops [49]. Although alginate is a non-toxic polysaccharide, the reported sperm motility after thawing was 20% lower compared to standard protocols. According to the study, decreased motility might be based on the adhesion of alginic acid to sperms surface.

Inactive and biologically sterile empty agarose microspheres of 100-μm in diameter were examined as carrier for the cryopreservation of one to ten sperm cells. The conducted post-thaw results in different studies show high recovery and motility rate (above 90% and above 80% respectively) and preserved membrane integrity of the cells [50, 51]. The hollow-core agarose capsule seems to be a promising substitute to ZP and *Volvox globator* algae.

Enzymatically fabricated hyaluronan (HA) microcapsules with thick membrane (30-μm) and 200 μm in diameter were also tested as carriers for cryopreservation of solitary spermatozoa. No differences according to recovery and motility rates after thawing of spermatozoa loaded into HA-Ph - microcapsules and ZP (95.5 vs. 93.9% and 13.6 vs. 15.1% respectively) were registered [48, 52].

Newly developed spherical analogues for rare sperm freezing would be of great benefit when ethical problems arise, and empty ZP could not be used for clinical or experimental application. No preliminary processing of the carrier is required and the procedure is less time consuming, but still highly qualified and trained embryologist as well as specialized technique is needed.

The inculcation of such promising non-biologically derived carriers in cryobiology needs further investigation and affirmation in regard to their safety and efficiency.

6.2 Non- biological carriers for rare sperm cryopreservation

6.2.1 Open-pulled straws

Open pulled straw (OPS) is a specially designed carrier for ultra-rapid vitrification. The tool was introduced in 1998 by Professor Gábor Vajta and it is considered to be highly efficient for single sperm cryopreservation. At considerably low risk of microbial contamination while in LN2, OPS could be incorporated for cryopreservation of very small volumes (1–5 μl), without the use of cryoprotectants. The reproductive cells are loaded in the end of the OPS by spontaneous capillary action when the straw is submerged into microdroplets of sperm suspension. The loaded straws, inserted into 90 mm straws, are hermetically closed and submerged in LN2 [53]. Preselection and loading of the sperm cells into the OPS could be performed via polar body biopsy (PBB) pipette [54]. In order to thaw the sperm cells, the outer straw is cut and the open pulled straw is drawn out. The tip should be immediately plunged into microcentrifuge tube containing media.

The OPS tool is of comparable efficiency to other systems and methods when rare sperm cells are cryopreserved. It is relatively easy to use and allows selection of sperm by its morphokinetic parameters prior cryopreservation.

6.2.2 Cryoloops

Cryoloops have been explored as a rare sperm freezing tool by Schuster et al. In 2002 [55]. Further investigation on nylon cryoloops with aspect to successful loading of preselected spermatozoa and cryopreserving oligozoospermic samples and surgically retrieved epididymal or testicular spermatozoa was conducted [56]. The open cryoloop should be dipped in small droplet of sperm suspension and placed into cryovial. Ultra-rapid freezing by either direct submersion in LN2, or 5 min of exposure to liquid nitrogen vapor prior submersion was performed. Standard slow freezing protocol could also be applied. Vitrification in cryoloops without additional cryoprotectants was also investigated and higher sperm motility compared to control group with cryoprotectants was reported (89.5 ± 7.1% vs. 77.5 ± 8.9%) [36].

Sperm samples were thawed by resuspendation in media immediately after the cryovial was taken out of the liquid nitrogen.

Sperm motility, viability, plasma membrane and acrosome integrity were assessed. Certain concerns according to acrosome damage and sperm cryo-capacitation after thawing have been arisen [57]. Cryo-injury is common consequence to different freezing protocols and cryoprotective media. When such small numbers of spermatozoa are frozen any structural or functional damage to the cell could be crucial to the overall treatment outcome.

This method would be convenient for sporadic sperm freezing due to its simplicity. It also provides a set of samples that could be used in multiple ART cycles for ICSI procedures. Cross-contamination should be considered as the cryoloop system is opened and allows liquid nitrogen flow.

6.2.3 Cryopreservation in microdroplets

Ultra-rapid cryopreservation of rare sperm cells in microdroplets results in high post thaw total motility and progressive motility rates compared to slow freezing technique. Sperm DNA fragmentation index (DFI) was also comparable to stated values in the fresh sample. On contrary, when standard slow freezing was conducted, DFI values increased significantly after cryopreservation in the post-thawed samples [58]. This method was adopted and resembles oocyte and embryo vitrification.

Suspension, obtained by the mixture of proceeded sperm and cryoprotective media (1: 1) added by drops in every 30 seconds, was prepared. Modified French mini straws, cut in half from the center to the end by its length, were loaded with 2 μl droplets of the suspension after it was equilibrated at room temperature for 10 minutes. Each hemi-straw (HS) was loaded by the extents of the open gutter with 10–15 droplets placed at equal distance of 2 mm in-between. The HS was placed in 0,5 ml straw and was secured through the two-stage stoppers which it has. After short exposure to LN2 vapor the straws were plunged into liquid nitrogen. Droplets carrying sperm cells were derived by gentle struck of the HS against the bottom of 1.5 ml Eppendorf tube. The samples were incubated at 37°C for 15 minutes. No additional centrifugation for enrichment of the sample was necessary. Washing the cryoprotective media was performed for the selected spermatozoa in droplets of the ICSI dish before sperm injection. This seems to be quite convenient when poor semen samples are frozen, as reduction of numerous centrifugation and washing steps increases the chance for higher number of sperm cells retrieved after thawing.

6.2.4 Cryotop

Cryotop, mainly used as embryo freezing and storage commercialized tool, has been adopted as a carrier for sperm vitrification. Different studies have been conducted in order to establish the most efficient protocol when Cryotop as a carrier is used. The most efficient protocol for the vitrification of rare sperm cells was setting 1 μl droplet of sperm suspension and sucrose as cryoprotectants on the strip. The Cryotop was immediately transferred over LN2 vapor (2 min at −120°C) and then plunged into liquid nitrogen. Reported recovery and motility rates after thawing sperm cells retrieved from the testes were 95% and 42.1%, and for single sperm cryopreservation obtained from ejaculates – 90% and 44.4% respectively [59]. Freezing semen samples on Cryotop and without cryoprotectants show higher viability after thawing and lower damage to DNA integrity compared to samples frozen with sucrose as adjuvant [60].

Cryotop is efficient tool for cryopreservation of embryos and rare sperm samples. It rises no ethical issues as it is of non-biological origin. The tool has been implemented in cryobiology and it has been randomly used resulting in successful pregnancies. In recent years, similar devices, based on knowledge cumulated from Cryotop examination, were developed. Moreover, due to its great performance, Cryotop has been used as a measure tool for newly developed sporadic sperm cells freezing devices and their efficiency [61].

6.2.5 Cell sleeper

Freezing small number of spermatozoa is still a challenge for modern cryobiology. In order to find not only the most reliable and efficient, but a carrier easy to use and relevantly less time consuming, different devices were fabricated, tested and compared.

Cell sleeper is a novel device with comparatively small use in practice. It is constructed of an inner tray as a sperm sample carrier and an outer vial. The system is closed and when the tray is placed inside the vial they are sealed together by a screw cap [62]. The device could be used as a cryopreservation carrier for preselected spermatozoa derived from ejaculates or from testicular tissue. Sperm cells were transferred from the proceeded samples in a microdroplet of freezing media on the tray of the Cell sleeper through ICSI needle. After placing the tray inside the vial and sealing it through the cup, the vial was positioned over LN2 vapor (2.5 min at −120°C) and then sunken into liquid nitrogen.

For thawing of the sample, the vial was warmed at room temperature for 1 minute. Afterwards the tray was drawn out of the vial and transfered in a petri dish then covered with oil. Following incubation period (37°C for 2 minutes) the recovery and motility rates were observed. Sperm recovery and motility rates of 94% and 56% were stated. Pregnancies were reported for both – ejaculated and retrieved from testicular tissue sperm cells [62, 63].

This device needs further investigation, but the comparatively large volume of the drop placed in the tray inevitably leads to time consuming search for the sperm cells. Since time for micromanipulation of the oocytes is important matter the latter could be considered as great disadvantage of the Cell Sleeper device.

6.2.6 Polydimethylsiloxane (PDMS) chip

Microfluidic devices for gamete handling have been incorporated in ART more than 20 years ago [64]. Since the initial study of the technology, the microfluidic systems developed specifically for sperm investigation, selection and cryopreservation, have been upgraded, improved and widely used in the clinical practice.

Polydimethylsiloxane (PDMS), silicone elastomer, chips for cryopreservation of single spermatozoa without cryoprotectants have been thoroughly investigated. Microfluidic two-layered chip was fabricated. The upper layer has two separate openings – inlet, transfusing into microchannel, and outlet. The smooth bottom layer is connected through plasma to the upper one. Different height of the microchannel were examined. For ultra-rapid freezing of rare sperm cells without cryoprotective media, best results were obtained when 10 μm height microchannel was tested [65].

Before cryopreservation the ejaculate should be processed by sperm gradient technique. The semen sample was loaded in the microchannel of the sterilized chip through the inlet. Approximately 5×10^{-3} μL medium containing 1000 sperm cells can be injected in the 10 μm channel by needle connected to micro-injector. The whole chip is covered in silver paper, so direct contact with liquid nitrogen could be avoided.

The chip containing sperm cells was thawed at 37°C for 10 min. The content was ejected in a culture petri dish through the outlet by applying pressure of a syringe connected with the input. Sperm viability, motility, DNA and acrosome integrity in post-thawed samples were researched. Comparison for PDMS chips with 10 μm height microchannel, where samples were frozen with ultra-rapid cryoprotectants-free protocol, and samples frozen through conventional slow freezing protocol was conducted. The compared post-thaw parameters for the investigated parameters were of comparable values. The most essential advantage of the on chip ultra-rapid cryoprotectants-free cryopreservation is the lack of cytotoxic cryoprotective media. The thawing of the sample, as no cryoprotectants were added, is simple and time and consumable saving [66].

6.2.7 Sperm vitrification device (sperm VD)

Sperm vitrification device (Sperm VD) is a novel tool specially designed for cryopreservation of small number of spermatozoa in microdroplets [67]. The device could be exclusively helpful when sperm cells are retrieved by means of TESE. Each Sperm VD plate carrier has three wells for placing sperm cells. Droplets of mixture 1:1 of cryoprotectants and washing media are placed individually for each well of the Sperm VD plate. Sperm VD should be transferred in a petri dish covered with oil. Using the injection needle of the micromanipulator, spermatozoa were transferred from neighboring droplets (PVP/washing media) into the droplets of the wells of the Sperm VD. As cryoprotective media has negative influence on sperm cells it is crucial to minimize the time of exposure to the media before freezing the sperm. Substantial freezing should be done within 10 minutes past the first sperm cell transfer [68]. After loading each well of the Sperm VD plate it is transferred in pre-cooled cryotube over liquid nitrogen. The tool should be handled with tweezers and the excess oil should be allowed to drain. The cryotube is sealed with cup.

Immediately after unfreezing (5 min in room temperature) the Sperm VD is placed in a pre-heated petri dish with PVP drops and sperm wash media covered with oil.

Sperm VD is quite convenient for rare sperm freezing and it gives the opportunity for direct sperm washing, selection and injection in the petri dish right after thawing.

7. Rare sperm freezing significance

Since the first attempts for freezing reproductive cells, a completely new horizon for fertility preservation has been discovered. The opportunity to cryopreserve, thaw and use gametes, embryos and reproductive tissue has given the unique chance to men and women to parent their biological child even when their reproductive functions have been lost.

Modern day society has invented and incorporated countless amenities in day to day life. Unfortunately, some of them have direct negative impact on health: polluted air as the result of factory overproduction, car exhaust gasses, overconsumption and large amount of waste contaminating water and agricultural lands, etc. Others tend to create bad habits: sedentary way of life and lack of physical activity, unhealthy and excessive eating, smoking, and drinking. Mental health, self-esteem and tension should also be considered when certain health issues arise. All of the above mentioned factors, including reproduction postpone and advanced paternal age, could disrupt fertility. Thus cryopreservation has great value in ART.

Cancer, the scourge of modern society, could affect reproduction and leave an indelible mark in one's life. Preserving fertility in cancer patients should be a priority as high as the treatment of the cancer itself – a guarantee for good quality of life after healing. Cancer by itself may affects fertility and alterations in spermatogenesis and low sperm quality could be registered even before treatment [69]. Rare sperm freezing of multiple samples for those patients is mandatory. The unique techniques developed for single sperm freezing and cryopreservation represent the chance for those patients to reproduce in future.

Rare sperm cryopreservation is of high value to patients with severe oligoasthenozoospermia, cryptozoospermia, retrograde ejaculation, and PESA or TESE procedures. All these conditions are associated with extremely low sperm count in the ejaculate and still creates difficulties for laboratory handling. Securing frozen samples through single sperm cryopreservation, inspires calm not only to the patient, but to the clinical and laboratory staff handling the gametes.

Rare sperm cryopreservation could be considered as opportunity beneficial to wildlife and endangered species preservation [70–72]. Breeding and assisted reproduction in animals has long-standing traditions and has been explored in husbandry for centuries. In times when hundreds of animal species are near extinction, rare sperm freezing is a key procedure for stock up of larger amount of samples for future breeding. Genetic diversity should be preserved and on time establishment of cryobanks conserving samples of different representatives of the species on Earth is of high importance [73].

8. Conclusion

Rare sperm freezing is a procedure with wide application and of high value in many aspects to ART, fertility preservation and endangered wildlife conservation. Freezing single sperm cells is still a challenge in modern laboratories. Incredible effort has been set and numerous devices and sperm freezing protocols have been investigated in order to establish the most reliable approach to rare sperm freezing. Despite the great achievements in the area, scientists continue the search for better results.

Conflict of interest

The authors declare no conflict of interest.

Thanks

The authors would like to express gratitude to their colleagues in the IVF Unit of SAGBAL "Dr. Shterev".

"Many ideas grow better when transplanted into another mind than the one where they sprang up."

Oliver Wendell Holmes

Abbreviations

AR	assisted reproduction
ART	assisted reproductive technology
AZF	azoospermic factor
DMSO	dimethyl sulfoxide
DFI	DNA fragmentation index
ICSI	intracytoplasmic sperm injection
HA	hyaluronan
HA-Ph	hyaluronan -phenolic hydroxyl
HS	hemi-straw
OPS	Open pulled straw
PESA	percutaneous epididymal aspiration
PDMS	Polydimethylsiloxane
PROH	1, 2 propanediol
PVP	polyvinylpyrrolidone
ROS	reactive oxygen species
Sperm VD	Sperm vitrification device
TESE	testicular sperm extraction
SMF	severe male factor
SCO	Sertoli cell only syndrome
YCMs	Y-chromosome microdeletions
ZP	zona pellucida

Author details

Desislava Dyulgerova-Nikolova[1*] and Tanya Milachich[2]

1 SAGBAL "Dr. Shterev", Sofia, Bulgaria

2 Institute of Biology and Immunology of Reproduction, Bulgarian Academy of Science, Sofia, Bulgaria

*Address all correspondence to: dess_ie@mail.bg

References

[1] Wolff, Michael & Andersen, Claus & Woodruff, Teresa & Nawroth, Frank. (2019). Ferti PROTEKT, Oncofertility Consortium and the Danish Fertility-Preservation Networks – What Can We Learn From Their Experiences?. Clinical Medicine Insights: Reproductive Health. 13. 117955811984586. 10.1177/1179558119845865.

[2] Polge, C., Smith, A. & Parkes, A. Revival of spermatozoa after Vitrification and dehydration at low temperatures. Nature 164, 666 (1949). https://doi.org/10.1038/164666a0

[3] Ombelet W, Van Robays J. Artificial insemination history: hurdles and milestones. Facts Views Vis Obgyn. 2015; 7(2):137-43. PMID: 26175891; PMCID: PMC4498171.

[4] Whittingham DG, Leibo SP, Mazur P. Survival of mouse embryos frozen to −196 degrees and −269 degrees C. Science. 1972 Oct 27; 178(4059):411-414. PMID: 5077328.

[5] Nakagata N. Cryopreservation of mouse spermatozoa. Mamm Genome. 2000; 11:572-576.

[6] Takeo, T., Nakao, S., Nakagawa, Y. et al. Cryopreservation of mouse resources. Lab Anim Res 36, 33 (2020). https://doi.org/10.1186/s42826-020-00066-w

[7] Ozkavukcu, S., Erdemli, E., Isik, A. *et al.* Effects of cryopreservation on sperm parameters and ultrastructural morphology of human spermatozoa. J Assist Reprod Genet 25, 403-411 (2008). https://doi.org/10.1007/s10815-008-9232-3

[8] Hezavehei M, Sharafi M, Kouchesfahani HM, Henkel R, Agarwal A, Esmaeili V, Shahverdi A. Sperm cryopreservation: A review on current molecular cryobiology and advanced approaches. Reprod Biomed Online. 2018 Sep; 37 (3):327-339. doi: 10.1016/j.rbmo.2018.05.012. Epub 2018 Aug 22. PMID: 30143329.

[9] Park JS, Kim J, Elghiaty A, Ham WS. Recent global trends in testicular cancer incidence and mortality. Medicine (Baltimore). 2018; 97 (37):e12390. doi:10.1097/MD.0000000000012390

[10] *S. Iacob, R. Vrînceanu, B. Novac*: **Asymptomatic complex testicular neoplasia associated with orchiepididymitis - case report.** Vol 121, No 4,page: 730 (2017): The Medical-Surgical Journal

[11] S. Jane Henley et al. Annual report to the nation on the status of cancer, part II: Progress toward Healthy People 2020 objectives for 4 common cancers. Cancer Volume 126, Issue10, May 15, 2020, Pages 2250-2266 DOI: 10.1002/cncr.32801 Published online March 12, 2020 in Wiley Online Library (wileyonlinelibrary.com)

[12] Biedka M, Kuźba-Kryszak T, Nowikiewicz T, Żyromska A. Fertility impairment in radiotherapy. Contemp Oncol (Pozn). 2016; 20 (3):199-204. doi:10.5114/wo.2016.57814

[13] Kimberly D. Miller et al. Cancer statistics for adolescents and young adults, 2020. CA a cancer journal for clinitians, Volume70, Issue6, November/December 2020. Pages 443-459.https://doi.org/10.3322/caac.21637

[14] Jefferys A, Siassakos D, Wardle P. The management of retrograde ejaculation: A systematic review and update. Fertil Steril. 2012 Feb; 97(2):306-312. doi: 10.1016/j.fertnstert.2011.11.019. Epub 2011 Dec 15. PMID: 22177462.

[15] Giuliano F, Clement P. Neuroanatomy and physiology of

ejaculation. Annu Rev Sex Res. 2005; 16:190-216. PMID: 16913292.

[16] Zhou J, Chen L, Li J, et al. The Semen pH Affects Sperm Motility and Capacitation. PLoS One. 2015; 10(7):e0132974. Published 2015 Jul 14. doi:10.1371/journal.pone.0132974

[17] Ding GL, Liu Y, Liu ME, et al. The effects of diabetes on male fertility and epigenetic regulation during spermatogenesis. Asian J Androl. 2015; 17(6):948-953. doi:10.4103/1008-682X.150844

[18] Miyamoto T, Minase G, Shin T, Ueda H, Okada H, Sengoku K. Human male infertility and its genetic causes. Reprod Med Biol. 2017 Apr; 16(2): 81-88. Published online 2017 Mar 26. doi: 10.1002/rmb2.12017

[19] Albrecht Röpke and Frank Tüttelmann. MECHANISMS IN ENDOCRINOLOGY: Aberrations of the X chromosome as cause of male infertility. European Journal of Endocrinology, Endocrinology 2017, Volume 177: Issue 5. DOI: https://doi.org/10.1530/EJE-17-0246

[20] Pointud JC, Mengus G, Brancorsini S, Monaco L, Parvinen M, Sassone-Corsi P, Davidson I. The intracellular localisation of TAF7L, a paralogue of transcription factor TFIID subunit TAF7, is developmentally regulated during male germ-cell differentiation. J Cell Sci. 2003 May 1; 116(Pt 9):1847-1858. doi: 10.1242/jcs.00391. PMID: 12665565.

[21] Bansal, S., Jaiswal, D., Gupta, N. *et al.* Gr/gr deletions on Y-chromosome correlate with male infertility: An original study, meta-analyses and trial sequential analyses. Sci Rep **6,** 19798 (2016). https://doi.org/10.1038/srep19798

[22] Yu XW, Wei ZT, Jiang YT, Zhang SL. Y chromosome azoospermia factor region microdeletions and transmission characteristics in azoospermic and severe oligozoospermic patients. Int J Clin Exp Med. 2015; 8(9):14634-14646. Published 2015 Sep 15.

[23] Akınsal EC, Baydilli N, Dündar M, Ekmekçioğlu O. The frequencies of Y chromosome microdeletions in infertile males. Turk J Urol. 2018; 44(5):389-392. doi:10.5152/tud.2018.73669

[24] Johnson M, Raheem A, De Luca F, Hallerstrom M, Zainal Y, Poselay S, Mohammadi B, Moubasher A, Johnson TF, Muneer A, Sangster P, Ralph DJ. An analysis of the frequency of Y-chromosome microdeletions and the determination of a threshold sperm concentration for genetic testing in infertile men. BJU Int. 2019 Feb; 123(2):367-372. doi: 10.1111/bju.14521. Epub 2018 Sep 9. PMID: 30113756.

[25] Krausz C, Rajpert-De Meyts E, Frydelund-Larsen L, Quintana-Murci L, McElreavey K, Skakkebaek NE, Double-Blind Y Chromosome Microdeletion Analysis in Men with Known Sperm Parameters and Reproductive Hormone Profiles: Microdeletions Are Specific for Spermatogenic Failure, The Journal of Clinical Endocrinology & Metabolism, Volume 86, Issue 6, 1 June 2001, Pages 2638-2642, https://doi.org/10.1210/jcem.86.6.7527

[26] Ilacqua, A., Izzo, G., Emerenziani, G.P. et al. Lifestyle and fertility: The influence of stress and quality of life on male fertility. Reprod Biol Endocrinol 16, 115 (2018). https://doi.org/10.1186/s12958-018-0436-9

[27] Gollenberg AL, Liu F, Brazil C, Drobnis EZ, Guzick D, Overstreet JW, et al. Semen quality in fertile men in relation to psychosocial stress. Fertil Steril. 2010; 93:1104-1111.

[28] Durairajanayagam D. Lifestyle causes of male infertility. Arab J Urol. 2018; 16(1):10-20. Published 2018 Feb 13. doi:10.1016/j.aju.2017.12.004

[29] Sharpe RM. Lifestyle and environmental contribution to male infertility. Br Med Bull. 2000; 56(3):630-642. doi: 10.1258/0007142001903436. PMID: 11255550.

[30] Bessonnat J, Brouillet S, Sintzel S, *et al*. In cryptozoospermia or severe oligozoospermia is sperm freezing useful? Basic and clinical andrology 2014 24(1):15, DOI: 10.1186/2051-4190-24-15

[31] Behrman SJ, Sawada Y. Heterologous and homologous inseminations with human semen frozen and stored in a liquid-nitrogen refrigerator. Fertil Steril. 1966 Jul-Aug; 17(4):457-466. doi: 10.1016/s0015-0282(16)36003-4. PMID: 5947006.

[32] Agarwal, Ashok & Tvrda, Eva. (2017). Chapter 5 slow freezing of human sperm. Methods in Molecular Biology. 1568. 10.1007/978-1-4939-6828-2_5.

[33] Mossad H, Morshedi M, Torner JP & Oehninger S 1994 Impact of cryopreservation on spermatozoa from infertile men – Implication for artificial insemination. Archives of Andrology 33 51-57.

[34] O'Connell M, McClure N, Lewis SE. The effects of cryopreservation on sperm morphology, motility and mitochondrial function. Hum Reprod. 2002 Mar; 17(3):704-709. doi: 10.1093/humrep/17.3.704. PMID: 11870124.

[35] Pabón D, Meseguer M, Sevillano G, Cobo A, Romero JL, Remohí J, M. Santos MJ. A new system of sperm cryopreservation: evaluation of survival, motility, DNA oxidation, and mitochondrial activity. Andrology, Volume7, Issue3, May 2019, Pages 293-301. https://doi.org/10.1111/andr.12607

[36] Isachenko E, Isachenko V, Katkov II, Rahimi G, Schöndorf T, Mallmann P, Dessole S, Nawroth F. DNA integrity and motility of human spermatozoa after standard slow freezing versus cryoprotectant-free vitrification. Hum Reprod 2004 a; 19:932-939.

[37] Wowk B. Thermodynamic aspects of vitrification. Cryobiology. 2010; 60:11-22.

[38] Schulz M, Risopatrón J, Uribe P, Isachenko E, Isachenko V, Sánchez R. Human sperm vitrification: A scientific report. Andrology, Volume8, Issue6; Special Issue on: Late onset Hypogonadism, November 2020, Pages 1642-1650. doi.org/10.1111/andr.12847

[39] Alemayehu Lemma. Effect of Cryopreservation on Sperm Quality and Fertility. www.intechopen.com; Artificial Insemination in Farm Animals. Submitted: October 13th 2010, Reviewed: April 10th 2011, published: June 21st 2011. DOI: 10.5772/16563

[40] Silber SJ, Ord T, Balmaceda J, Patrizio P, Asch RH. Congenital absence of the vas deferens. The fertilizing capacity of human epididymal sperm. N Engl J Med. 1990 Dec 27; 323(26):1788-1792. doi: 10.1056/NEJM199012273232602. PMID: 2247117.

[41] Silber SJ, Nagy Z, Liu J, Tournaye H, Lissens W, Ferec C, Liebaers I, Devroey P, Van Steirteghem AC. The use of epididymal and testicular spermatozoa for intracytoplasmic sperm injection: The genetic implications for male infertility. Hum Reprod. 1995 Aug; 10(8):2031-2043. doi: 10.1093/oxfordjournals.humrep.a136231. PMID: 8567837.

[42] Devroey P, Liu J, Nagy Z, Goossens A, Tournaye H, Camus M, et al. Pregnancies after testicular sperm extraction and intracytoplasmic sperm injection in nonobstructive azoospermia. Hum Reprod. 1995; 10(6):1457-1460.

[43] Cohen J, Garrisi GJ, Congedo-Ferrara TA, Kieck KA, Schimmel TW, Scott RT. Cryopreservation of single human spermatozoa. Hum Reprod. 1997 May; 12(5):994-1001. doi: 10.1093/humrep/12.5.994. PMID: 9194653.

[44] Hsieh YY, Tsai HD, Chang CC, Lo HY. Sperm cryopreservation with empty human or mouse zona pellucidae. A comparison. J Reprod Med. 2000 May; 45(5):383-386. PMID: 10845170.

[45] Levi-Setti PE, Albani E, Negri L, Cesana A, Novara P, Bianchi S. Cryopreservation of a small number of spermatozoa in yolk-filled human zonae pellucidae. Arch Ital Urol Androl. 2003 Dec; 75(4):195-198. PMID: 15005492.

[46] Ye Y, Xu C, Qian Y, Jin F, Huang H. Evaluation of human sperm function after being cryopreserved within the zona pellucida. Fertility and Sterility, Volume 92, Issue 3, 2009, Pages 1002-1008, ISSN 0015-0282, https://doi.org/10.1016/j.fertnstert.2008.07.1737.

[47] Just A, Gruber I, Wöber M, Lahodny J, Obruca A, Strohmer H. Novel method for the cryopreservation of testicular sperm and ejaculated spermatozoa from patients with severe oligospermia: A pilot study. Fertil Steril. 2004;82:445-447 DOI:https://doi.org/10.1016/j.fertnstert.2003.12.050

[48] Liu, Shasha & Li, Fuping. (2020). Cryopreservation of single-sperm: Where are we today?. Reproductive Biology and Endocrinology. 18. 10.1186/s12958-020-00607-x.

[49] Herrler A, Eisner S, Bach V, Weissenborn U, Beier HM. Cryopreservation of spermatozoa in alginic acid capsules. Fertil Steril. 2006 Jan; 85(1):208-213. doi: 10.1016/j.fertnstert.2005.06.049. PMID: 16412755.

[50] Isaev DA, Zaletov SY, Zaeva VV, Zakharova EE, Shafei RA, Krivokharchenko IS. Artificial microcontainers for cryopreservation of solitary spermatozoa. Hum Reprod 2007; 22:i154.

[51] Araki Y, Yao T, Asayama Y, Matsuhisa A, Araki Y. Single human sperm cryopreservation method using hollow-core agarose capsules. Fertil Steril. 2015 Oct; 104(4):1004-1009. doi: 10.1016/j.fertnstert.2015.06.043. Epub 2015 Jul 21. PMID: 26207962.

[52] Tomita K, Sakai S, Khanmohammadi M, Yamochi T, Hashimoto S, Anzai M, Morimoto Y, Taya M, Hosoi Y. Cryopreservation of a small number of human sperm using enzymatically fabricated, hollow hyaluronan microcapsules handled by conventional ICSI procedures. J Assist Reprod Genet. 2016 Apr; 33(4):501-11. doi: 10.1007/s10815-016-0656-x. Epub 2016 Jan 19. PMID: 26781440; PMCID: PMC4818628.

[53] Isachenko V, Isachenko E, Montag M, Zaeva V, Krivokharchenko I, Nawroth F, Dessole S, Katkov II, van der Ven H. Clean technique for cryoprotectant-free vitrification of human spermatozoa. Reprod Biomed Online. 2005 Mar; 10(3):350-354. doi: 10.1016/s1472-6483(10)61795-6. PMID: 15820041.

[54] Kuznyetsov V, Moskovtsev S, Crowe M, Lulat A, & Librach C. Vitrification of a small number of spermatozoa in normozoospermic and severely oligozoospermic samples. Systems Biology in Reproductive Medicine, Volume 61, 2015 - Issue 1, Pages 13-17. https://doi.org/10.3109/19396368.2014.987855

[55] Schuster TG, Keller LM, Dunn RL, Ohl DA, Smith GD. Ultra-rapid freezing of very low numbers of sperm using cryoloops. Hum Reprod. 2003; 18:788-795.

[56] Desai NN, Blackmon H, Goldfarb J. Single sperm cryopreservation on

cryoloops: An alternative to hamster zona for freezing individual spermatozoa. Reprod BioMed Online. 2004; 9:47-53.

[57] Isachenko V, Maettner R, Petrunkina AM, Sterzik K, Mallmann P, Rahimi G, Sanchez R, Risopatron J, Damjanoski I, Isachenko E. Vitrification of human ICSI/IVF spermatozoa without cryoprotectants: New capillary technology. J Androl. 2012 May-Jun; 33(3):462-468. doi: 10.2164/jandrol.111.013789. Epub 2011 Jun 30. PMID: 21719694.

[58] Huang WJ, Zhang D, Hong ZW, Chen ZB, Dong LH, Zhang Y, Chen GY, Li Y, Yao B. Sequential interval micro-droplet loading in closed hemi-straw carrier system: A convenient and efficient method for ultra-rapid cryopreservation in extreme oligozoospermia. Cryobiology, Volume 93, 2020, Pages 75-83, ISSN 0011-2240, https://doi.org/10.1016/j.cryobiol.2020.02.005.

[59] Endo Y, Fujii Y, Shintani K, Seo M, Motoyama H, Funahashi H. Single spermatozoon freezing using cryotop. J Mamm Ova Res. 2011; 28:47-52.

[60] Li, Lin & Qian, Y. & Xu, C. & Zhu, Y. & Huang, H. & Jin, F. & Ye, Yangyang. (2014). Small-volume vitrification for human spermatozoa in the absence of cryoprotectants by using Cryotop. Andrologia 47. 10.1111/and.12320.

[61] Nakata K, Yoshida K, Yamashita N. Preclinical evaluation of a new cryopreservation container for a limited number of human spermatozoa. J Reprod Dev. 2019; 65(4):297-304. doi:10.1262/jrd.2017-086

[62] Endo Y, Fujii Y, Kurotsuchi S, Motoyama H, Funahashi H. Successful delivery derived from vitrified-warmed spermatozoa from a patient with nonobstructive azoospermia. Fertil Steril. 2012; 98:1423-1427.

[63] Coetzee K, Ozgur K, Berkkanoglu M, Bulut H, Isikli A. Reliable single sperm cryopreservation in cell sleepers for azoospermia management. Andrologia. 2016; 48:203-210.

[64] Vajta G, Peura TT, Holm P, Páldi A, Greve T, Trounson AO, Callesen H. New method for culture of zona-included or zona-free embryos: The well of the well (WOW) system. Mol Reprod Dev. 2000 Mar; 55(3):256-264. doi: 10.1002/(SICI)1098-2795(200003)55:3<256::AID-MRD3>3.0.CO;2-7. PMID: 10657044.

[65] Zou Y, Yin T, Chen S, Yang J, Huang W (2013) On-Chip cryopreservation: A novel method for ultra-rapid Cryoprotectant-free cryopreservation of small amounts of human spermatozoa. PLoS ONE 8(4): e61593. https://doi.org/10.1371/journal.pone.0061593

[66] Zhao G, Fu J. Microfluidics for cryopreservation. Biotechnol Adv. 2017; 35(2):323-336. doi:10.1016/j.biotechadv.2017.01.006

[67] Berkovitz, Arie & Miller, Netanella & Silberman, Michal & Belenky, Michael & Itsykson, Pavel. (2018). A novel solution for freezing small numbers of spermatozoa using a sperm vitrification device. Human reproduction (Oxford, England). 33. 10.1093/humrep/dey304.

[68] Belenky M, Itzhakov D, Freger V, et al. Optimizing the protocol for vitrification of individual spermatozoa by adjusting equilibration time. Systems Biology in Reproductive Medicine. 2020 Jun; 66(3):223-228. DOI: 10.1080/19396368.2020.1737271.

[69] Agarwal A, Allamaneni SS. Disruption of spermatogenesis by the cancer disease process. J Natl Cancer Inst Monogr. 2005; (34):9-12. doi: 70. 10.1093/jncimonographs/lgi005. PMID: 15784813.

[70] Fickel, Joerns & Wagener, Asja & Ludwig, Arne. (2007). Semen cryopreservation and the conservation of endangered species. European Journal of Wildlife Research. 53. 81-89. 10.1007/s10344-007-0089-z.

[71] Hermes R, Hildebrandt TB, Göritz F (2018) Cryopreservation in rhinoceros—Setting a new benchmark for sperm cryosurvival. PLOS ONE 13(7): e0200154. https://doi.org/10.1371/journal.pone.0200154

[72] Cardoso B, Sánchez-Ajofrín I, Castaño C, et al. Optimization of Sperm Cryopreservation Protocol for Peregrine Falcon (*Falco peregrinus*). Animals (Basel). 2020; 10(4):691. Published 2020 Apr 16. doi:10.3390/ani10040691

[73] Pierre Comizzoli. Biobanking and fertility preservation for rare and endangered species. Animal Reproduction, vol.14, n1, p.30-33, 2017. http://dx.doi.org/10.21451/1984-3143-AR889

Chapter 11

A Method for Small Number of Human Sperm Cryopreservation

Xiangli Niu, Hua Huang, Yi Mo, Yan Sun and Wei-Hua Wang

Abstract

Recently, some sperm vitrification devices were developed to simplify the procedures to freeze small number of human sperm. In the present study, we used these devices to further examine some factors that affect sperm motility after fast freezing. Experiments were designed to examine the effects of 1) direct immersion of the devices to liquid nitrogen and indirect immersion of the devices to liquid nitrogen in which the devices were sealed in cryogenic storage vials; 2) different freezing volumes (1–5 μl); 3) different equilibration times (1–5 min); and 4) different ratio of freezing solution (0,1-5,1) on post thawing sperm motility. It was found that fast sperm freezing in the sealed vials had high post thawing sperm motility (91.3–93.7% of recovered sperm motility rates) while direct immersion of the devices to liquid nitrogen had 0% post thawing sperm motility. No differences in the recovered sperm motility rates were observed between different freezing solution volumes (87.4–90.5%), different equilibration times (89.5–94.0%), and different freezing solution ratios (90.8–94.6%). However, only 6.8% of recovered sperm motility rate was obtained if sperm were frozen in the medium without sperm freezing solution. These results indicate that human sperm can be rapidly frozen after the devices are sealed in the vials with different equilibration time in the medium containing sperm freezing solution. High post thawing sperm motility can be recovered with this method so that ~90% of sperm are usable after freezing.

Keywords: cryopreservation, fast freezing, human, motility, sperm

1. Introduction

Vitrification, as a fast cryopreservation method, has been used to cryopreserve human oocytes and embryos for many years and has become the routine and major method for cryopreservation of human oocytes and embryos as high survival rates can be obtained after warming [1, 2] However, for human sperm freezing, the current methods still mainly rely on slow freezing [3, 4]. Various methods for vitrification or fast freezing of human sperm have been tested, especially for cryopreservation of small number of sperm [5–12]. However, so far, no standard and practical vitrification/fast freezing method has been developed. This may be due to the facts that the number of sperm is quite large in most semen samples and current slow-programmed sperm freezing method can provide acceptable post recovery rate and survival rate. Furthermore, vitrification did not offer significantly superior results than slow freezing for sperm cryopreservation in the previous study [13].

Clinical uses of rare sperm or small number of sperm in human in vitro fertilization (IVF) are very common, especially when sperm are collected from testicle biopsy. Due to very small number of sperm in these samples, many clinics chose to freeze the sperm during the initial semen analysis or testicle biopsy. However, sperm numbers and/or sperm motility may decrease after the traditional slow freezing. Occasionally, there are not enough sperm survival to inseminate all oocytes from a cycle. Therefore, methods for cryopreservation of small number of human sperm with high recovery and survival rates need to be investigated.

Currently, there are two methods for cryopreservation of small number of human sperm. One is to freeze all tissue or samples in cryogenic storage vials (1–2 ml) or straws (0.25–0.5 ml) by slow freezing [3]. Another is to find motile sperm and then the sperm were placed in some small devices to perform fast freezing or vitrification [5–8]. However, most protocols do not offer satisfactory recovery and motility rates after thawing. Because sperm are very small, it is difficult to process sperm for freezing. Devices and methods for oocyte and embryos vitrification are not suitable to freeze sperm. Therefore, it is necessary to develop devices and methods that are easy to use, and can also provide high recovery rate and good motility, to freeze small number of human sperm. Recently, a SpermVD, a sperm vitrification device, has been reported to freeze small number of human sperm from men with non-obstructive azoospermia [13]. Although it has been reported that high sperm recovery rates can be obtained with this device, sperm motility rates after thawing varied from 0 to 100% among samples from different patients [14]. It is still unknown whether the big differences between samples were resulted from freezing method, different samples, or technical difficulties. Therefore, in the present study, to avoid the differences among different samples, we used normal sperm samples to examine some factors that affect the post thawing sperm motility after fast freezing.

2. Materials and methods

2.1 Ethical statement

All patients undergoing sperm cryopreservation signed informed consents and the research was approved by ethics committee at the Reproductive Hospital of Guangxi Zhuang Autonomous Region.

2.2 Samples and devices

Semen samples were obtained from patients who were requested to freeze their semen for later IVF. A small portion of samples was used for fast freezing after swim-up for the study and the remaining was frozen by slow programmed freezing method. Samples were used after swim-up to obtain high percentage of motile sperm so that motility assessment is more accurate with swim-up samples than the original samples in which there were more immotile sperm and debris.

Two devices, as shown in **Figure 1**, SpermVD (MFC Global, Israel) and Microdevice (Xinchang Medical, China) were used in the experiments. For device holding, 2.0 ml externally threaded cryogenic storage vials (Fisher Scientific, USA) were used.

Sperm were washed and processed for swim-up with sperm washing medium (Fujifilm-Irvine Scientific, CA, USA) and then were frozen after being mixed with different ratios of Quinn's advantage sperm freezing medium (Origio, CT, USA). In the present study, to avoid the result variations between good samples and poor samples, we used normal sperm samples for all experiments. For loading the sperm to devices, we used 140 μl flexible pipette to add different volumes of samples to the devices and then processed the freezing.

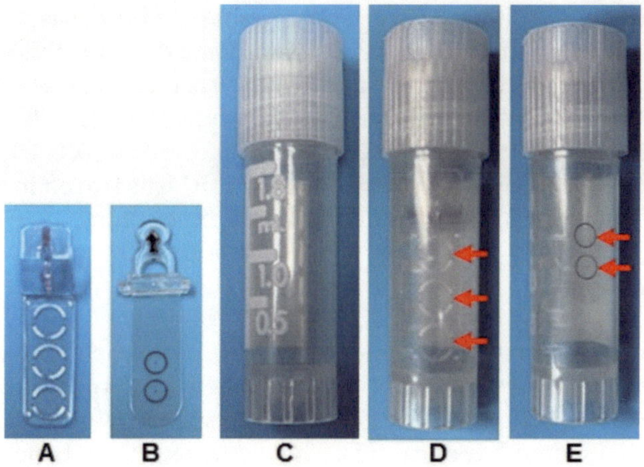

Figure 1.
Fast sperm freezing devices and set up for freezing. A: SpermVD, B: Microdevice, C: 2 ml externally threaded cryogenic storage vial. D: SpermVD in the vial, and E: Microdevice in the vial. Red arrows indicate the location of sperm drops in the devices.

2.3 Fast sperm freezing

Two methods were used for fast sperm freezing. Method I: after sperm were loaded to the devices and equilibrated in the sperm freezing solution for different times, the devices were directly immersed to liquid nitrogen and then each device was inserted to the cryogenic storage vial for storage. Method II: after sperm were loaded to the device, the device was inserted to the vial, the vial was tightly closed with the cap and then immersed to liquid nitrogen.

2.4 Sperm thawing and motility assessment

For sperm thawing, cryogenic vials were removed from liquid nitrogen, and the devices were taken out of the vials with forceps, placed on a 60 mm culture dish. After the frozen drop was thawed or melted within ~1 min at room temperature, the device was directly placed in a 60 mm culture dish with warm oil for sperm motility assessment. Because the volume is very small, it is not necessary to transfer sperm to other sperm count chamber to do motility assessment. Motility was assessed under a phase contrast microscope at ×200 magnifications.

2.5 Experiment design

In experiment 1, post thawing sperm motility was compared between Method I and Method II as well as between two devices, SpermVD and Microdevice. Each 1 μl of micro drop of equilibrated sperm for 5 min in 1:1 of sperm washing solution and sperm freezing medium was frozen in the SpermVD and Microdevice with either Method I or Method II. Three replications were done for this experiment. Temperature changes for two methods during sperm cooling were measured with a digital thermometer.

In experiment 2, post thawing sperm motility was compared among different volumes of micro drops. Each 1 μl, 2 μl and 5 μl of micro drops of equilibrated sperm (5 min in 1:1 of sperm washing solution and sperm freezing medium) was frozen in the SpermVD with the Method II. Five replications were done for this experiment.

In experiment 3, post thawing sperm motility was compared after different equilibration times. Each 1 μl of micro drop of sperm equilibrated for 1, 2 and 5 min in 1:1 of sperm washing solution and sperm freezing medium was frozen in the SpermVD with the Method II. Three replications were done for this experiment.

In experiment 4, post thawing sperm motility was compared among different ratios of sperm freezing solutions. Each 1 µl of micro drop of equilibrated sperm for 5 min with different proportions of sperm freezing solution (0:1, 1:1, 2:1 and 5:1 of sperm freezing medium and sperm washing solution) was frozen in SpermVD with the Method II. Five replications were done for this experiment.

2.6 Statistical analysis

Each experiment was repeated three to five times, and each time with a different semen sample being used. For motility assessment, 100 sperm in each sample were counted. Mean ± SD of percentages of motile sperm before freezing and after thawing were obtained with replications. The recovered rates of sperm motility were calculated after dividing the post thawing sperm motility by the original sperm motility. All data were analyzed by ANOVA. If there were differences among groups, the differences between groups were further compared with chi-square test. If the P value was less 0.05, the difference was considered statistically significant.

3. Results

3.1 Effects of direct and indirect exposure of sperm to liquid nitrogen on the post thawing sperm motility

In the first study, we compared sperm motility after freezing with the Method I and Method II, i.e. direct and indirect immersion of sperm freezing devices (**Figure 1**) to liquid nitrogen and found that no sperm were motile if the devices were directly immersed to liquid nitrogen, while indirect immersion had high post thawing sperm motility. As shown in **Table 1**, the original motility was 85.0 ± 1.0%, and post thawing motilities were 79.7 ± 1.5% and 77.7 ± 2.1% with SpermVD and Microdevice, respectively. The recovery rates (post thawing motility/original motility) of motility were 93.7 ± 0.7% and 91.3 ±1.4% with SpermVD and Microdevice, respectively. No statistical differences were found between the devices (**Table 1**). Based on these findings, all following experiments were done in the SpermVD with the Method II.

After temperature changes were examined during direct and indirect immersion of devices to liquid nitrogen, as shown in **Figure 2**, we found that direct immersion has a 107°C/second cooling rate, or 2 seconds from 25°C to −190°C, while indirect

Devices	Methods	Original motility	Post thawing motility	Recovered motility***
SpermVD	I*	85.0 ± 1.0	0^{a}	0^{a}
	II**	85.0 ± 1.0	79.7 ± 1.5^{b}	93.7 ± 0.7^{b}
Microdevice	I*	85.0 ± 1.0	0^{a}	0^{a}
	II**	85.0 ± 1.0	77.7 ± 2.1^{b}	91.3 ± 1.4^{b}

**Method I: Direct immersion of sperm freezing devices to liquid nitrogen.*
***Method II: Sperm freezing devices were placed cryogenic storage vial, vials were sealed and then immersed to liquid nitrogen.*
****Percentage of post thawing sperm motility/original motility.*
[ab]Values are significantly different in the same column, P < 0.00001.

Table 1.
Effects of direct and indirect exposure of sperm to liquid nitrogen on the post thawing sperm motility.

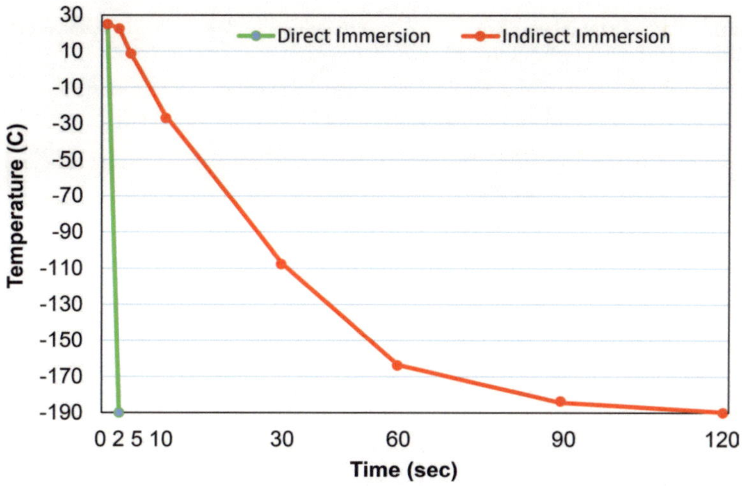

Figure 2.
Temperature changes during direct and indirect immersion of sperm freezing devices to liquid nitrogen. Times were recorded at 0, 2, 5, 10, 30, 60, 90 and 120 seconds during cooling from room temperature (25°C) to −190°C.

immersion has slow cooling rates with a 2 min of total cooling time from 25°C to −190°C. However, the cooling rates were further examined during this period and we found that it was 1.2°C/second during the first 2 seconds (25°C to 22.6°C), 4.6°C/second from 22.6°C to 8.7°C, 7.1°C/second from 8.7°C to −27°C, 4.03°C/second from −27°C to −107.6°C, 1.87°C/second from −107.6°C to −163.8°C, 0.66°C/second from −163.8°C to −183.6°C and 0.22°C/second from −183.6°C to −190°C. The temperature and time were not examined after the temperature reached to −190°C as it showed very slow changes after −190°C.

3.2 Effects of freezing volumes on the post warming sperm motility

As shown in **Table 2**, we found that there were no significant differences in the post thawing sperm motility between 1, 2 and 5 μl of freezing volumes. The original motility was 95.6 ± 1.7%, and post thawing motilities were 83.5 ± 5.5%, 88.9 ± 1.3%, and 86.4 ± 5.0%, respectively. The recovery rates of motility were 87.4 ± 6.2, 93.0 ± 1.9 and 90.5 ± 5.2%, respectively.

Volume (μl)	Original motility	Post thawing motility	Recovered motility**
1	95.6 ± 1.7	83.5 ± 5.5	87.4 ± 6.2
2	95.6 ± 1.7	88.9 ± 1.3	93.0 ± 1.9
5	95.6 ± 1.7	86.4 ± 5.0	90.5 ± 5.2

**Method II and SpermVD were used to freeze sperm.*
***Percentage of post thawing sperm motility/original motility.*

Table 2.
Effects of freezing volumes on the post warming sperm motility.*

3.3 Effects of equilibration times on post thawing sperm motility

As shown in **Table 3**, we found that equilibration of 1, 2 and 5 minutes of sperm in the freezing solution had similar post thawing sperm motility. Original motility was 94 ± 2%, and post thawing motilities were 88.3 ± 2.1, 85.4 ± 1.6 and 84.1 ± 0.9%, respectively. The recovery rates of motility were 94.0 ± 1.6, 90.9 ± 3.0 and 89.5 ± 2.4%, respectively.

Time (min)**	Original motility	Post thawing motility	Recovered motility***
1	94.0 ± 2.0	88.3 ± 2.1	94.0 ± 1.6
2	94.0 ± 2.0	85.4 ± 1.6	90.9 ± 3.0
5	94.0 ± 2.0	84.1 ± 0.9	89.5 ± 2.4

*Method II and SpermVD were used to freeze sperm.
**Sperm equilibration time in the freezing solution before freezing.
***Percentage of post thawing sperm motility/original motility.*

Table 3.
Effects of equilibration times on post thawing sperm motility.*

3.4 Effects of freezing solution ratios on the post warming sperm motility

In this experiment, no differences were observed in the post thawing sperm motility between different ratios of sperm freezing medium (1:1, 2:1 and 5:1). As shown in **Table 4**, the original sperm motility was 91.4 ± 2.4%, and post thawing motility was 83.0 ± 3.7, 86.8 ± 2.8 and 85.2 ± 1.8%, respectively. The recovery rates of sperm motility were 90.9 ± 5.4, 94.6 ± 3.7 and 93.1 ± 4.2%, respectively. However, if sperm were frozen in the solution without sperm freezing medium (0:1), only 6.2 ± 1.1% motility, or 6.8 ± 1.2% of recovery rate of motility was obtained (**Table 4**).

Ratio**	Original motility	Post thawing motility	Recovered motility***
0:1	91.4 ± 2.4	6.2 ± 1.1^{a}	6.8 ± 1.2^{a}
1:1	91.4 ± 2.4	83.0 ± 3.7^{b}	90.9 ± 5.4^{b}
2:1	91.4 ± 2.4	86.8 ± 2.8^{b}	94.6 ± 3.7^{b}
5:1	91.4 ± 2.4	85.2 ± 1.8^{b}	93.1 ± 4.2^{b}

*Method II and SpermVD were used to freeze sperm.
**Ratio of sperm freezing solution to sperm washing medium.
***Percentage of post thawing sperm motility/original motility.
^{ab}Values are significantly different in the same column, $P < 0.00001$.*

Table 4.
Effects of freezing solution ratios on the post warming sperm motility.*

4. Discussion

Vitrification has been used to cryopreserve human oocytes and embryos in human infertility clinics for many years. For oocyte and embryo cryopreservation, vitrification requires high concentration (30%) of cryoprotectants in the vitrification solutions [1, 2]. Cryoprotectants are macromolecules added to the freezing medium to protect cells from the detrimental effects of intracellular ice crystal formation during the process of freezing and thawing. When embryo vitrification solution is cooled to −196°C in liquid nitrogen, substances in the solution is transformed into a glass, not ice crystal. However, in the present study, we used slow sperm freezing solution with low concentration of cryoprotectant (7.5% glycerol) and sperm still survived after freezing. It is still unknown whether ice crystal is formed inside sperm or not.

Although the procedure used in the present study is similar to vitrification, cooling time from room temperature to −196°C is longer (~2 minutes) than vitrification, thus the cooling rate is lower than vitrification. In fact, direct immersion of sperm to liquid nitrogen (that is similar as vitrification) did not support sperm survival, which is completely different from vitrification of oocytes and embryos. Our data indicate that this fast sperm freezing method with regular concentration of cryoprotectant in the freezing solution can bring about ~90% recovered rate of sperm motility after thawing. This rate is higher than those reported in the previous studies with other methods [4–12]. The results in our study were very stable after freezing of a total of 16 semen samples, further indicating that this method is practicable in human IVF clinics.

A few previous publications indicated that vitrification or fast sperm freezing with different concentrations of sucrose as cryoprotectant also supported sperm motility after thawing, but the overall sperm motility rates were less than 40% [4–12]. Reduced sperm motility after freezing/thawing is mainly caused by the injury of sperm membrane [12–15]. Sperm DNA can also be further damaged by different cryopreservation methods or cryopreservation medium [12, 16, 17]. We did not examine sperm DNA fragmentation before vitrification and after warming in the present study, it remains necessary to further examine whether high survival rate is correlated with low DNA fragmentation.

Some devices for embryo vitrification have been used for vitrification/fast freezing of sperm but they are not the ideal devices for sperm freezing [5, 6]. Cryogenic storage vials may be suitable for normal sperm freezing because large volume is required for these kinds of freezing, but not suitable for small number of sperm freezing [10, 12–15]. Recently, a report indicated that direct pellet vitrification of human sperm with 0.25 M sucrose and thawing at 42°C increased sperm motility to ~70% and the authors considered that their high post thawing survival rate was resulting from a higher thawing temperature [10]. However, this method may not be suitable for freezing of small number of sperm.

Based on our study, we found that the following technical aspects are important to obtain high rates of sperm motility after fast freezing:

First, the traditional slow sperm freezing solution containing glycerol and sucrose works well for fast sperm freezing. It is not necessary to use higher concentrations of cryoprotectants, like those used for oocyte and embryo vitrification. However, cryoprotectants are still necessary for fast sperm freezing because very low motile sperm was obtained in the solution without cryoprotectants. This result indicates that the current commercial sperm freezing solution is appropriate for fast sperm freezing.

Second, time for equilibration of sperm in the freezing solution and volume of solution did not affect the post thawing sperm motility. These advantages allow this fast sperm freezing procedure to be easily used in human infertility clinics. For example, if there are very few sperm, freezing solution drop can be as small as 1 μl, and if there are more sperm, the volume of micro drop can be increased to 5 μl. However, it may not be necessary to freeze more than 20 sperm (if there is small number of sperm in a sample) in one device as high recovery and survival rates can be obtained with this method. Also, the time range (1–5 min) for equilibration of sperm in the sperm freezing solution allows laboratory technicians to process the freezing without rushing. We did not examine whether longer equilibration time has similar post thawing sperm motility or not, but it appears that up to 5 minutes is sufficient for technicians to load and freeze sperm.

Third, direct immersion of sperm to liquid nitrogen does not support post thawing sperm motility. This result indicates that fast cooling rate, like that for embryo vitrification, does not work for sperm freezing. By contrast, slow cooling rate is better than rapid cooling rate. When the devices are sealed in the cryogenic storage vial and then immersed to liquid nitrogen, cooling rate is reduced 60 times (120 sec vs. 2 sec) as compared with direct immersion of device to liquid nitrogen. These results indicate that vitrification does not work for human sperm freezing with the current sperm freezing solutions. When the device was placed in the vial and then immersed to liquid nitrogen, the cooling rate was much slower than vitrification.

High survival rates (>90%) can be obtained when human oocytes and embryos were vitrified [1, 2]. Here we provide evidence that ~90% of recovered sperm motility can also be obtained with this fast sperm freezing method. In the present study, we examined sperm motility, but did not examine sperm vitality because ~90% of sperm were motile after thawing. Usually, sperm survival rates after freezing and thawing are higher than motility, indicating that sperm membrane has been injured in some sperm and these sperm cannot move but they are still live [4–12]. However, in the present study, high post thawing sperm motility indicates that sperm membrane was not injured during freezing and thawing, thus the current method may have less injury to sperm and/or sperm membrane than the previous methods [4–12].

The advantage of the devices used in the present study is that these devices can be directly placed in a culture dish, so sperm loading before freezing and sperm picking up after thawing can be done directly under a phase contrast microscope. Therefore, it is not necessary to transfer sperm between devices or wash sperm by centrifugation.

Furthermore, this method is a closed system. The vials must be closed tightly before immersion to liquid nitrogen to avoid liquid nitrogen entering the vials. Therefore, this method not only guarantees high rate of sperm motility after freezing, but also ensures samples not to have cross contamination during freezing and storage.

5. Conclusion

In conclusion, our data indicate that high post thawing sperm motility can be obtained after fast sperm freezing with the current commercial sperm freezing solution and commercially available devices, such as SpermVD and Microdevice. Our results also indicate that this method is safe as the devices are sealed in the storage vials during freezing and storage, which can avoid cross contamination. Furthermore, this method is simple and easy to learn.

Acknowledgements

This research was supported by a grant from Nanning Scientific Research and Technology Development project, (20173017-8) and Guangxi Medical and Health Department (20190862).

Conflict of interest

The authors declare that they have no conflict of interests.

Age	30.88 ± 0.57
BMI(kg/m2)	23.91 ± 0.51
Basal E2	297.2 ± 69.45
Basal FSH	6.53 ± 0.46
Duration of infertility (y)	5.4 ± 0.62
Antral follicle count(≥14 mm)	10 ± 2.22
No. of oocytes collected	23.56 ± 1.05
No. of matured oocytes	18.6 ± 0.65
No. of embryo transferred	1.63 ± 0.08

Note: data showed mean ± SEM.

Table 1.
Characteristics of patients in this study.

To avoid frequent opening/closing of the incubator door, the 'one patient one incubator' strategy was conducted in our study, which means COCs or embryos from one patient were cultured separately in one incubator.

2.2 Incubators and parameters monitoring

As showed in **Figure 1A** and **B**, the air jacket incubator (EC9 triple gas bench-top incubator, ASTEC CO., LTD. Japan) and a conventional water jacket incubator (Penguin AQ series/APM30D, triple gas incubator, ASTEC CO., LTD. Japan) were used in our research. The specifications of different incubators were listed in **Figure 1C**. A range of 12–15 repeated opening/closing processes were conducted in a single ART cycle (from oocyte collection to blastocyst transfer).

For temperature monitoring, a handheld temperature measuring equipment with a long and soft linear sensor (TES 1310 TYPE-K, China) was used to monitor the variation of temperature in a center-well organ culture dish (FALCON, 353037) with 1 ml medium covered with 1 ml mineral oil in the dishes. Briefly, according to the length of time consuming in routine embryo culture, we made a single 10-seconds door opening/closing process, after which the temperature of incubator chambers was detected. It should be noted that 5-seconds door opening/closing was enough for air jacket incubator, in which only one dish was usually placed. Considering the consistency of this study, 10-seconds opening/closing treatment was accepted for two kinds of incubators. CO2 and 02 recovering times were recorded according to the corresponding display panels.

For pH measurement, 5 ml medium was poured into a tube and equilibrated for overnight. At the second day, we tested the initial pH values (initial state) by a pH meter (PB-10 Sartorius). As temperature monitoring, after a 3 min holding on the thermostatic desk, pH values were recorded again (out for 3 min), after which the medium was put back into incubators and detected at 10 min, 30 min and 1 hour (showed 'in for 10 min', 'in for 30 min' and 'in for 1h' respectively).

2.3 Sperm preparation, fertilization and embryo culture

After semen liquefaction (nearly 30 minutes), density gradient centrifugation combined with swim-up was used to sort sperm with normal morphology and high motility [7]. G-IVF (vitrolife) was used to wash sperm and120,000 motile sperm/ml was used for short-time in vitro fertilization. After 4 hours co-culture, oocyte denudation was performed using mechanical method and the remaining

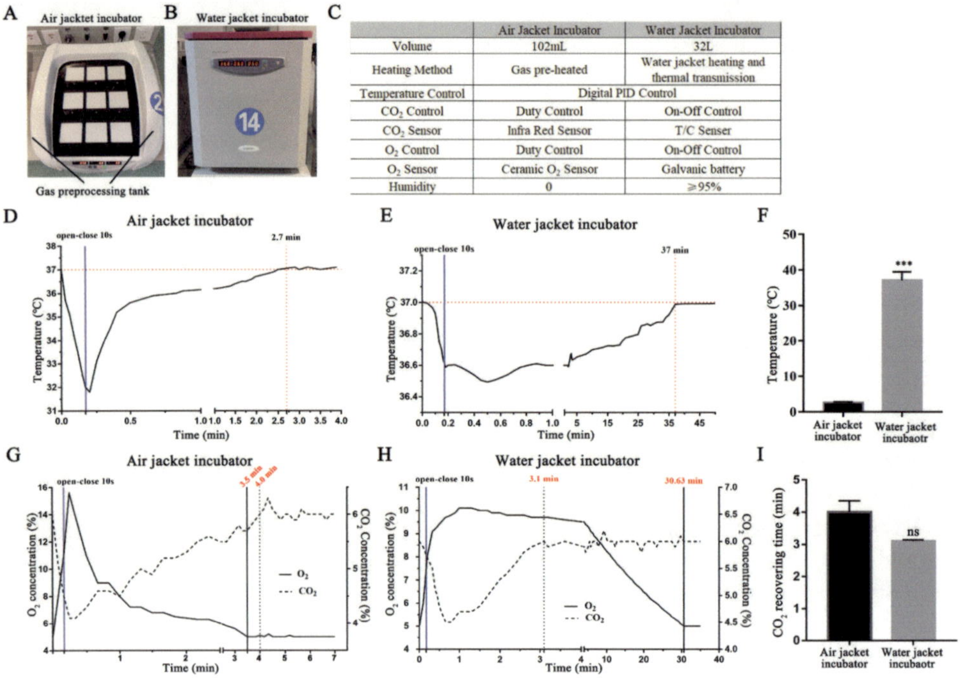

	Air Jacket Incubator	Water Jacket Incubator
Volume	102mL	32L
Heating Method	Gas pre-heated	Water jacket heating and thermal transmission
Temperature Control	Digital PID Control	
CO_2 Control	Duty Control	On-Off Control
CO_2 Sensor	Infra Red Sensor	T/C Senser
O_2 Control	Duty Control	On-Off Control
O_2 Sensor	Ceramic O_2 Sensor	Galvanic battery
Humidity	0	≥95%

Figure 1.
*Comparison of the air jacket incubator and water jacket incubator. (A) and (B): Photograph of the air jacket incubator (A) and the water jacket incubator (B). (C): Physical parameters of different types of incubators. (D) and (E): Incubator temperature recovering process after a 10 seconds opening/closing process. The solid line and right vertical axis represented the changing process of the air jacket incubator. The dotted line and left vertical axis represented the change of temperature in the water jacket incubator. (F): Statistical data of temperature in different incubators. ***: $P < 0.001$. (G) and (H): CO2 and O2 recovering process in different incubators (G was the air jacket incubator; H was the water jacket incubator). (I): CO2 recovering time in different incubators. Ns: no significant differences.*

sperm was also removed. Depending on the presence of the second polar body, we judged if oocytes were fertilized and only these oocytes with two polar bodies were then transferred into cleavage culture medium (G1 medium, vitrolife). At day 1 (16–18 hours after fertilization), the number of pronucleus (PN) was recorded and 2PN-gametes were identified as normal fertilization, after which these gametes were transferred into new G1 medium. At day 3 and day 5, embryos were transferred into G2 medium (vitrolife) for blastocyst culture.

2.4 Embryo and blastocyst scoring

Embryos and blastocysts were graded according to the Istanbul consensus and Gardner criteria [8, 9]. Briefly, embryos (day 3) with 7–9 cells, less than 10% fragmentation by volume and symmetric blastomeres were identified the good. Blastocysts (day 5) graded 4BB or even better were identified the good, including 4BB, 4AB, 4BA and 4AA. Embryos on day 3 or blastocysts on day 5 were assessed by three experienced embryologists and the assessments were recorded individually. Although most of the results were consistent between embryologists, the lowest score (when exist) was accepted.

2.5 Embryo transfer and clinical follow-up

Using abdominal ultrasound guidance, one or two embryos (fresh or frozen–thawed embryos) were transferred to each woman. In some situations, such as the patient with ovarian hyper-stimulation syndrome (OHSS), embryos were cryo-preserved and the frozen–thawed embryos were transferred later. Serum β-hCG levels were monitored on day 14 after embryo transfer, which was used to confirm biochemical pregnancy. When the gestational sac (should have heartbeat) was observed using ultrasound one month after embryo transfer, clinical pregnancy was confirmed. Considering the possibility of failure in one cycle, we calculated the successful rate of every transfer cycles to compare the clinical outcomes in two groups. For example, if one patient was conducted two times of frozen–thawed embryo transfer (FET) (all embryos from the air jacket incubator) and was verified pregnant at last, the clinical pregnancy rate would be 50%.

2.6 Statistical analysis

Statistical analysis was performed using Student's t-test or Fisher's exact test with GraphPad Prism 7 software. Data were expressed as mean ± SEM. As for comparing the proportion of pregnancies, dichotomous outcomes data were showed as frequency and percentage. The differences between two groups were represented by computing the odds ratio with 95% confidence interval, and Fisher's exact tests was used. $P < 0.05$ was considered statistically significant.

3. Results

3.1 Microenvironment in air jacket incubators recovers faster than that in water jacket incubators

As shown in **Figure 1A** and **B** the gas preprocessing tank takes up a large space of the incubator, which is used to heat and mix the gas (6% CO_2, 5% O_2, and 89% N_2). After that, the warmed and mixed gas was released into culture chamber. The volume, heating method, gas control system and humidity are main differences between two kinds of incubators (**Figure 1C**). Besides, the gas control system of air jacket incubators is duty control, which provide better fault-tolerant capabilities than the on–off control system (**Figure 1C**).

During embryo culture, the door of an incubator was opened and closed frequently. We monitored the temperature recovering process after a 10s-opening/closing procedure. As shown in **Figure 1D**, after an opening-10s-closing procedure, the chamber temperature of air jacket incubators decreased steeply (the lowest temperature was 31.8°C). However, in less than 3 min (2.7 ± 0.12 min, n = 4), the chamber temperature of air jacket incubators recovered to the normal. On the contrary, despite the gentle decline of temperature in water jacket incubators (the lowest temperature was 36.5°C), it taken nearly 37 min to recover its intra-environment temperature (37 ± 2.48 min, n = 4; $P < 0.0001$) (**Figure 1E** and **F**). For gas recovering process, as shown in **Figure 1G** and **H**, CO_2 recovering time was 4 min and O_2 recovering time was 3.5 min in air jacket incubators. However, O_2 recovering time was more than 30 min in water jacket incubators. There was no significant difference in the CO_2 recovering time between two types of incubators (air jacket incubator vs. water jacket incubator: 4 ± 0.35 min vs. 3.1 ± 0.15 min, n = 4; $P > 0.5$)) (**Figure 1I**).

The temperature of culture medium in air jacket incubators recovers faster than in water jacket incubators, but there are no differences in pH values between two groups.

We also detected the change of medium temperature over time. Simulating the observation and operation of embryos, we taken out the dishes from the incubator and placed on a 37°C thermostatic desk for 3 min (**Figure 2A**). As shown in

Figure 2B, we found that the temperature of medium covered with mineral oil recovered to 37°C within 31.5 min in air jacket incubators. However, more than 65 min were taken for temperature recovering in the conventional water jacket incubator. As shown in **Figure 2C**, the pH values of G-IVF, G1 and G2 (Vitrolife) represented similar changing trends between two groups and no significant differences were observed.

3.2 There are no differences in short time IVF and embryo development between two types of incubators

Since the differences in intra-incubator micro-environment regulating method between two types of incubators, we investigated if the fertilization and embryo development were affected due to the factors of culture environment fluctuating. As shown in **Table 2**, there were no differences in fertilization rate between two groups (water jacket incubator group: 77.84 ± 2.15%, n = 498 vs. air jacket incubator group: 74.57 ± 2.24%, n = 478; $P > 0.05$). The normal fertilization rates (2PN rates) at day 1 were also similar between two groups (water jacket incubator group: 53.99 ± 3.04%, n = 498 vs. air jacket incubator group: 52.18 ± 2.74%, n = 478; $P > 0.05$) (**Table 2**). Meanwhile, there were also no significant statistical differences in the abnormal fertilization rates (≥3PN for IVF, 1 PN or ≥ 3PN for ICSI) between two groups (water jacket incubator group: 8.04 ± 1.65%, n = 498 vs. air jacket incubator group: 7 ± 1.77%, n = 478; $P > 0.05$).

On day 3, we assessed the quality of embryos in two groups and found that there were also no differences in good quality of embryos that with 7–9 symmetric blastomeres and less than 10% fragmentation by volume (water jacket incubator

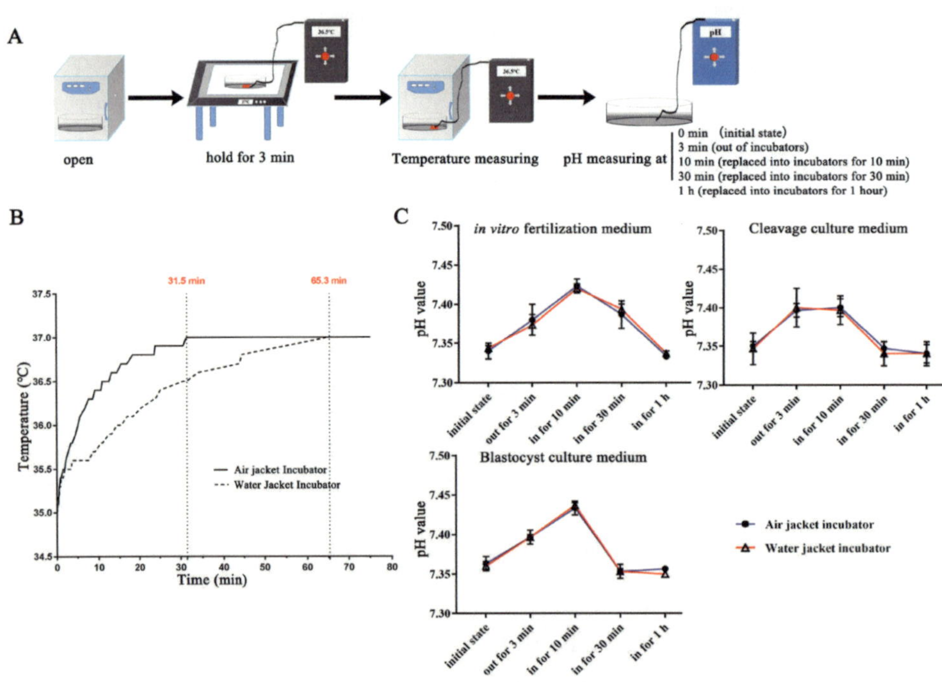

Figure 2.
Temperatures and pH values of culture medium recovering process in different incubators. (A): The cartoon indicating the timing of temperature and pH monitoring. (B): Temperature variation of culture medium covered with oil in incubators after a 3-min-handling outside the incubator. The solid line represented the changing process of air jacket incubators, the dotted line represented the water jacket incubator. (C): pH values of G-IVF, G1 and G2 recovering processes in different types of incubators.

	Air jacket incubator	Water jacket incubator	P value
Fertilization rate	74.57 ± 2.24% (n = 478)	77.84 ± 2.15% (n = 498)	0.14
Normal fertilization rate	67.57 ± 2.61% (n = 478)	69.8 ± 2.51% (n = 498)	0.47
Abnormal fertilization rate	7 ± 1.77% (n = 478)	8.04 ± 1.65% (n = 498)	0.61
D3 good embryo rate	49.48 ± 4.18% (n = 315)	50.97 ± 3.32% (n = 336)	0.7
Blastocyst formation rate	60.74 ± 3.82% (n = 269)	65.54 ± 3.97% (n = 288)	0.33
Good blastocyst rate	43.97 ± 4.92% (n = 166)	48.14 ± 4.67% (n = 191)	0.52

Note: Data presented as mean ± SEM (n). Paired t test was used for the statistical analysis between two groups. P values >0.05 indicated there were no differences between two groups.

Table 2.
Fertilization and embryo development in different types of incubators.

	Air jacket incubator	Water jacket incubator	Odds ratio (95% Cl)	P value
Biochemical pregnancy	14/26(53.85%)	22/33(66.67%)	1.71(0.62–4.92)	0.42
Clinical pregnancy	11/26(42.31%)	18/33(54.55%)	1.64(0.58–4.52)	0.43
Implantation	15/37(40.54%)	20/46(43.48%)	1.13(0.46–2.63)	0.83
Live birth	9/26(34.62%)	11/33(33.33%)	0.94(0.32–2.92)	>0.99

Note: Data presented as proportions, n(%). Fisher's exact test was used for between-group data comparisons. Odds ratio with 95% confidence interval (Cl) were also listed. P values>0.05 indicated there were no differences between two groups.

Table 3.
Clinical outcome comparisons between two types of incubators.

group: 50.97 ± 3.32%, n = 336 vs. air jacket incubator group: 49.48 ± 4.18%, n = 315; P > 0.05) (**Table 2**). As for blastocyst formation rate, the water jacket incubator group was 65.54 ± 3.97% (n = 288), compared to 60.74 ± 3.82% (n = 269) blastocyst formation of the air jacket incubator group (P > 0.05). There were no significant differences observed in good blastocyst formation (water jacket incubator group: 48.14 ± 4.67%, n = 191 vs. air jacket incubator group: 43.97 ± 4.92%, n = 166; n = 43, P > 0.05). All these results indicated that intra-incubator microenvironment regulating method does not affect fertilization and embryo development.

3.3 The clinical outcomes were also similar between two groups

As shown in **Table 3**, the rates of biochemical pregnancy and clinical pregnancy were 53.85% and 42.31% respectively in air jacket incubators, which were similar as that in water jacket incubator (rates of biochemical pregnancy and clinical pregnancy were 66.67% and 54.55% respectively). No statistically significant differences were observed between two groups (P > 0.05). The implantation rate and live-birth rate of the air jacket incubator were 40.54% and 34.62% respectively, which were also similar with that in the water jacket incubator (the implantation rate was 43.48% and the live-birth rate was 33.33%, P > 0.05).

4. Discussion

Although many types of incubators have been successfully applied for human IVF, there were few studies compared the effects of the incubators with different features on embryo development and clinical outcomes. We noticed two related reports about the effects of intra-incubator environment on embryo development; however, their results were inconsistent [5, 6]. Besides, it is worth noting that previous conclusions were based on 'one patient, one incubator' and strictly paired comparisons ('one patient, two types of incubators') were lacking. We allocated COCs from one patient equally and non-selectively to either incubator from fertilization to day-6-embryo-culture and found that the microenvironment of air jacket incubator could recover quickly, but there were no significant differences for embryo development and clinical outcomes between two types of incubators.

The pH levels, temperature, osmolality and humidity of embryo culture microenvironment are maintained by the incubator [6]. However, different incubators have different methods to heat, control gas and humidity. In our study, we found that the air jacket incubator represented a better performance in temperature recovering (including the atmosphere temperature and culture medium temperature) and O2 recovering. For air jacket incubators, the gas pre-processing tank was used to heat and mix different gas, after which the warmed and mixed gas (37°C, 6% CO2, 5% O2, and 89% N2) was released into the culture chamber. Besides, with a smaller volume and heated lid, the parameters of incubator micro-environment are easy to recover. On the contrary, for the conventional water jacked incubator, due to the large volume, the distance of thermal transmission to dishes is relatively long, which leads to a long time needed for temperature recovering. On the other hand, the gas control system is different between two types of incubators (**Figure 1C**). On–off control is a simple form of gas feedback control in conventional water jacket incubators, which drives CO2/O2 from fully closed to full open depending on the set point. Therefore, during the process of steady state recovering, the related parameters could fluctuate around the set point. However, the duty control is a stricter and precise method for gas control in air jacket incubators.

Although air jacket incubators have better properties than water jacket incubators, there were no significant differences in fertilization, embryo development and clinical outcomes observed in our study (**Tables 2** and **3**). As shown in **Figure 2B**, after 3 min operation outside of the incubator (still placed on a 37°C thermostatic platform), the temperature of culture medium dropped to 35°C. It appears that this low temperature in a short time might not affect embryo development. Actually, the temperatures in the cervix, oviduct and the ovary are between 36°C and 37°C [10]. Therefore, although a temperature recovering in water jacket incubators is longer, the short duration of limited low temperature did not affect embryo development and clinical outcomes. It was reported that incubator door openings could lead to measurable, significant changes in mouse embryo morphokinetics [11], suggesting that frequent disruption of intra-incubator environment is harmful for embryo development.

Overall, we concluded that, types of incubators could not affect embryo developmental competence and clinical outcomes as long as the intra-incubator environments are maintained to be stable and it should avoid frequent and prolonged door openings.

Acknowledgements

We thank the other members of the Affiliated Weihai Second Municipal Hospital of Qingdao University for their kind discussions about this study.

Conflict of interest

The authors declare no conflict of interest.

Author details

Ji Liu[1,2,3*†], Yan-Hua Zhou[1,2†], Xiao-Xiao Wang[1,2], Ling-Xi Tong[1,2], Yan-Hong Li[1,2], Ling Liu[1,2], Zhi-Yan Xu[1,2] and Hong-Hui Wang[1,2,3,4*]

1 The Affiliated Weihai Second Municipal Hospital of Qingdao University, Weihai, Shandong, China

2 Weihai Maternal and Child Health Hospital, Weihai, Shandong, China

3 WEGO Ruisheng Medical Devices CO., LTD, Weihai, Shandong, China

4 WEGO Holding Company Limited, Weihai, Shandong, China

*Address all correspondence to: lljj361@163.com and honghui1223@163.com

† These authors are contribute equally to this study.

References

[1] Swain JE, Carrell D, Cobo A, Meseguer M, Rubio C, Smith GD. Optimizing the culture environment and embryo manipulation to help maintain embryo developmental potential. Fertil Steril. 2016;105(3):571-587. doi:10.1016/j.fertnstert.2016.01.035.

[2] Wale PL, Gardner DK. The effects of chemical and physical factors on mammalian embryo culture and their importance for the practice of assisted human reproduction. Hum Reprod Update. 2016;22(1):2-22. doi:10.1093/humupd/dmv034.

[3] Swain JE. Decisions for the IVF laboratory: comparative analysis of embryo culture incubators. Reprod Biomed Online. 2014;28(5):535-547. doi:10.1016/j.rbmo.2014.01.004.

[4] Esteves SC, Bento FC. Implementation of air quality control in reproductive laboratories in full compliance with the Brazilian Cells and Germinative Tissue Directive. Reprod Biomed Online. 2013;26(1):9-21. doi:10.1016/j.rbmo.2012.10.010.

[5] Fujiwara M, Takahashi K, Izuno M, Duan YR, Kazono M, Kimura F et al. Effect of micro-environment maintenance on embryo culture after in-vitro fertilization: comparison of top-load mini incubator and conventional front-load incubator. J Assist Reprod Genet. 2007;24(1):5-9. doi:10.1007/s10815-006-9088-3.

[6] Fawzy M, AbdelRahman MY, Zidan MH, Abdel Hafez FF, Abdelghafar H, Al-Inany H et al. Humid versus dry incubator: a prospective, randomized, controlled trial. Fertil Steril. 2017;108(2):277-283. doi:10.1016/j.fertnstert.2017.05.036.

[7] Rappa KL, Rodriguez HF, Hakkarainen GC, Anchan RM, Mutter GL, Asghar W. Sperm processing for advanced reproductive technologies: Where are we today? Biotechnol Adv. 2016;34(5):578-587. doi:10.1016/j.biotechadv.2016.01.007.

[8] Alpha Scientists in Reproductive M, Embryology ESIGo. The Istanbul consensus workshop on embryo assessment: proceedings of an expert meeting. Hum Reprod. 2011;26(6):1270-1283. doi:10.1093/humrep/der037.

[9] Gardner DK, Lane M, Stevens J, Schlenker T, Schoolcraft WB. Blastocyst score affects implantation and pregnancy outcome: towards a single blastocyst transfer. Fertil Steril. 2000;73(6):1155-1158. doi:10.1016/s0015-0282(00)00518-5.

[10] Ng KYB, Mingels R, Morgan H, Macklon N, Cheong Y. In vivo oxygen, temperature and pH dynamics in the female reproductive tract and their importance in human conception: a systematic review. Hum Reprod Update. 2018;24(1):15-34. doi:10.1093/humupd/dmx028.

[11] Nguyen Q, Sommer S, Greene B, Wrenzycki C, Wagner U, Ziller V. Effects of opening the incubator on morphokinetics in mouse embryos. Eur J Obstet Gynecol Reprod Biol. 2018;229:64-69. doi:10.1016/j.ejogrb.2018.08.003.

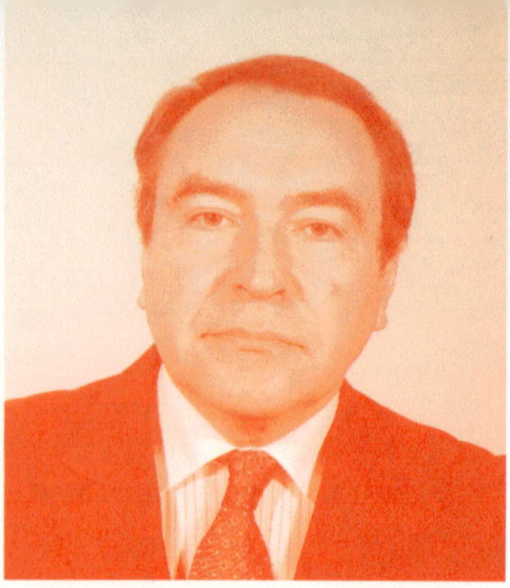
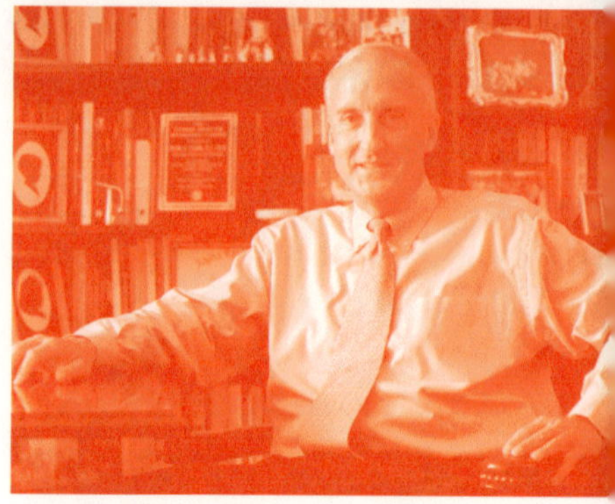
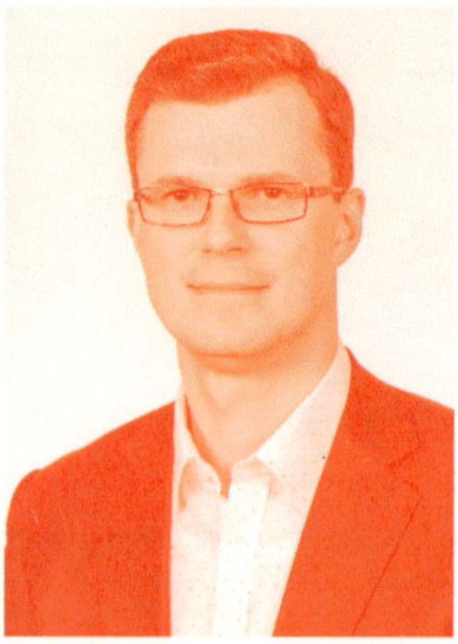
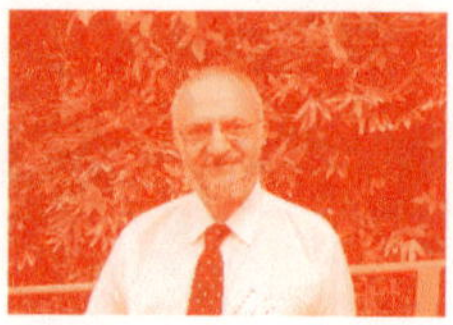
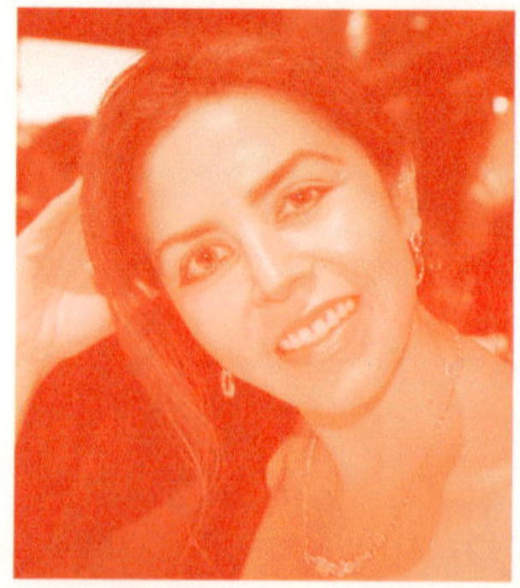

Supporting open minds since 2005

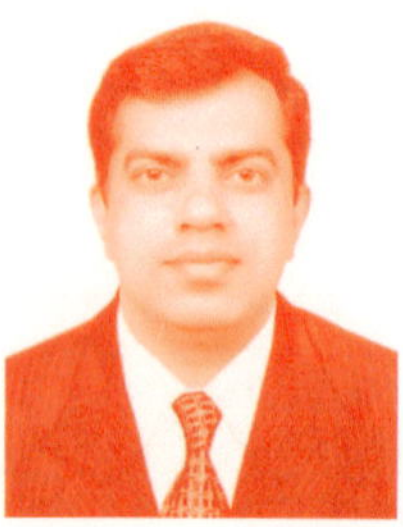
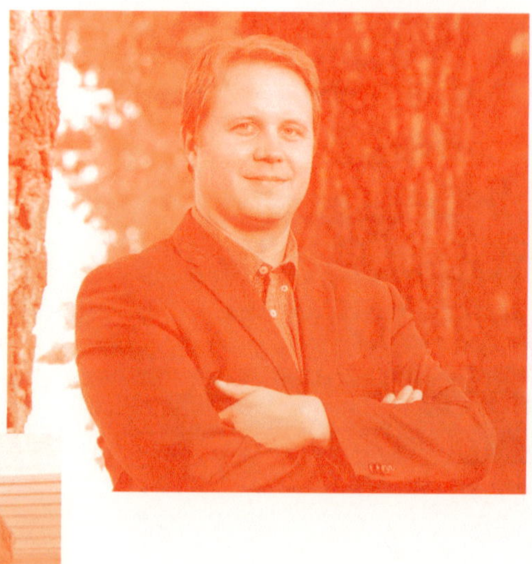
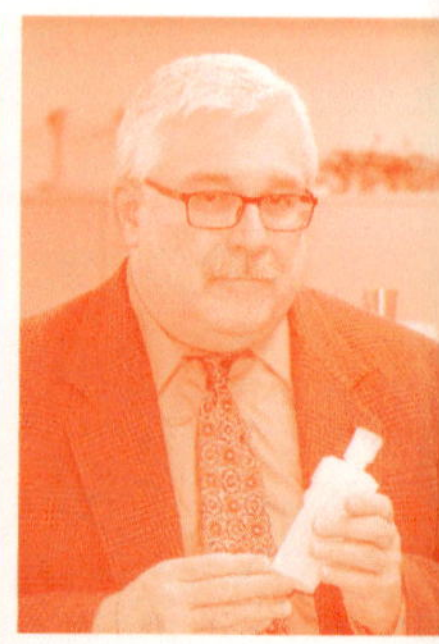
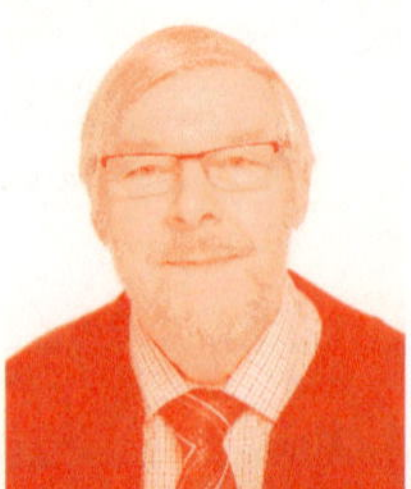
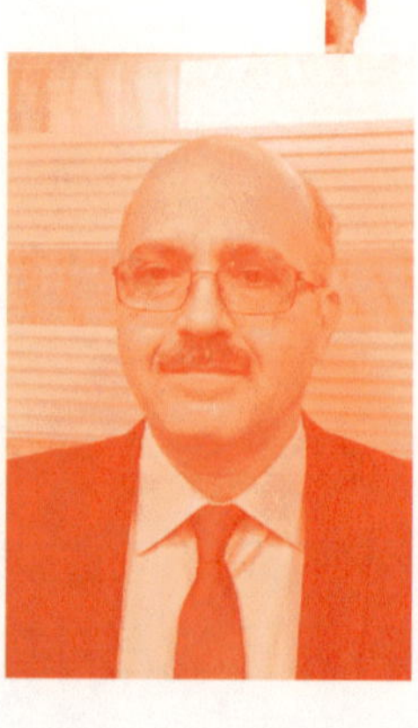
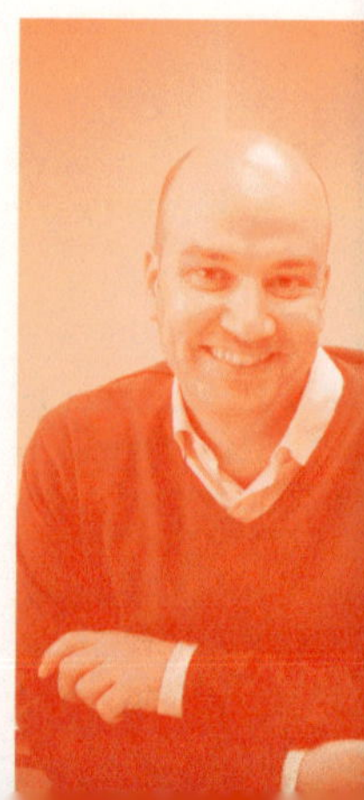
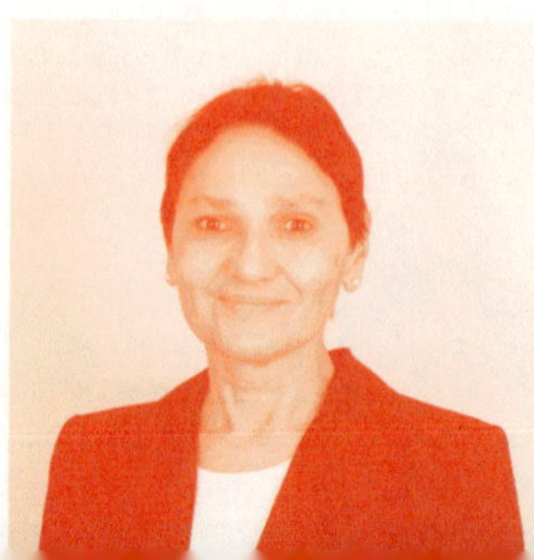

Infertility and Assisted Reproduction
http://dx.doi.org/10.5772/intechopen.95184
Edited by Wei-Hua Wang

Contributors
Bhawna Kushawaha, Rohit Beniwal, Lava Kumar Surarapu, Aradhana Mohanty, Ajay Kumar Singh, Satish Kumar Garg, Desislava Dyulgerova-Nikolova, Tanya Milachich, Leila Mohammadi, Silvia Martinez, Erin Ahart, Courtney Marsh, Michael Wolfe, Elaine Phillips, Juris Erenpreiss, Violeta Fodina, Alesja Dudorova, Mariana Fonseca Roller Barcelos, Jean Pierre B. Brasileiro, Natalia I. Zavattiero Tierno, Murilo C. Souza-Oliveira, Tatianna Q. F. Ribeiro, Amanda Evelyn C. Goulart, Aluisio Mendes R. Filho, Vinicius M. Lopes, Anna Luiza Moraes Souza, Isadora Manzi Novais Theodoro, Gabriela Galdino De F. Barros, Daniely Toledo Costa, Valeria Leal Mathias, Alice Ioana Albu, Dragos Albu, Ji Liu, Hong-Hui Wang, Yan-Hua Zhou, Xiao-Xiao Wang, Ling-Xi Tong, Yan-Hong Li, Ling Liu, Zhi-Yan Xu, Wei-Hua Wang, Cassie T. Wang, Xiangli Niu, Qiuyan Ruan, Yi Mo, Hua Huang, Yan Sun, yaxin Yao, Yan Zhou, Jun Ren, Sijia Lu, Jing Wang, Jin Huang, Ping Liu, Mahruk Hameed Zargar, Faisel Ahmad, Tahir Mohuidin Malla, Mohammad Lateef Khaliq, Juan Luis Giraldo, Susana Salazar López, Jialin Jia, Daniel Aranda

First published in London, United Kingdom, 2021 by IntechOpen
IntechOpen is the global imprint of INTECHOPEN LIMITED, registered in England and Wales, registration number: 11086078, 5 Princes Gate Court, London, SW7 2QJ, United Kingdom
Printed in Croatia

British Library Cataloguing-in-Publication Data
A catalogue record for this book is available from the British Library

Additional hard and PDF copies can be obtained from orders@intechopen.com

Infertility and Assisted Reproduction
Edited by Wei-Hua Wang
p. cm.
Print ISBN 978-1-83962-824-5
Online ISBN 978-1-83962-825-2
eBook (PDF) ISBN 978-1-83962-829-0

For EU product safety concerns:
IN TECH d.o.o., Prolaz Marije Krucifikse Kozulić 3, 51000 Rijeka, Croatia, info@intechopen.com or visit our website at intechopen.com.

Meet the editor

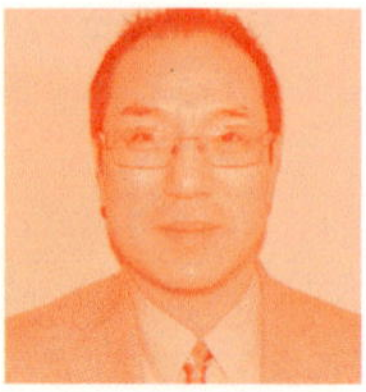

Wei-Hua Wang is laboratory director at Aspire-Houston Fertility Institute, Prelude Fertility/Inception, Texas. He has twenty-five years of experience in in vitro fertilization (IVF) services. He has established one of the largest frozen donor egg banks in the United States. He was also an adjunct professor at the Chinese Academy of Sciences, Lanzhou University, and Guangzhou Medical University. His research has been recognized internationally and has received numerous awards including a General Program Prize (meiotic spindle imaging in living human oocytes) from the American Society for Reproductive Medicine in 1999. He has published more than 100 research papers in peer-reviewed journals and books, and these papers have been cited more than 7000 times. Dr. Wang also serves as an active reviewer for about twenty international journals.

Contents

Chapter 12

The Role of Kisspeptin in the Ovarian Cycle, Pregnancy, and Fertility

Erin Ahart, Elaine Phillips, Michael Wolfe and Courtney Marsh

Abstract

Kisspeptins are a group of neuropeptides with regulatory functions related to puberty, fertility, and reproduction. They are primarily produced by hypothalamic nuclei and are thought to regulate the activity of neurons that produce gonadotropin-releasing hormone. They are also expressed by placental syncytiotrophoblasts in developing pregnancies and are likely involved in the processes of trophoblast invasion and placentation. Similarly to beta-hCG, kisspeptins are found in maternal plasma during the first trimester of pregnancy and increase proportionately with gestational age. Because of their role in implantation, there is currently interest in the use of kisspeptins as minimally invasive biomarkers. It is suspected that maternal kisspeptin levels have diagnostic potential in identifying viable early pregnancies.

Keywords: kisspeptin, reproduction, fertility, placentation, biomarker

1. Introduction

Kisspeptins are a family of neuropeptides with diverse functions in humans. They are cleaved from a precursor peptide encoded by the *KISS-1* gene, which was originally identified in melanoma cells as a metastasis suppressor gene [1]. Expression of KISS-1 has subsequently been identified in many other cell lines, including those of the placenta, ovaries, and testes [2]. It is now known that kisspeptin plays a critical role in reproduction and fertility [3]. Kisspeptin is believed to regulate the secretion of gonadotropin-releasing hormone (GnRH) by integrating central and peripheral signals [4]. During the menstrual cycle, gonadal sex steroid concentrations impact the secretion of GnRH from neurons located in the hypothalamus. It is hypothesized that kisspeptin mediates this hypothalamic feedback because 1) GnRH neurons lack gonadal sex steroid receptors but some express kisspeptin receptors [5–7] and 2) kisspeptin neurons express sex steroid receptors [8, 9]. This review will focus on the role of kisspeptins throughout the menstrual cycle and their potential use as a biomarker of viable pregnancy.

2. Kisspeptin in the follicular phase and periovulation

Kisspeptin neurons are primarily located in the preoptic area and hypothalamic arcuate nucleus and function as upstream regulators of GnRH neurons [10]. In

both of these anatomic locations, serum estrogen and progesterone concentrations have been shown to regulate kisspeptin-mediated GnRH secretion [11]. During the early follicular phase of the menstrual cycle, estrogen exerts negative feedback on GnRH stimulation of luteinizing hormone (LH) secretion. As the follicular phase progresses, rising estrogen levels result in pulsatile secretion of GnRH, which then stimulates the pulsatile release of follicle-stimulating hormone (FSH) and LH [10]. This pulsatile secretion pattern is likely mediated by kisspeptin through regulation of GnRH neurons. Involvement of kisspeptin in this regulatory pathway is suspected because GnRH neurons lack estrogen and progesterone receptors, and thus cannot directly respond to serum sex steroid concentrations [12, 13]. The absence of a direct biochemical connection between the gonads and hypothalamus suggests the presence of an intermediary signal. This "missing link" is thought to be kisspeptin neurons, which express estrogen receptors and secrete a ligand that can bind to GnRH [12].

During the early follicular phase when follicles are underdeveloped, kisspeptin levels are low [4, 14]. A study by Zhai et al. showed that kisspeptin levels sharply increase when the dominant follicle reaches 1.2 cm in diameter [14]. Kisspeptin levels during the periovulatory period are then high [4, 14, 15], and may have potential in predicting development of the dominant ovarian follicle [14]. A study by Dhillo et al. demonstrated that administration of exogenous kisspeptin to healthy women results in increased gonadotropin secretion; this response is most potent during the preovulatory phase [16].

A study by Meczekalski et al. demonstrated that kisspeptin and LH are co-secreted (i.e. each kisspeptin pulse is accompanied by a pituitary LH pulse in response to a hypothalamic GnRH pulse) [11]. Another study demonstrated that blockade of the kisspeptin receptor (GPR54) resulted in blockade of pulsatile LH secretion [17]. There is also topographical evidence of the connection between GnRH and kisspeptin neurons – in several species, it has been shown that GnRH neuronal axons extend from the arcuate nucleus, where kisspeptin neurons are located, to the median eminence, where GnRH is secreted [12]. Human studies have not reproducibly demonstrated this neuroanatomy for all GnRH neurons, which may suggest that kisspeptin neuronal connections in humans are more complex [11, 18].

3. Kisspeptin in ovulation

At mid-cycle, estrogen secreted by the preovulatory follicle eventually triggers GnRH neurons to transition from pulsatile GnRH secretion to sustained secretion. The mechanism by which estrogen transforms from a negative to positive feedback signal on the hypothalamus still remains unclear. Estrogen binds to the ERα receptor on kisspeptin neurons in the arcuate nucleus, inhibiting kisspeptin secretion and subsequent GnRH secretion [15]. In the anteroventral periventricular nucleus, estrogen binds kisspeptin ERα receptors and exerts positive feedback, which ultimately initiates the LH surge associated with ovulation.

The sustained secretion of high concentrations of GnRH (GnRH surge) occurs for over 24 hours and triggers the pituitary gland to secrete high levels of LH (LH surge) [19]. The LH surge is what ultimately triggers ovulation [7]. The LH surge is also the target of at-home ovulation predictor kits [14]. This cascade of hormone surges is thought to be primarily regulated by kisspeptin; in fact, kisspeptin is the most potent activator of GnRH neurons discovered to date [5]. It is suspected that rising estrogen levels during the follicular phase stimulate kisspeptin neurons, which then activate GnRH neurons to initiate the GnRH surge [7]. In contrast,

administration of a monoclonal antibody that blocks kisspeptin has been shown to prevent ovulation in rat models [20].

It is postulated that kisspeptin could be useful as a biomarker of the periovulatory/ovulatory phase [14]. This would be clinically useful because kisspeptin surges prior to LH and therefore could predict the time of ovulation before it happens (rather than as it happens). The target of most ovulation prediction kits is LH, which surges at the time of ovulation. According to Zhai et al., the probability of ovulation is increased when kisspeptin surges on the 11th day and LH surges on the 14th day [14]. In comparison, a study by Goto et al. showed that administration of a kisspeptin antagonist resulted in shrinkage of ovarian follicles and delayed ovulation [21].

4. Kisspeptin in the luteal phase and implantation

Kisspeptin is not only expressed in the central nervous system – it also performs peripheral functions. Expression of kisspeptin and its receptor KISS-1 has been demonstrated in the human ovary, fallopian tube, uterus, and placenta [22]. It is thought that kisspeptin primarily functions in the hypothalamus, but also interacts between the signaling pathways of the central and peripheral reproductive systems [23]. In fact, several studies have supported the idea that kisspeptin exerts direct effects on ovarian tissue via ovarian kisspeptin receptors [24–26].

A number of studies have demonstrated that kisspeptin is expressed at the maternal-fetal interface of many species, including humans [27]. In the human uterus, kisspeptin is expressed in the endometrial epithelial and stromal cells, but not in the myometrium [28]. In the early placenta, kisspeptin is initially produced by villous cytotrophoblast cells, then villous syncytiotrophoblast cells and the placental bed [29, 30]. As pregnancy progresses, placental production of kisspeptin declines [31, 32].

Kisspeptin expression in the endometrium is absent during the proliferative and early secretory phases but becomes abundant during the late secretory phase [27, 33]. This indicates a potential role of kisspeptin in the preparation of endometrial tissue for implantation. Kisspeptin knockout mice exhibit thin, weak uteri with almost no endometrial glands, suggesting kisspeptin is an important regulator of normal endometrial development [34]. Kisspeptin may also act as a mediator that facilitates implantation of the growing embryo to the uterine wall. It has been shown that exogenous kisspeptin administration strengthens adhesion of kisspeptin-expressing trophoblast cells to collagen present in uterine tissue [34]. Immediately after implantation, kisspeptin levels are known to rise; this suggests involvement of kisspeptin during the decidualization process [35]. A study by Wu et al. demonstrated a dose-dependent relationship between kisspeptin expression and inhibition of cell invasion/migration in human decidualized endometrial cells [29]. In contrast, a kisspeptin antagonist called kisspeptin 234 stimulates the process of decidual invasion and migration [29]. Similarly, when small interfering RNAs that antagonize kisspeptin are introduced, stromal decidualization is impaired [35]. In a study by Calder et al., ablation of the KISS-1 gene and subsequent absence of kisspeptin expression resulted in infertile mice [36]. Even in mice that received rescue gonadotropins and estradiol, which restored ovulation, the mice embryos could not implant in the mice that lacked KISS-1. These embryos were, however, able to implant in wildtype mice [36].

Kisspeptin was originally identified as a suppressor of cancer metastasis; its function in the regulation of cellular proliferation and growth is also integral to the

process of placentation. The early placenta expresses high levels of kisspeptin, perhaps to tame the invasive and migratory capability of trophoblasts [32]. Kisspeptin decreases the activity of collagenases, matrix metalloproteinases, and vascular endothelial growth factor, which are all signaling proteins involved in trophoblast proliferation [31, 37]. Kisspeptin also supports the adhesion of extravillous trophoblasts to the endometrium, which inhibits migration [38]. This careful balance between invasion and the prevention of invasion is essential to the placentation process as well as the appropriate remodeling of the maternal uterine wall [34]. As the placenta develops throughout pregnancy, it exhibits a pattern of kisspeptin expression that follows a circadian rhythm [39]. The term placenta demonstrates kisspeptin surges at 0400 and 1200 daily. This rhythm correlates with circadian expression of other proteins involved in placental physiology, including TNFα, melatonin, and oxytocin [39].

5. Kisspeptin in pregnancy

Maternal kisspeptin levels rise dramatically during pregnancy, then return to normal within 15 days of delivery [28]. Unlike β-hCG, kisspeptin levels rise steadily and do not plateau [40]. It is thought that the primary source of maternal kisspeptin is placental tissue [27], and that maternal kisspeptin levels reflect the volume of viable placental tissue [41]. Kisspeptin may be useful as a biomarker of pregnancy due to its association with placental invasion and apoptosis [42]. It also has potential utility as a biomarker of miscarriage.

Spontaneous abortion (SAB) is a common experience, seen in 10–20% of clinically recognized pregnancies [43]. A study by Jayasena et al. showed that maternal plasma kisspeptin is significantly lower in women with early pregnancies who later develop SAB compared to women who have a viable intrauterine pregnancy (IUP) [44]. Maternal kisspeptin levels also had higher diagnostic performance than β-hCG in detecting SAB [44]. Wu et al. demonstrated that women with recurrent SAB have decreased decidual kisspeptin expression compared to women with IUP [45]. Kavvasoglu also showed decreased maternal kisspeptin levels in women with SAB compared to healthy IUPs [46]. Sullivan et al. validated a serum kisspeptin-54 assay as well as confirmed that maternal kisspeptin levels are positively correlated with fetal gestational age and pregnancy viability [40].

There is currently no established clinical test for early miscarriage; diagnosis relies on serial β-hCG measurements and correlation with ultrasound. This requires multiple maternal encounters with the healthcare system, a prolonged timeframe, and can involve considerable distress of the patient and partner. Jayasena et al. describes the current diagnostic pathway for establishing fetal viability as having limited clinical utility due to delay and a high degree of uncertainty [44]. Thus, there is interest in establishing a more accurate and streamlined diagnostic marker of viable IUP vs. SAB.

Kisspeptin has been shown to be massively downregulated in the case of ectopic pregnancy [47]. Ectopic pregnancy occurs when a fertilized ovum implants and develops outside the uterine cavity. Similarly to SAB, ectopic pregnancy is currently diagnosed by serial β-hCG measurements in correlation with ultrasound. Definitive diagnosis may require direct visualization via laparoscopy [48]. A study by Romero-Ruiz et al. explored the roll of kisspeptin in individuals with ectopic pregnancy. They found that maternal circulating kisspeptins gradually increased during the first trimester of pregnancy in healthy controls. However, in those with ectopic

pregnancy, kisspeptin levels were suppressed. The study correlated these results to levels of microRNAs (miRNA) (small noncoding RNAs that can modulate gene and protein expression). In particular, miR-324-3p is known to inhibit kisspeptin function. Romero-Ruiz et al. found that in ectopic pregnancies, miR-324-3p was significantly increased in placental tissue (though maternal circulating levels were low). This finding suggests defective export of the miRNA from its embryonic/placental source in ectopic pregnancy, which may further contribute to the local suppression of kisspeptin. The authors suggested that correlation of maternal miR-324-3p with kisspeptin and β-hCG levels could provide a better modality for timely diagnosis of ectopic pregnancy, especially considering the stability of miRNA in maternal serum [46].

Kisspeptin could also have diagnostic utility in identifying women at risk of preeclampsia. A study by Qaio showed that the placentas of term preeclamptic pregnancies express significantly lower kisspeptin levels compared to healthy pregnancies [49]. These findings were reproduced by Farina et al., which demonstrated lower KISS-1 expression in preeclamptic patients compared to healthy pregnant patients [50]. The study also suggested KISS-1 cell-free mRNA has potential to serve as a predictive biomarker of preeclampsia [50]. Matjila et al. investigated the relationship between maternal kisspeptin levels and placental kisspeptin expression in preeclamptic pregnancies – they found that preeclamptic placentas demonstrated high kisspeptin expression but low maternal kisspeptin levels [30]. It is speculated that elevated kisspeptin expression in diseased placentas may inhibit trophoblast invasion and contribute to the development of preeclampsia [30, 34]. Kisspeptin therefore has potential to offer predictive information about the risk of preeclampsia.

6. Kisspeptin in in vitro fertilization

Because of its apparent role in reproduction and fertility, there is interest in the use of kisspeptin as a tool to aid in assisted reproductive technology. Exogenous kisspeptin has been used to trigger oocyte maturation in women undergoing in vitro fertilization (IVF) with very low rates of ovarian hyperstimulation syndrome (OHSS) [41, 51]. Oocyte maturation is the process during which an oocyte transitions from metaphase I to metaphase II; at this time, it is capable of becoming fertilized [51]. Jayasena et al. demonstrated that a single kisspeptin bolus was capable of producing an LH surge that induced oocyte maturation in women undergoing IVF [41]. This was an important study, as it was the first to label kisspeptin as an effective maturation trigger. 92% of the study participants who received kisspeptin had at least one embryo available for transfer [41]. A study by Owens et al. then demonstrated that when kisspeptin is administered as an oocyte trigger during IVF cycles, granulosa cell gene expression is altered in such a way that increases FSH and LH receptor expression [52]. This altered gene expression is postulated to augment downstream signaling, resulting in increased sex steroid synthesis [52]. In fact, kisspeptin is currently considered to be the most potent stimulator of GnRH secretion [53, 54].

OHSS is considered a serious adverse event during IVF treatment and is typically related to the use of hCG as a trigger for oocyte maturation. This syndrome is characterized by extreme vascular permeability, which can result in pleural effusions, ascites, renal impairment, and in severe cases, death [51]. This vascular permeability is a downstream effect of hCG-mediated release of vascular endothelial growth factor (VEGF) from the ovary [55]. Kisspeptin has been shown to

directly inhibit ovarian VEGF production, which significantly decreases the risk of OHSS when used as a trigger for ovulation induction [56]. Moreover, kisspeptin acts to release endogenous GnRH, which triggers an LH surge dependent on the individual's own GnRH reserves, and is unlikely to excessively or pathologically stimulate the ovaries [57].

7. Kisspeptin in puberty

In addition to its role in pregnancy and fertility, kisspeptin is also implicated in sexual development in humans. The target of the kisspeptin molecule is G-protein coupled receptor 54 (GPR54) [58]. A study by de Roux et al. demonstrated that humans with a defect in the *GPR54* gene exhibit isolated hypogonadotrophic hypogonadism, suggesting that kisspeptin is an important regulator of gonadal axis development [59]. This finding was then reproduced by an independent study by Seminara et al., who evaluated a large family with idiopathic hypogonadotrophic hypogonadism and generated *GPR54* knockout mice, which failed to undergo adult sexual development and had low serum gonadotropin levels [47]. In contrast, exogenous kisspeptin administration in prepubertal rodents and primates has been shown to induce precocious puberty [60]. Furthermore, Teles et al. describes a female with an activating mutation of *GPR54* who exhibited idiopathic central precocious puberty [61].

Kisspeptin is thought to be imperative in all phases of sexual development, beginning in the embryonic phase. During the second trimester of pregnancy, GnRH secretion first occurs and is required for normal testicular development [62]. Aberrant gonadal pathways can result in male infants born with microphallus or cryptorchidism [63]. Kisspeptin is suspected to be crucial in the stimulation of GnRH secretion in both infancy and puberty [62].

8. Conclusion

Kisspeptins have a multitude of regulatory neuroendocrine functions that span the sexual life cycle. Though its mechanisms are not entirely characterized, there is strong evidence supporting its involvement in puberty and development, ovulation, implantation, and pregnancy. Because of their role in these reproductive processes, kisspeptins have potential to be useful as biomarkers in a variety of contexts, such as ovulation prediction and diagnosis of viable IUP. Kisspeptins may also be useful in the advancement of assisted reproductive technology. Continued exploration of kisspeptin function will help to develop and standardize practices that harness its diagnostic and therapeutic potential.

Author details

Erin Ahart*, Elaine Phillips, Michael Wolfe and Courtney Marsh
University of Kansas Medical Center, Kansas City, KS, USA

*Address all correspondence to: eahart@kumc.edu

References

[1] Kotani M, Detheux M, Vandenbogaerde A, Communi D, Vanderwinden JM, Le Poul E, et al. The metastasis suppressor gene KiSS-1 encodes kisspeptins, the natural ligands of the orphan G protein-coupled receptor GPR54. J Biol Chem. 2001;276(37):34631-34636.

[2] Horikoshi Y, Matsumoto H, Takatsu Y, Ohtaki T, Kitada C, Usuki S, et al. Dramatic elevation of plasma metastin concentrations in human pregnancy: metastin as a novel placenta-derived hormone in humans. J Clin Endocrinol Metab. 2003;88(2):914-919.

[3] Harter CJL, Kavanagh GS, Smith JT. The role of kisspeptin neurons in reproduction and metabolism. Journal of Endocrinology. 2018;238(3): R173-RR83.

[4] R. Latif NR. Serum kisspeptin levels across different phases of the menstrual cycle and their correlation with serum oestradiol The Netherlands Journal of Medicine 2015;74(4):175-179.

[5] Han SK, Gottsch ML, Lee KJ, Popa SM, Smith JT, Jakawich SK, et al. Activation of gonadotropin-releasing hormone neurons by kisspeptin as a neuroendocrine switch for the onset of puberty. J Neurosci. 2005;25(49): 11349-11356.

[6] Huang X, Harlan RE. Absence of androgen receptors in LHRH immunoreactive neurons. Brain Research. 1993;624(1-2):309-311.

[7] Herbison AE, D'Anglemont De Tassigny X, Doran J, Colledge WH. Distribution and Postnatal Development of Gpr54 Gene Expression in Mouse Brain and Gonadotropin-Releasing Hormone Neurons. Endocrinology. 2010;151(1):312-321.

[8] Franceschini I, Lomet D, Cateau M, Delsol G, Tillet Y, Caraty A. Kisspeptin immunoreactive cells of the ovine preoptic area and arcuate nucleus co-express estrogen receptor alpha. Neuroscience Letters. 2006;401(3):225-230.

[9] Greenwald-Yarnell ML, Marsh C, Allison MB, Patterson CM, Kasper C, Mackenzie A, et al. ERα in Tac2 Neurons Regulates Puberty Onset in Female Mice. Endocrinology. 2016;157(4): 1555-1565.

[10] Katulski K, Podfigurna A, Czyzyk A, Meczekalski B, Genazzani AD. Kisspeptin and LH pulsatile temporal coupling in PCOS patients. Endocrine. 2018;61(1):149-157.

[11] Meczekalski B, Katulski K, Podfigurna-Stopa A, Czyzyk A, Genazzani AD. Spontaneous endogenous pulsatile release of kisspeptin is temporally coupled with luteinizing hormone in healthy women. Fertil Steril. 2016;105(5):1345-1350 e2.

[12] Hrabovszky E. Neuroanatomy of the human hypothalamic kisspeptin system. Neuroendocrinology. 2014;99(1):33-48.

[13] Leonardi CEP, Dias FCF, Adams GP, Araujo ER, Singh J. Kisspeptin induces ovulation in heifers under low plasma progesterone concentrations. Theriogenology. 2020;141:26-34.

[14] Zhai J, Ding L, Zhao S, Li W, Sun Y, Su S, et al. Kisspeptin: a new marker for human pre-ovulation. Gynecol Endocrinol. 2017;33(7):560-563.

[15] Smith JT, Popa SM, Clifton DK, Hoffman GE, Steiner RA. Kiss1 neurons in the forebrain as central processors for generating the preovulatory luteinizing hormone surge. J Neurosci. 2006;26(25):6687-6694.

[16] Dhillo WS, Chaudhri OB, Thompson EL, Murphy KG,

Patterson M, Ramachandran R, et al. Kisspeptin-54 stimulates gonadotropin release most potently during the preovulatory phase of the menstrual cycle in women. J Clin Endocrinol Metab. 2007;92(10):3958-3966.

[17] Roseweir AK, Kauffman AS, Smith JT, Guerriero KA, Morgan K, Pielecka-Fortuna J, et al. Discovery of potent kisspeptin antagonists delineate physiological mechanisms of gonadotropin regulation. J Neurosci. 2009;29(12):3920-3929.

[18] Genazzani ADML, BM, Claudia Strucchi, Stefano Luisi1, EC, , Bernardi1 F, ARGaFP. Pulsatile secretory characteristics of allopregnanolone, a neuroactive steroid, during the menstrual cycle and in amenorrheic subjects. European Journal of Endocrinology 2002;146:347-356.

[19] Caraty A. Nature and bioactivity of gonadotropin-releasing hormone (GnRH) secreted during the GnRH surge. 1995;136(8):3452-3460.

[20] Kinoshita M, Tsukamura H, Adachi S, Matsui H, Uenoyama Y, Iwata K, et al. Involvement of central metastin in the regulation of preovulatory luteinizing hormone surge and estrous cyclicity in female rats. Endocrinology. 2005;146(10): 4431-4436.

[21] Goto Y, Endo N, Nagai K, Ohkura S, Wakabayashi Y, Tanaka A, et al. Ovarian and hormonal responses to follicular phase administration of investigational metastin/kisspeptin analog, TAK-683, in goats. Reprod Domest Anim. 2014;49(2):338-342.

[22] Cejudo Roman A, Pinto FM, Dorta I, Almeida TA, Hernandez M, Illanes M, et al. Analysis of the expression of neurokinin B, kisspeptin, and their cognate receptors NK3R and KISS1R in the human female genital tract. Fertil Steril. 2012;97(5):1213-1219.

[23] Jamil Z, Fatima SS, Arif S, Alam F, Rehman R. Kisspeptin and embryo implantation after ICSI. Reprod Biomed Online. 2017;34(2):147-153.

[24] Castellano JM, Tena-Sempere M. Animal modeling of early programming and disruption of pubertal maturation. 2016. p. 87-121.

[25] Byri P, Gangineni A, Reddy KR, Raghavender KBP. Effect of kisspeptin on in vitro maturation of sheep oocytes. Vet World. 2017;10(3):276-280.

[26] Abbara A, Clarke S, Islam R, Prague JK, Comninos AN, Narayanaswamy S, et al. A second dose of kisspeptin-54 improves oocyte maturation in women at high risk of ovarian hyperstimulation syndrome: A Phase 2 randomized controlled trial. Human Reproduction. 2017;32(9):1915-1924.

[27] Hu KL, Chang HM, Zhao HC, Yu Y, Li R, Qiao J. Potential roles for the kisspeptin/kisspeptin receptor system in implantation and placentation. Human Reproduction Update. 2019;25(3): 326-343.

[28] Cao Y, Li Z, Jiang W, Ling Y, Kuang H. Reproductive functions of Kisspeptin/KISS1R Systems in the Periphery. Reproductive Biology and Endocrinology. 2019;17(1).

[29] Wu HM, Huang HY, Soong YK, Leung PCK, Wang HS. Kisspeptin regulation of human decidual stromal cells motility via FAK-Src intracellular tyrosine kinases. Hum Reprod. 2019;34(7):1291-1301.

[30] Matjila M, Millar R, van der Spuy Z, Katz A. Elevated placental expression at the maternal-fetal interface but diminished maternal circulatory kisspeptin in preeclamptic pregnancies. Pregnancy Hypertens. 2016;6(1):79-87.

[31] Bilban M, Ghaffari-Tabrizi N, Hintermann E, Bauer S, Molzer S,

Zoratti C, et al. Kisspeptin-10, a KiSS-1/metastin-derived decapeptide, is a physiological invasion inhibitor of primary human trophoblasts. Journal of Cell Science. 2004;117(8):1319-1328.

[32] Janneau JL, Maldonado-Estrada J, Tachdjian G, Miran I, Motté N, Saulnier P, et al. Transcriptional expression of genes involved in cell invasion and migration by normal and tumoral trophoblast cells. J Clin Endocrinol Metab. 2002;87(11): 5336-5339.

[33] Baba T, Kang HS, Hosoe Y, Kharma B, Abiko K, Matsumura N, et al. Menstrual cyclic change of metastin/GPR54 in endometrium. Med Mol Morphol. 2015;48(2):76-84.

[34] Radovick S, Babwah AV. Regulation of Pregnancy: Evidence for Major Roles by the Uterine and Placental Kisspeptin/KISS1R Signaling Systems. Seminars in Reproductive Medicine. 2019;37(4): 182-190.

[35] Zhang P, Tang M, Zhong T, Lin Y, Zong T, Zhong C, et al. Expression and function of kisspeptin during mouse decidualization. PLoS One. 2014;9(5): e97647.

[36] Calder M, Chan YM, Raj R, Pampillo M, Elbert A, Noonan M, et al. Implantation failure in female Kiss1-/- mice is independent of their hypogonadic state and can be partially rescued by leukemia inhibitory factor. Endocrinology. 2014;155(8):3065-3078.

[37] Francis VA, Abera AB, Matjila M, Millar RP, Katz AA. Kisspeptin regulation of genes involved in cell invasion and angiogenesis in first trimester human trophoblast cells. PLoS One. 2014;9(6):e99680.

[38] Taylor J, Pampillo M, Bhattacharya M, Babwah AV. Kisspeptin/KISS1R signaling potentiates extravillous trophoblast adhesion to type-I collagen in a PKC- and ERK1/2-dependent manner. Mol Reprod Dev. 2014;81(1):42-54.

[39] de Pedro MA, Moran J, Diaz I, Murias L, Fernandez-Plaza C, Gonzalez C, et al. Circadian Kisspeptin expression in human term placenta. Placenta. 2015;36(11):1337-1339.

[40] Sullivan-Pyke C, Haisenleder DJ, Senapati S, Nicolais O, Eisenberg E, Sammel MD, et al. Kisspeptin as a new serum biomarker to discriminate miscarriage from viable intrauterine pregnancy. Fertil Steril. 2018;109(1):137-41.e2.

[41] Jayasena CN, Abbara A, Comninos AN, Nijher GM, Christopoulos G, Narayanaswamy S, et al. Kisspeptin-54 triggers egg maturation in women undergoing in vitro fertilization. J Clin Invest. 2014;124(8):3667-3677.

[42] Torricelli M, Novembri R, Conti N, De Falco G, De Bonis M, Petraglia F. Correlation with placental kisspeptin in postterm pregnancy and apoptosis. Reprod Sci. 2012;19(10):1133-1137.

[43] Ammon Avalos L, Galindo C, Li DK. A systematic review to calculate background miscarriage rates using life table analysis. Birth Defects Res A Clin Mol Teratol. 2012;94(6): 417-423.

[44] Jayasena CN, Abbara A, Izzi-Engbeaya C, Comninos AN, Harvey RA, Gonzalez Maffe J, et al. Reduced levels of plasma kisspeptin during the antenatal booking visit are associated with increased risk of miscarriage. J Clin Endocrinol Metab. 2014;99(12):E2652-E2660.

[45] Wu S, Zhang H, Tian J, Liu L, Dong Y, Mao T. Expression of kisspeptin/GPR54 and PIBF/PR in the first trimester trophoblast and decidua of women with recurrent spontaneous

abortion. Pathol Res Pract. 2014;210(1):47-54.

[46] Kavvasoglu S, Ozkan ZS, Kumbak B, Simsek M, Ilhan N. Association of kisspeptin-10 levels with abortus imminens: A preliminary study. Archives of Gynecology and Obstetrics. 2012;285(3):649-653.

[47] Romero-Ruiz A, Avendaño MS, Dominguez F, Lozoya T, Molina-Abril H, Sangiao-Alvarellos S, et al. Deregulation of miR-324/KISS1/kisspeptin in early ectopic pregnancy: mechanistic findings with clinical and diagnostic implications. Am J Obstet Gynecol. 2019;220(5):480.e1-.e17.

[48] Barnhart KT. Ectopic Pregnancy. New England Journal of Medicine. 2009;361(4):379-387.

[49] Qiao C, Wang C, Zhao J, Liu C, Shang T. Elevated expression of KiSS-1 in placenta of Chinese women with early-onset preeclampsia. PLoS One. 2012;7(11):e48937.

[50] Farina A, Sekizawa A, Purwosunu Y, Rizzo N, Banzola I, Concu M, et al. Quantitative distribution of a panel of circulating mRNA in preeclampsia versus controls. Prenat Diagn. 2006;26(12):1115-1120.

[51] Abbara A, Clarke SA, Dhillo WS. Novel Concepts for Inducing Final Oocyte Maturation in In Vitro Fertilization Treatment. Endocr Rev. 2018;39(5):593-628.

[52] Owens LA, Abbara A, Lerner A, O'Floinn S, Christopoulos G, Khanjani S, et al. The direct and indirect effects of kisspeptin-54 on granulosa lutein cell function. Hum Reprod. 2018;33(2):292-302.

[53] Roa J, Castellano JM, Navarro VM, Handelsman DJ, Pinilla L, Tena-Sempere M. Kisspeptins and the control of gonadotropin secretion in male and female rodents. Peptides. 2009;30(1):57-66.

[54] Quaas AM, Legro RS. Pharmacology of medications used for ovarian stimulation. Best Pract Res Clin Endocrinol Metab. 2019;33(1):21-33.

[55] Hunjan T, Abbara A. Clinical Translational Studies of Kisspeptin and Neurokinin B. Semin Reprod Med. 2019;37(3):119-124.

[56] Zhai J, Liu J, Zhao S, Zhao H, Chen ZJ, Du Y, et al. Kisspeptin-10 inhibits OHSS by suppressing VEGF secretion. Reproduction. 2017;154(4):355-362.

[57] Abbara A, Jayasena CN, Christopoulos G, Narayanaswamy S, Izzi-Engbeaya C, Nijher GM, et al. Efficacy of Kisspeptin-54 to Trigger Oocyte Maturation in Women at High Risk of Ovarian Hyperstimulation Syndrome (OHSS) During In Vitro Fertilization (IVF) Therapy. J Clin Endocrinol Metab. 2015;100(9): 3322-3331.

[58] Franssen D, Ioannou YS, Alvarez-real A, Gerard A, Mueller JK, Heger S, et al. Pubertal timing after neonatal diethylstilbestrol exposure in female rats: Neuroendocrine vs peripheral effects and additive role of prenatal food restriction. Reproductive Toxicology. 2014;44:63-72.

[59] de Roux N, Genin E, Carel JC, Matsuda F, Chaussain JL, Milgrom E. Hypogonadotropic hypogonadism due to loss of function of the KiSS1-derived peptide receptor GPR54. Proc Natl Acad Sci U S A. 2003;100(19): 10972-10976.

[60] Navarro VM, Fernandez-Fernandez R, Castellano JM, Roa J, Mayen A, Barreiro ML, et al. Advanced vaginal opening and precocious activation of the reproductive axis by KiSS-1 peptide, the endogenous ligand

of GPR54. J Physiol. 2004;561(Pt 2):379-386.

[61] Teles MG, Bianco SD, Brito VN, Trarbach EB, Kuohung W, Xu S, et al. A GPR54-activating mutation in a patient with central precocious puberty. N Engl J Med. 2008;358(7):709-715.

[62] Chan YM, Broder-Fingert S, Seminara SB. Reproductive functions of kisspeptin and Gpr54 across the life cycle of mice and men. Peptides. 2009;30(1):42-48.

[63] Grumbach MM. A window of opportunity: the diagnosis of gonadotropin deficiency in the male infant. J Clin Endocrinol Metab. 2005;90(5):3122-3127.

Chapter 13

Effects of Different Types of Incubators on Embryo Development and Clinical Outcomes

Ji Liu, Yan-Hua Zhou, Xiao-Xiao Wang, Ling-Xi Tong, Yan-Hong Li, Ling Liu, Zhi-Yan Xu and Hong-Hui Wang

Abstract

Main differences of incubators are humidity, temperature and gas control ways, which play important roles in regulating the steady state of culture media. In this study, we compared the effects of different types of incubators (air jacket incubators and water jacket incubators) on embryo development and clinical outcomes in human assisted reproduction. We found that temperature recovery time in air jacket incubators was significantly shorter than that in water jacket incubators. Although the O_2 recovering time was also significantly shorter in air jacket incubators as compared with the water jacket incubator, no significant differences were observed in CO_2 recovering time between two groups, which was also verified by pH recovering time of culture media. Besides, the temperature of culture medium in the dish covered with oil recovered more quickly in the air jacket incubators. However, there were no significant differences observed in the fertilization rate, Day 3 high-quality embryo rate, blastocyst rate, good blastocyst rate and clinical outcomes between two groups. These results indicate that the microenvironment, especially the temperature, in air jacket incubator recover faster than that in water jacket incubators, however, there were no significant differences in embryo development and clinical outcomes between two types of incubators.

Keywords: Embryo culture, Incubator, Temperature, CO2

1. Introduction

For most kinds of cell culture, a suitable culture condition depending on the cell type is used. Human embryos are usually cultured in incubators in a humidified condition with 5–7% CO2 with or without reduced oxygen at 37°C condition. Although culture media are very important for embryo development, the environment of embryo culture is also a critical factor, which provides stable conditions for embryo development by controlling pH and temperature of the culture media.

During oocyte fertilization and embryo development, maintaining an appropriate and stable culture environment for gametes and embryos is the guarantee for protecting the developmental competence of embryos. The primary functions of

incubators are to maintain stable temperature, optimal pH levels for embryo growth and stable osmolality of the media [1, 2]. Different types of incubators based on these principles have been developed in the past few years, which include water jacket incubators, benchtop incubators, drawer incubators and time-lapse incubators [3]. The main differences of these incubators are temperature control system, gas control system (the gas premixed incubator, the conventional gas incubator with CO2 only) and humidity. For the air jacket incubator, the gas is pre-heated. While the warming process of culture medium in the water jacket incubator is thermal conductivity by gas, which is heated by the water jacket.

As for embryo culture, the culture medium is usually covered by mineral oil for maintaining a normal range of osmolarity for embryo development. Besides, with the development of CO2 sensors, conventional thermal conductivity sensors were replaced by infrared sensors [3]. Therefore, the dry incubator becomes a new choice for embryo culture. Compared with the conventional incubator, the dry incubator is easier to clean due to its smaller size and the risk of contamination is also reduced significantly under the moisture-free environment [4].

Although dry incubators have been widely applied to the field of human IVF, their effects, especially the clinical outcomes, are reported rarely. It was reported that the early stage embryo and blastocyst formation rates in top-load mini-incubators are superior to that in front-load conventional incubators [5]. However, Mohamed Fawzy and colleagues reported that embryos cultured in dry incubators showed significantly decreased implantation and clinical ongoing pregnancy rates [6]. However, in their study, live-birth rate was not reported and the paired comparison for embryos derived from the same patient was also of lack.

In the present study, we compared the effects of the air jacket incubator and conventional water jacket incubator on embryo development and the final clinical outcomes. We found that the temperature and gas concentration in air jacket incubators recovered more quickly than conventional water jacket incubators, but there were no significant differences observed for embryo development and clinical outcomes.

2. Materials and methods

2.1 Patients

Ethical approval was obtained from the Medical Ethics Committee of Weihai Maternal and Child Health Hospital (WFEY-QR-CR-825, 3 January 2017). The written cognitive and approval consents were also signed by patients. Patients undergoing routine IVF treatment (the number of COCs acquired ≥10) at the Reproductive Medical Center of Weihai Second Municipal Hospital between Jun 2017 and Aug 2019 were treated as candidates for this study. The characteristics of patients were listed in **Table 1**, including age, body mass index (BMI), basal sex hormone levels, duration of infertility. Women with endometriosis, poor endometrium (<8 mm diameter), premature ovarian insufficiency on the hCG trigger day or the transfer day were excluded. Samples from their husbands were also excluded if they had severe asthenospermia/oligospermia and aspermia.

The follicles of women receiving gonadotropin releasing hormone agonist (GnRH-a) long protocol were monitored by ultrasound. When 10 or more follicles had reached a mean diameter of ≥14 mm, the women were given appropriate dose of hCG to induce oocyte meiotic maturation. Cycles with more than 10 COCs retrieved were assigned in this study and all COCs were allocated equally and non-selectively to either incubator.

Author details

Xiangli Niu[1], Hua Huang[1], Yi Mo[1], Yan Sun[1] and Wei-Hua Wang[2*]

1 Research Center for Reproductive Medicine, Reproductive Hospital of Guangxi Zhuang Autonomous Region, Nanning, Guangxi, China

2 Prelude-Houston Fertility Laboratory, Houston, TX, USA

*Address all correspondence to: wangweihua11@yahoo.com

References

[1] Rienzi L, Gracia C, Maggiulli R, LaBarbera AR, Kaser DJ, Ubaldi FM, Vanderpoel S, Racowsky C. Oocyte, embryo and blastocyst cryopreservation in ART: systematic review and meta-analysis comparing slow-freezing versus vitrification to produce evidence for the development of global guidance. Hum Reprod Update 2017; **23:**139-155.

[2] Levi-Setti PE, Patrizio P, Scaravelli G. Evolution of human oocyte cryo-preservation: slow freezing versus vitrification. Curr Opin Endocrinol Diabetes Obes 2016; **23:**445-450.

[3] Dupesh S, Rasappan P, Shila S, Gunasekaran. Human sperm freezing: Mini update. Advances in Reprod Sci 2018; **6:**59-69.

[4] Just A, Gruber I, Wober M, Lahodny J, Obruca A, Strohmer H. Novel method for the cryopreservation of testicular sperm and ejaculated spermatozoa from patients with severe oligospermia: A pilot study. Fertil Steril 2004; 82:445-447.

[5] Desai NN, Blackmon H, Goldfarb J. Single sperm cryopreservation on cryoloops: An alternative to hamster zona for freezing individual spermatozoa. Reprod Biomed Online 2004; 9:47-53.

[6] Liu F, Zou, SS, Zhu Y, Sun C, Liu YF, Wang SS, Shi WB, Zhu JJ, Huang YH, Li Z. A novel micro-straw for cryopreservation of small number of human spermatozoon. Asian J Androl 2017; 19:326-329.

[7] Desai N, Goldberg J, Austin C, Sabanegh E, Falcone T. Cryo-preservation of individually selected sperm: Methodology and case report of a clinical pregnancy. J Assist Reprod Genet 2012; 29:375-379.

[8] Borini A, Sereni E, Flamigni C. Freezing a few testicular spermatozoa retrieved by TESA. Mol Cell Endocrinol 2000; 169:27-32.

[9] AbdelHafez F, Bedaiwy M, El-Nashar SA, Sabanegh E, Desai N. Techniques for cryopreservation of individual or small numbers of human spermatozoa: A systematic review. Hum Reprod Update 2009; 15:153-164.

[10] Dupesh S, Rasappan P, Shila S, Gunasekaran. A simple method of human sperm vitrification. MethodsX 2019; **6:**2198-2204.

[11] Isachenko V, Isachenko E, Petrunkina Am, Sanchesz R. Human sperm vitrified in the absence of permeable cryoprotectants: Birth of two healthy babies. Reprod Fertil Dev 2012; **24:**323-326.

[12] Aizpurua J, Medrano L, Enciso M, Sarasa J, Romero A, Fernandez MA, Gomez-Torres MJ. New permeable cryoprotectant-free vitrification method for native human sperm. Hum Reprod 2017; **32:**2007-2015.

[13] Agha-Rahimi A, Khalili MA, Nabi A, Ashourzadeh S. Vitrification is not superior to rapid freezing of normozoo-spermic spermatozoa: Effects on sperm parameters, DNA fragmentation and hyaluronan binding. Reprod Biomed Online 2014: **28:**352-358.

[14] Berkovitz A, Miller N, Silberman M, Belenky M, Itsykson P. A novel solution for freezing small numbers of spermatozoa using a sperm vitrification device. Hum Reprod 2018; 33:1975-1983.

[15] Ozkavukcu S, Erdemli E, Isik A, Oztuna D, Karahuseyinoglu S. Effects of cryopreservation on sperm parameters and ultrastructural morphology of human sperm. J Assist Reprod Genet 2008; **25:**403-411.

[16] Lusignan MF, Li X, Herrero B, Delbes G, Chan PTK. Effects of different cryopreservation methods on DNA

integrity and sperm chromatin quality in men. Andrology 2018; 6:829-835.

[17] Raad G, Lteif L, Lahoud R, Azoury J, Azoury J, Tanios J, Hazzouri M, Azoury J. Cryopreservation media differentially affect sperm motility, morphology and DNA integrity. Andrology 2018; 6:836-845.